Clinical Nutrition

A Functional Approach

Contributing Authors and Editors
(2004 Revision)

> DeAnn Liska, PhD, Technical Editor
> Sheila Quinn, Managing Editor
> Dan Lukaczer, ND
> David S. Jones, MD
> Robert H. Lerman, MD, PhD

Contributing Authors and Reviewers
(1999 Edition)

> Jeffrey S. Bland, PhD
> Linda Costarella, ND
> Buck Levin, PhD, RD
> DeAnn Liska, PhD
> Dan Lukaczer, ND
> Barbara Schiltz, MS, RN, CN
> Michael A. Schmidt, PhD
> Robert H. Lerman, MD, PhD

©2004

The Institute for Functional Medicine
A Nonprofit Educational Organization
P.O. Box 1697
Gig Harbor, Washington 98335, USA
www.functionalmedicine.org
800-228-0622

ACKNOWLEDGMENTS

Contributions from the following generous individuals
provided vital support for the 2004 *Clinical Nutrition* revision project.
IFM offers its warmest thanks and appreciation.

Kathi A. Bowen-Jones and David Jones
Ron Kurtz and Terry Toth
Robert and Gay MacLellan
Bill and Barbara Patridge
John and Cathy Schleining
Dan and Virginia Shapiro
Fredrick and JoAnn Soued
Mark and Donna Eisenstein
Brady C. Davis
Arnold B. Freiman
Karl and Carole Hesse

TABLE OF CONTENTS

Preface   *xi*

About the Authors and Editors   *xiii*

List of Figures   *xvii*

List of Tables   *xix*

Chapter 1: Nutrition from a Functional Perspective   **1**

Why a "Functional" Approach to Clinical Nutrition?   2

What is Functional Medicine?   3

    Biochemical Individuality in Nutrition   5

    Patient-Centered Nutrition   7

    Dynamic Balance and Nutrition   8

    Weblike Interconnections and Nutrition   9

    How Nutrition Supports Health as a Positive Vitality   11

    Promotion of Organ Reserve with Nutrition and Conditionally Essential Nutrients   13

Summary   14

References   14

Chapter 2: Carbohydrates   **17**

Classes of Carbohydrates   18

    Fructose   19

    High Fructose Corn Syrup (HFCS)   21

    Inulin and Fructooligosaccharides   22

    Nondigestible or "Resistant" Starch   24

    Dietary Fibers   26

Evaluating Fiber Intake   27

    Increasing Fiber in the Diet   29

A Functional Approach to Carbohydrates   29
    Carbohydrate Metabolism and Maldigestion   29
    Carbohydrate Metabolism and Blood Sugar Regulation   31
        Glycemic index   *31*
        Factors affecting glycemic response   *34*
        Second meal effect   *35*
        Clinical conclusions about carbohydrates and glycemic index   *35*
Carbohydrate Research: Future Directions   36
Summary   36
References   37

Chapter 3: Proteins and Amino Acids   **41**
Amino Acids   42
    Essential and Nonessential Amino Acids   42
    Amino Acids and Amino Acid Derivatives: Examples   45
        The sulfation cycle: cysteine, methionine, and betaine   *45*
        Amino acid conjugation: taurine and glycine   *45*
        The urea cycle and signal transduction: arginine, ornithine, and citrulline   *47*
        The branched-chain amino acids: leucine, isoleucine, and valine   *49*
        Mitochondrial metabolism: creatine and carnitine   *50*
        Glutamine   *51*
        Excitatory amino acid: glutamate   *52*
Proteins and Peptides   53
    Biologically Active Peptides   53
    Glycoproteins and Proteoglycans   55
    Soy Protein   56
    Rice Protein   57
A Functional Approach to Amino Acids, Proteins, and Peptides   58
    Oxidative Stress and N-Acetylcysteine   58
    Glutamine and the NMDA Receptor Pathway   58
    Detoxification, Sulfate Reserves, and Neurodegenerative Diseases   61
    Food Intolerance, Allergies, and the Elimination Diet   62
Summary   64
References   64

Chapter 4: Fats   **69**

Fats and Cell Membranes   70
    Fat Classification   70
Fatty Acid Classification   71
    Fatty Acids in the Laboratory   73
    Omega Family Fatty Acid Ratios   74
Arachidonic Acid Cascade   74
    Arachidonic Acid, Omega Ratios, and Inflammation   77
    Plant Oil Supplementation and the AA Cascade   79
    Trans Fatty Acids   79
    Fats and Oxidative Insult   80
    Lipid Peroxides and Antioxidant Protection of Cell Lipids   80
    Vitamin E and Lipid Protection   83
    Vitamin C and Lipid Protection   83
    Coenzyme Q10 and Lipid Protection   84
Sterols: The Second Major Category of Lipids   85
    Cholesterol   85
    Fatty Acids and Thyroid Function   87
Short-Chain Fatty Acids   87
Medium-Chain Fatty Acids and Medium-Chain Triglycerides (MCFAs and MCTs)   89
    Clinical Use of MCTs   89
    Commercial Preparation of MCT Oils   89
    Clinical Effectiveness of 8-Carbon and 10-Carbon MCFAs within MCT Oils   90
    Hypercholesterolemic Effects of Lauric and Myristic Acids   90
Fats and Dietary Macronutrient Balance   91
Food Fats and Plant Oils   92
    Nuts, Seeds, and Their Oils   92
    Fat and Physical Performance   93
Summary   93
References   94

Chapter 5: Vitamins   **97**

Vitamin Structure and Function   98
Vitamin Classification   98
Vitamin Insufficiency, Deficiency, and Biochemical Individuality   98
Dietary Reference Intakes (DRIs): Relevance to Clinical Therapeutics   100
A Functional Approach to Vitamins   101

Each of the following vitamin subsections includes the following elements: Structure,
  Absorption, Functions, Sources, Therapeutic considerations, Safety and toxicity, and
  Functional medicine considerations.

The Water-Soluble Vitamins   105
    Vitamin B1 (Thiamin)   105
    Vitamin B2 (Riboflavin)   109
    Vitamin B3 (Niacin)   112
    Vitamin B5 (Pantothenic Acid)   115
    Vitamin B6 (Pyridoxine)   117
    Vitamin B12 (Cobalamin)   119
    Folic Acid   122
    Biotin   126
    Vitamin C (Ascorbate)   128
The Fat-Soluble Vitamins   131
    Vitamin E   131
    Vitamin A   134
    Vitamin D   139
    Vitamin K   142
Summary   144
References   **145**

Chapter 6: Minerals   **151**

Each of the following mineral subsections includes the following elements:
  Absorption and regulation, Functions, Sources, Therapeutic considerations,
  Safety and toxicity, and Functional medicine considerations.

Mineral Classification   152
    Calcium   152
    Phosphorus   160
    Magnesium   161
    Sodium, Chloride, and Potassium   165
    Chromium   169
    Zinc   171
    Copper   172
    Iodine   175
    Iron   176
    Manganese   179
    Molybdenum   181
    Selenium   182
    Vanadium   184
    Boron   186
Summary   186
References   **187**

Chapter 7: Digestion, Absorption, and Gut Ecology   **191**

Gastrointestinal Function   192
    Digestion   192
    Lifestyle Factors Affecting Proper Digestion   192
    The Brain and Gut: Cephalic Phase of Digestion   192
    Physiology of Digestion   193
    Digestion in the Mouth   193
    Digestion in the Stomach   194
    Clinical Issues: Gastritis, Ulcers, and *Helicobacter Pylori* Infection   196

Digestion in the Small Intestine   197
    Pancreatic enzyme secretion   197
    Bile secretion   197
Clinical Issues: Impaired Digestion and Disease   197
Digestion in the Colon   199
A Functional Approach to Digestion, Absorption, and Intestinal Permeability   200
  Permeability in Healthy Individuals: Basic Physiology and Pediatric Gastroenterology   201
  Permeability and Bacterial Imbalance   203
  Bacterial Imbalance and the Development of Chronic Disease   204
    Direct promotion of bacterial balance through probiotics   205
    Indirect support of bacterial balance through prebiotic supplementation   206
    Nutritional support of intestinal mucosal cells   207
      L-glutamine   207
      Butyric Acid   207
      EPA and GLA   208
      Gamma-oryzanol   208
  Permeability and the 4R Gastrointestinal Support Program   208
    Remove   209
    Replace   210
    Reinoculate   210
    Repair   211
Summary   211
References   212

Chapter 8: Energy   **215**

Energy   216
  Mitochondria and Energy Production   216
  Structure Influences Function   219
  Anaerobic vs. Aerobic Metabolism   219
  The Krebs Cycle   219
  Oxidative Phosphorylation   222
Energy and Nutrition   223
  Mitochondria and Nutrition   223
  Energy and Absorption of Nutrients   224

Key Cofactors in Mitochondrial Metabolism 225

    Mitochondrial Free Radicals and Oxidative Stress 225

        Uncoupling 226

    Clinical Issues: Mitochondrial Dysfunction 226

    Clinical Issues: Mitochondrial Energy Crisis and Parkinson's Disease 228

A Functional Approach to Energy 229

    Mitochondrial Resuscitation 229

    Reducing Mitochondrial Oxidative Stress 230

    Specific Nutrient Substances Useful in Improving Mitochondrial Efficiency 230

        Coenzyme Q10 232

        Lipoic Acid 232

        Vitamin E 233

        L-carnitine 233

        B-Complex vitamins 233

        Vitamin K 233

        N-Acetylcysteine and/or glutathione 234

        Creatine 234

Summary 234

References 234

Chapter 9: Environment and Toxicity **237**

Total Load 238

Endogenous Toxicants 240

    Inborn Errors of Metabolism 240

    Imbalanced Metabolism 240

    Polymorphisms, Biochemical Individuality, and Toxicity 240

    Gastrointestinal Microbial Metabolism 242

Exogenous Toxicants 243

    Heavy Metals 244

    Food Additives 246

    The Excitotoxin Concept 247

    Prescription Drugs 247

A Functional Approach to Toxicity   248
   Decrease Toxic Load   249
   Promote Bacterial Balance   249
   Promote Healthy Detoxification   249
     The biochemistry of detoxification   249
   Clinical Relationships   252
     Drugs and detoxification pathways   252
     Idiopathic disease and detoxification   256
     Neurologic disease and detoxification   256
   Nutritional Support for Detoxification   256
   Assessment of Detoxification   257
Summary   258
References   259

Chapter 10: Assessment of Nutritional Status   **263**
Clinical Assessment of Nutritional Status   264
A Functional Approach to Laboratory Assessment of Nutrient Status   265
   Static Level Determination of a Nutrient or Metabolite 268
   Box A: Clinical and Laboratory Assessment of Fatty Acid Insufficiencies 269
   Challenge Tests   270
   Indirect Nutrient Assessment   271
Key Considerations in a Functional Medicine Assessment   272
   Assessment of Food Allergy and Intolerance   272
   Box B: Assessment of Oxidative Stress   273
   Box C: Assessment of Insulin Resistance and Metabolic Syndrome 276
   The Gastrointestinal Milieu   278
     Evaluating digestion and absorption   278
     Intestinal barrier function   278
     Gastrointestinal microecology   279
Summary   280
References   280

Index   283

PREFACE

Clinicians and researchers today are still following the exciting path carved out by the four intrepid pioneers of what we now call functional medicine. Their contributions so advanced our understanding of molecular nutrition, that our intellectual debt to them is permanent. Linus Pauling, PhD, gave birth to the field of molecular medicine; Roger Williams, PhD, developed the concept of biochemical individuality; Abram Hoffer, MD, PhD, introduced biomolecular psychiatry; and Bruce Ames, PhD, extended research connecting single-nucleotide polymorphisms and increased need for enzyme vitamin cofactors. The fields of inquiry that grew out of their work have focused on biomolecular nutrition as the foundation of health, and the scientific evidence for that view is very compelling.

The Institute for Functional Medicine is dedicated to integrating a comprehensive approach to clinical nutrition into our healthcare system. Such a change is vital to the health of every human being, for three reasons:

- Nutrition is a pervasive environmental factor that influences gene expression and contributes heavily to the phenotypic expression of every human being.
- Nutrients act as important biological response modifiers at every level of human biochemistry and physiology.
- The health of the molecular milieu of the body *depends on* the interaction of an individual's genes with macronutrients, micronutrients, and conditionally essential nutrients.

Many of today's most challenging, costly, and debilitating conditions, including a variety of age-related diseases, are now recognized as being closely tied to the mismatch between dietary and lifestyle habits and genetic predisposition. Heart disease, stroke, type 2 diabetes, and many cancers, digestive disorders, autoimmune and atopic diseases, osteoporosis, neurodegenerative conditions, and numerous endocrine and immune problems have all been linked to inappropriate nutrition. "Inappropriate," of course, is different for each of us because we are each unique, both genetically as well as in the environmental context of our lives.

As many readers of this book already know, most contemporary health practitioners have little formal education in clinical nutrition beyond recognizing deficiency diseases (although there certainly are exceptions). Even when a great deal of nutritional information has been absorbed, many clinicians still do not know how to apply it effectively *for the individual patient*. *Clinical Nutrition: A Functional Approach* helps to close that knowledge gap.

This book will advance your understanding beyond the traditional emphasis on isolated nutrient deficiencies and RDA guidelines by focusing on underlying metabolic patterns and nutrient interactions. Combined with a functional medicine focus on the unique biochemistry, genetics, and environment of the individual patient, the innovative approach of this text helps clinicians make the vital connection between nutritional theory and practice.

Originally authored by a multidisciplinary team of scientists and clinicians, the first edition took an integrated approach to nutrition. The current edition was revised and edited by key members of IFM's Curriculum Development Committee—likewise a multidisciplinary team—and contains a significant emphasis on integrating the concepts and applications of functional medicine with essential knowledge in clinical nutrition and biochemistry.

In this spirit, we believe *Clinical Nutrition: A Functional Approach* (2004) will advance the mission of creating a healthcare system founded on solid evidence about the real basis of health. The vision that drives this mission has been developing for more than 100 years; our efforts would not have been possible without the great thinkers who have shown us the path.

Jeffrey S. Bland, PhD, Founder and Chairman, Board of Directors

David S. Jones, MD, President
The Institute for Functional Medicine

April 2004

Jeffrey Bland, PhD, is an international authority on human biochemistry, nutrition, and health. After receiving his PhD from the University of Oregon in 1971, Dr. Bland was professor of chemistry for 13 years at the University of Puget Sound in Tacoma, Washington. He also served as senior research scientist at the Linus Pauling Institute of Science and Medicine and directed the Bellevue-Redmond Medical Laboratory in Washington. He is the author of over 50 original papers and books on nutrition and its relationship to health and disease. For the past 20+ years, Dr. Bland has produced *Functional Medicine Update*, a monthly audiotape series, now published by IFM, in which he reviews and synthesizes the medical literature, and conducts interviews of noted clinicians and researchers. Dr. Bland's distinguished career in nutritional biochemistry has earned him international acclaim as educator, research professor, leader in the natural products industry, recognized expert in human nutrition and functional medicine, and visionary for the future of health care. He serves on IFM's Curriculum Development Committee and is a core faculty member for the Institute's annual *International Symposium* and its six-day intensive course, *Applying Functional Medicine in Clinical Practice (AFMCP)*. Dr. Bland is President and Chief Science Officer of Metagenics, Inc., and Chairman of the Board of Directors for The Institute for Functional Medicine.

DeAnn Liska, PhD, received her PhD in biochemistry from the University of Wisconsin-Madison in 1987, where her research focused on the function of vitamin K. From 1988 to 1994, she was a Senior Fellow and, subsequently, Research Assistant Professor at the University of Washington. While there, she investigated the influence of nutrients and cytokines in the regulation of gene expression. Dr. Liska has authored numerous papers in peer-reviewed journals, contributed to textbooks on nutrition, is on the Biotechnology and Biomedical Device Advisory Board for the Washington Technology Center, and holds several U.S. patents. She has been an invited speaker at national and scientific meetings, Chair of the Nutrition Division and a member of the Scientific Advisory Panel for the American Association of Cereal Chemists (AACC), and is a member of the National Science Teachers Association and the American Medical Writers Association. Dr. Liska serves on IFM's Curriculum Committee, is Technical Editor for *Functional Medicine Update*, and has served as core faculty for *AFMCP* in the past. She is Director of Research Information Services at the Functional Medicine Research Center at Metagenics, Inc., Gig Harbor, WA.

Dan Lukaczer, ND, received his doctorate in naturopathic medicine from Bastyr University in 1991 and maintained a family practice from 1991 to 1995 in Seattle, WA. In 1996, Dr. Lukaczer served as the Assistant Director for Educational Services at Great Smokies Diagnostic Laboratory in Asheville, North Carolina. Dr. Lukaczer has co-authored journal articles and frequently lectures on topics relating to GI function, insulin resistance, detoxification, botanical medicine, and the influence of specific nutrients on illness. He serves on IFM's Curriculum Development Committee, has lectured at many IFM Symposia, and is a core faculty member for the Institute's six-day intensive course, *Applying Functional Medicine in Clinical Practice (AFMCP)*. He is the Director of Clinical Research for the Functional Medicine Research Center, in Gig Harbor, WA.

David S. Jones, MD is the President of The Institute for Functional Medicine. He has practiced as a family physician with emphasis in functional and integrative medicine for over 25 years. He is a recognized expert in the areas of nutrition, lifestyle changes for optimal health, and managed care, as well as the daily professional functions consistent with the modern specialty of Family Practice. Dr. Jones is the recipient of the 1997 Linus Pauling Award in Functional Medicine. He is a Past President of PrimeCare, the Independent Physician Association of Southern Oregon (IPASO) representing the majority of physicians in the Southern Oregon area. Dr. Jones is the author of *Healthy Changes* and

other publications, the Course Director for the Institute's annual International Symposium, core faculty for AFMCP, and chairs the Curriculum Development Committee.

Sheila Quinn, BS, Hon. ND, was a co-founder of Bastyr University and served as its initial Vice President for Finance and Administration Affairs (1978–1990). Subsequently, she was Executive Director for the American Association of Naturopathic Physicians (1993-2000), and then Vice President for Content and Public Policy for AlternativeDr.com. She has an extensive writing and editing background in the natural medicine field, and has been active in many public policy initiatives, including currently serving as Chair for the Board of Directors and Executive Committee of the Integrated Healthcare Policy Consortium. She is on the Advisory Board for the North American Board of Naturopathic Examiners. Ms. Quinn has been IFM's Senior Editor since late 2000.

Linda Costarella, ND, formerly Director of Curriculum at The Institute for Functional Medicine, received her doctorate in Naturopathic Medicine from Bastyr University in 1990, and has practiced naturopathic medicine for many years. Dr. Costarella was a faculty member in the Naturopathic Medicine program at Bastyr and at the Northwest Institute for Acupuncture and Oriental Medicine. Dr. Costarella served on the Advisory Council developing the academic programs at the North East College of Healing Arts and Science in Saxtons River,

VT, and from 1996 to 1997 she served as their Academic Dean. She was also a faculty member of Vermont College of Norwich University in Montpelier from 1995 to 1998. She began her career at HealthComm International, Inc., in 1997 as Manager of Clinical Education. Dr. Costarella has authored several articles published in the *Protocol Journal of Botanical Medicine* and co-authored *Herbs for Women's Health*.

Robert H. Lerman, MD, PhD, received his MD from Jefferson Medical College, a PhD in Nutritional Biochemistry from MIT, is Board-Certified in Internal Medicine, and has completed fellowships in Nephrology and Clinical Nutrition. He was formerly an Adjunct Clinical Associate Professor of Medicine at Boston University School of Medicine and Director of Clinical Nutrition at Boston Medical Center. Before joining IFM and the Functional Medicine Research Center in 1998, he was a faculty member in Nutritional Sciences at the Henry M. Goldman School of Graduate Dentistry and Director of Clinical Nutrition at Boston Medical Center for more than 15 years. He has completed fellowships in Nephrology and Clinical Nutrition and has been Chief of Medicine at U.S. Army Hospitals in Berlin, Germany and Vicenza, Italy as well as acting Chief of Nephrology at Soroka Medical Center in Beer Sheba, Israel. He has authored and co-authored numerous journal articles and book chapters in addition to lecturing on such topics as parenteral nutrition, obesity, fatty acid metabolism, healing and repair of acute my-

ocardial infarction, and trace element deficiency. He serves as IFM's Director of Medical Education, has lectured at many of the Institute's Symposia, is a member of the Curriculum Development Committee and is a core faculty member for *AFMCP*. He is Medical Director for Metagenics, Inc.

Buck Levin, PhD, MA, RD is Adjunct Associate Professor of Nutrition at Bastyr University, where he has been teaching since 1990, as well as Director of Health Science for SaluGenecists, Inc., a start-up company that is developing artificial intelligence tools for use in healthcare settings. In 1997, Dr. Levin founded HingePin Integrative Learning Materials (www.hingepin.com), a company that published his textbook, *Environmental Nutrition*, as well as his 21-credit self-study course on that topic for registered dietitians. Dr. Levin sees patients in private practice and publishes regularly in the field of nutrition. He also serves as Associate Editor for *Integrative Medicine – A Clinician's Journal* and sits on the Advisory Board of *Nutrition Science News*.

Barbara Schiltz, RN, MS, has been a Registered Nurse for 35 years, and since receiving a BS in Foods and Nutrition in 1986, she has been practicing as a nutritionist in private practice. She worked with Serafina Corsello, MD in New York City for 8 years, and after moving to Seattle in 1995 began working with David Buscher, MD at the Northwest Center for Environmental Medicine, and HealthComm Inc.. Ms. Schiltz has had extensive experience working with patients who have food allergies, ADHD, insulin resistance and diabetes, fibromyalgia, irritable bowel disease, and Multiple Chemical Sensitivities. Ms. Schiltz received her Master's Degree in Nutrition at Bastyr University in June 1997, having completed a thesis on *The Unique Role of Carbohydrate Metabolism in Regulation of Glycemic Index*. She has been Clinical Research Associate at the Functional Medicine Research Center in Gig Harbor, WA since 1996.

Michael A. Schmidt, PhD, did his doctoral research in nutritional biochemistry and molecular medicine at NASA Ames Research Center in Mountainview, CA. He is a Research Associate with the Psychophysiology Research Laboratory at NASA Ames Research Center and works in collaboration with the Cellular Environmental Toxicology and Neurophysiology Laboratory at NASA Lyndon B. Johnson Space Center in Houston. Dr. Schmidt has also been part of a working group at the National Institutes of Health developing validation models for biological response modifiers. Dr. Schmidt is a principal scientist and Research Fellow at Living Longer and ProScan Imaging in Cincinnati, OH, which combines metabolic profiling with CT scan, MRI, and functional MRI. As part of the Living Longer/ProScan group, Dr. Schmidt is also director of the Clinical Genomics program. Dr. Schmidt is a former Fellow in Clinical Research and Education at the Functional Medicine Research Center in Gig Harbor, WA.

LIST OF FIGURES

Figure No.	Figure Title
1.1	Nutrition and functional medicine: A simplified model
2.1	Structure of three major monosaccharides
2.2	Oligosaccharides having physiological activity include fructooligosaccharides, galactooligosaccharides, and soybean oligosaccharides
2.3	Bifidobacteria benefits
2.4	Some fructooligosaccharides
2.5	Starch: Amylose (a) and amylopectin (b) molecules
2.6	Calculation of glycemic index (GI)
3.1	Formulas of the 20 common amino acids
3.2	Trans sulfuration-sulfate pathways
3.3	Atherogenic mechanisms of homocysteine and their modulation by nitrogen oxides
3.4	Detoxification in the liver
3.5	Hepatic urea cycle—nitric oxide synthase relationship
3.6	The multiple influences of nitric oxide on immune, vascular, and nervous systems
3.7	Pathophysiologic consequences of the activation of cellular enzyme systems by excitatory amino acid-evoked increases in intracellular calcium
3.8	Overview of glutathione function and metabolism
3.9	Energy failure
4.1	Types of fatty acids
4.2	Arachidonic acid (AA) cascade
4.3	Nutritional, botanical, and synthetic inhibitors in the AA cascade
4.4	Dietary sources and the AA cascade
4.5	Configuration of *cis* fatty acid and *trans* fatty acid
4.6	The formation of F_2-isoprostanes
4.7	Electron transport chain of the mitochondrion
4.8	Some sterols
4.9	Hormone synthesis from cholesterol
4.10	The formation of a monoglyceride
5.1	Vitamin B1 (thiamin) molecule
5.2	Vitamin B2 (riboflavin) and flavin mononucleotide (FMN) as components of flavin-adenine dinucleotide (FAD)
5.3	Glutathione redox cycle
5.4	Vitamin B3 (niacin) molecule
5.5	Vitamin B5 (pantothenic acid) molecule
5.6	Vitamin B6 (pyridoxine) molecule

Figure No.	Figure Title
5.7	Vitamin B12 (cobalamin) molecule
5.8	Folic acid molecule (5-methyl-tetrahydropteroyl-glutamate)
5.9	Homocysteine metabolism in animals
5.10	Biotin molecule
5.11	Ascorbic acid molecule
5.12	Vitamin E molecules (tocopherols)
5.13	Role of vitamin E in oxidative stress reactions
5.14	Vitamin A (all-*trans* retinol) molecule
5.15	Vitamin D3 molecule
5.16	Vitamin D metabolism
5.17	Vitamin K molecule
6.1	Chemical structure of heme
7.1	Nutrient absorption
7.2	Permeability dynamics
7.3	Type and activity of intestinal bacteria
7.4	Common bacteria in the GI tract
7.5	4R GI support program
8.1	Mitochondrial energy production (from food)
8.2	Mitochondria and energy production
8.3	Role of vitamins in early energy production (pre-mitochondria)
8.4	The Krebs Cycle
8.5	Proton pumps in oxidative phosphorylation [Electron transport chain]
8.6	Carnitine biosynthetic pathway in mammals
8.7	Structural formula of carnitine
8.8	The creatine phosphate energy shuttle
8.9	Mitochondrion
8.10	The glutathione redox cycle
9.1	Managing problems of GI permeability, hepatic detoxification, and oxidative stress
9.2	Overview of detoxification
9.3	Liver detoxification pathways and supportive nutrients
10.1	Body mass index (BMI) calculation
10.2	Continuum of nutrient sufficiency/ insufficiency
10.3	Glycination of benzoic acid

LIST OF TABLES

Table No.	Table Title
2.1	Physiologically Important Classes of Carbohydrates
2.2	Classification of Certain Carbohydrates as Colonic Foods and Prebiotics
2.3	Inulin in Food
2.4	Fructooligosaccharides and Food
2.5	Differential Digestion of Starch Complexes
2.6	Dietary Fibers
2.7	Physiological Effects of Soluble/Insoluble Fibers
2.8	Glycemic Index Table of Commonly Eaten Foods
3.1	Carnitine in Detoxification
3.2	Carnitine Content of Selected Foods
3.3	Chronic Neurodegenerative Diseases Thought to be Mediated in Part through Stimulation of Glutamate Receptors
3.4	Modified Elimination Diet Summary
4.1	Examples of Short-, Medium-, and Long-Chain Fatty Acids
4.2	List of Nutritional, Botanical, and Synthetic Inhibitors in the Arachidonic Acid Cascade
4.3	Fatty Acids in Certain Oils
4.4	Formation of Certain Free Radicals
4.5	Molecular Redox Agents and Oxidative Enzymes
4.6	Preferred Cooking Techniques of Selected Oils
5.1	Classification of B Vitamins by Function
5.2	The Four Daily Reference Standards Used to Develop the Dietary Reference Intakes (DRIs)
5.3	Summary Table of the DRIs for Vitamins
5.4	Thiamin Content of Certain Foods
5.5	Riboflavin Content of Certain Foods
5.6	Niacin Content of Certain Foods
5.7	Pantothenic Acid Content of Certain Foods
5.8	Pyridoxine Content of Certain Foods
5.9	Cobalamin Content of Certain Foods
5.10	Folic Acid Content of Certain Foods
5.11	Biotin Content of Certain Foods
5.12	Ascorbic Acid Content of Certain Foods
5.13	Vitamin E Content of Certain Foods
5.14	Vitamin A Content of Certain Foods
5.15	Vitamin D Content of Certain Foods
5.16	Vitamin K Content of Certain Foods

Table No.	Table Title
6.1	Major and Minor Minerals
6.2	Summary Table of the Dietary Reference Intakes (DRIs) for Minerals
6.3	Food Sources of Calcium
6.4	Nondairy High-Calcium Foods
6.5	Food Sources of Phosphorus
6.6	Food Sources of Magnesium
6.7	Conditions that May Involve Magnesium Deficiency
6.8	Food Sources of Potassium
6.9	Food Sources of Sodium
6.10	Food with High Amounts of Added Sodium Chloride
6.11	Food Sources of Chromium
6.12	Food Sources of Zinc
6.13	Food Sources of Copper
6.14	Food Sources of Iodine
6.15	Food Sources of Iron
6.16	Food Sources of Manganese
6.17	Food Sources of Molybdenum
6.18	Food Sources of Selenium
6.19	Food Sources of Vanadium
7.1	Major Digestive Enzymes
7.2	Common Signs and Symptoms of Low Gastric Acidity
7.3	Diseases Associated with Low Gastric Acidity
7.4	Enzymatic Secretions of the Pancreas
7.5	Lactose Intolerance in Ethnic Populations
7.6	Common Sources of Dairy
7.7	Symptoms Associated with Increased Intestinal Permeability
7.8	Diseases Associated with Increased Intestinal Permeability
8.1	Clinical Conditions Related to Mitochondrial Dysfunction
8.2	Mitochondria-related Symptoms and Dysfunction
8.3	Nutritional Modulators of Mitochondrial Oxidative Phosphorylation
9.1	Diseases Attributable to One or More Mutations in a Single Gene
9.2	Signs and Symptoms Associated with Toxic Element Exposure
9.3	Detoxification: Bio-reactive Mechanisms
9.4	Inhibitors and Substrates of P450 Enzymes
10.1	Common Features of Nutritional Deficiencies
10.2	Terms Used to Describe Food Allergy and Food Intolerance
10.3	Clinical Conditions Associated with Increased Antigen Uptake by the Intestine
10.4	Stool Markers Suggestive of Intestinal Dysbiosis

1

Nutrition from a Functional Perspective

AS A PRACTITIONER WHO RELIES ON nutrition in clinical practice, you may find conventional methods for integrating nutrition into your practice to be limited. Perhaps you have tried analyzing dietary intake using computer software and found it time consuming and not even relevant to all the nutritional issues you are interested in. You may feel frustrated that reliable laboratory tests to assess nutrient status are often unavailable. You may not even have a nutritional strategy for your patients because you are concerned there is still too much debate about the role of nutritional support for specific conditions, or you worry that nutritional intervention might not have a timely impact on the health of your patient. If any of these thoughts and concerns are familiar to you,

then you probably wish that clinical nutrition could be a more accessible treatment modality and that a "blueprint" or "map" could be developed to help clarify ways of bringing nutrition into clinical practice.

We believe such a roadmap exists. Functional medicine can provide a context for understanding the role of nutrition in clinical practice, because one of the key elements of functional medicine is nutrition.

This chapter is designed to introduce you to fundamental concepts in clinical nutrition as it is applied within a functional medicine model. We will also preview subsequent chapters of the book in which we address very specific clinical issues. With that in mind, we welcome you to the new edition of *Clinical Nutrition—*nutrition from a functional perspective.

You will notice many changes and updates to this new edition of Clinical Nutrition. *Several new tables have been developed to provide more useful clinical tools. For example, tables showing the various suggested levels of vitamins and minerals with upper limits identified are valuable resources for developing individualized nutrition-based interventions. Many other tables and figures have been reorganized to more clearly document the influence of nutrition on health and disease. The functional medicine perspective is integrated more completely throughout each chapter with updated sections identifying and defining key concepts important to understanding the role of nutrition in promoting optimal health. The laboratory chapter is also reorganized around getting started in nutrition, and identifies the tests a clinician might first consider in bringing nutrition into clinical practice.*

WHY A "FUNCTIONAL" APPROACH TO CLINICAL NUTRITION?

"Function" is a simple word, but using it to guide how nutrition is applied in the clinic can make a substantial difference in promoting optimal health for your patients. Similarly, failing to learn and apply nutrition as a therapeutic and prevention-oriented modality can deprive your patients of the maximum benefit of your services. Functional medicine is more than a step-by-step approach; it is a conceptual guide, a way of putting all the pieces together.

Clinically, the study of function tells us that every naturally occurring nutrient, naturally occurring food, and naturally evolving dietary pattern likely has (or, at least, originally had) a purpose and design. Looking at food and nutrients in terms of function means adopting a broader perspective than the classical one: there's far more to be understood than calories, macronutrients, and defined essential vitamins and minerals.

Functional medicine also means looking at the conventionally acknowledged nutrients as multipurpose molecules. We don't assume they fill only (or even primarily) one very specific role in the body. Instead, we look at the many functions these key substances perform throughout the body, and identify the body's need based on that evaluation. For example, a conventional approach may say a person needs X grams of fiber a day, presuming that one fiber is like any other. A functional approach, however, asks more questions: What are the many roles of fiber? What is the type of fiber in this particular food source? Most important, is this particular fiber doing what this particular person actually needs? (What is its function?)

The functional approach assumes that food contains molecules that are necessary, purposeful, and designed to support life, promote well-being and optimal health. Looking at clinical nutrition from a functional perspective means understanding the roles of these molecules in human beings, and then adapting the applications of those molecules to meet the unique genetic and environmental needs of each particular patient. Enabling you to use the entire arsenal of foods components on behalf of your patient's health is the purpose of this book, and one of the main goals of functional medicine.

WHAT IS FUNCTIONAL MEDICINE?

Functional Medicine is a science-based field of healthcare that is grounded in the following principles:

- Biochemical individuality
- Patient-centered care
- Dynamic balance of internal and external factors
- Web-like interconnections of physiological factors
- Health as a positive vitality
- Promotion of organ reserve

Functional medicine involves examining the core clinical imbalances that underlie a disease or condition—looking beyond signs and symptoms to a deeper understanding of functionality. These imbalances arise as environmental inputs, such as diet and nutrients (including water), exercise, and trauma are processed by a patient's body, through his or her unique metabolism. (We also keep in mind that literally everything about that patient is also affected by his/her mind, spirit, attitudes, and beliefs.) The principles of functional medicine present a different context for identifying and understanding these imbalances.

Fundamental physiological processes that support healthy balance and optimal functioning include:

- communication (intra- and intercellular);
- bioenergetics, or the transformation of food into energy;
- replication and maintenance of structural integrity, from the cellular to the whole body level;
- elimination of wastes and defense; and
- circulation and transport of nutrients in the body.

From a functional medicine standpoint, imbalances in these processes can lead to changes in many different physiological systems that then become precursors to the signs and symptoms that we diagnose as organ system disease. Figure 1.1 provides a simplified model of the system described briefly in this chapter.

Approaching clinical nutrition from a functional medicine perspective also means identifying the core metabolic imbalances that most often result from system breakdowns at any point. The main categories of metabolic imbalances include:

- digestive, absorptive, and microbiological imbalances;
- detoxification and biotransformation imbalances;
- oxidation-reduction imbalances and mitochondropathies;

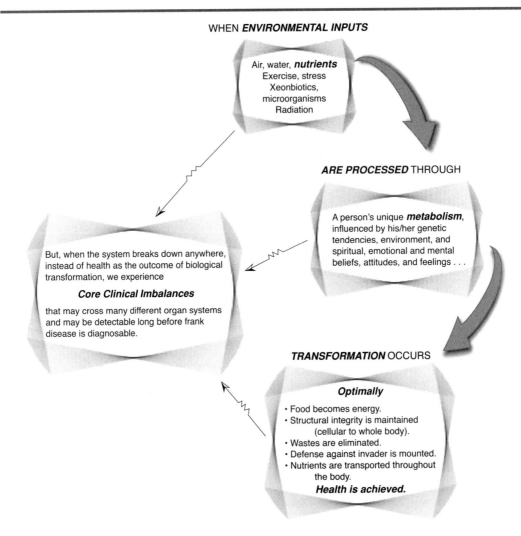

WHEN **ENVIRONMENTAL INPUTS**

Air, water, **nutrients**
Exercise, stress
Xeonbiotics,
microorganisms
Radiation

ARE PROCESSED THROUGH

A person's unique **metabolism**,
influenced by his/her genetic
tendencies, environment, and
spiritual, emotional and mental
beliefs, attitudes, and feelings . . .

But, when the system breaks down anywhere,
instead of health as the outcome of biological
transformation, we experience

Core Clinical Imbalances

that may cross many different organ systems
and may be detectable long before frank
disease is diagnosable.

TRANSFORMATION OCCURS

Optimally
• Food becomes energy.
• Structural integrity is maintained
    (cellular to whole body).
• Wastes are eliminated.
• Defense against invader is mounted.
• Nutrients are transported throughout
    the body.
Health is achieved.

FIGURE 1.1   *Nutrition and functional medicine—a simplified model*

- hormonal and neurotransmitter imbalances;
- immune imbalances and inflammatory imbalances; and
- structural imbalances, from cellular membrane function to musculoskeletal system.

A concise discussion of the relationship between nutrition and each of these areas is beyond the scope of this textbook; however, several areas are directly involved in how the body absorbs (takes in) and processes nutrients, which influences overall nutriture. These areas, which include the function of the gastrointestinal system as related to digestion and absorption, detoxification and the environment, energy (oxidation-reduction), and hormonal balance will be reviewed in detail in this text.

Consider just one example of how the complex system we have just briefly described can be influenced by nutrition. We now recognize that several factors affect the amount of estrogen that is produced in and flows through a woman's body at any given time. In particular, in the postmenopausal years, estrogen is no longer produced by the ovaries, but is still produced in other cells in her body.[1] The production of estrogen by adipose tissue in postmenopausal women is now understood to be one of the mechanisms linking obesity and the increased risk of postmenopausal, hormone-dependent cancers.[2] Diet and lifestyle choices that affect adiposity can, therefore, influence the amount of estrogen produced in a postmenopausal woman's body; excess estrogen, in turn, can create imbalances that influence the development of many problematic conditions. However, we need to know more than this to be effective with the patient.

Science has also recognized that "estrogen" is more than just estrone, estriol, and estradiol—it is a whole class of molecules that includes many metabolites of estrone and estradiol.[3] Some of these metabolites are extremely active and have been linked to increased risk of postmenopausal, hormone-dependent cancers. On the other hand, some of these metabolites appear to be protective to the body and are linked to a lower incidence of postmenopausal, hormone-dependent can-

cers.[4] We know that dietary substances, including vitamin and non-vitamin components, can modify how much of these estrogenic metabolites are made in the body, and which ones predominate. Therefore, diet can influence health in more ways than just the amount of adipose tissue; it can also affect the balance of metabolites in the body, and thus we believe it has a key role to play in hormone-dependent breast cancer prevention.[5]

Data are continuing to accumulate showing that dietary influences have repercussions on the development of many diseases. Research is now focusing on how to assess these imbalances earlier in life, and then readjust the metabolic balance to decrease the risk those conditions and diseases pose to the well-being and quality of life for our patients.

As this brief introduction demonstrates, nutrition is one of the key environmental inputs that can be reviewed with a patient and modified to support optimal health and function. The following section describes each of the principles of functional medicine from the perspective of nutrition. These principles are reflected throughout subsequent chapters of the book, as well as in the basic nutritional information presented and the discussions of key physiological and metabolic areas to be considered as you incorporate nutrition into your clinical practice and continue to improve your effectiveness.

Biochemical Individuality in Nutrition

A core principle in functional medicine is biochemical individuality. As children, we were told that all snowflakes are a little different: no two are exactly alike. As clinical scientists, we learn about the role of individuality in our voluntary activities—how we make decisions, how we develop our personalities, how we evolve our style of doing things. But, what about our everyday bodily processes?

Unfortunately, science has sometimes given the message that our bodily processes, those involuntary activities like metabolism, cellular information processing, and internal communication systems, are "all in our genes." That is to say, they are all predetermined, static, defined by our DNA and out of our control. At some point, clinical science lost the inclination to distinguish how individuality can impact everyday involuntary physical functions as well as voluntary ones.

A functional perspective does not differentiate so abruptly between voluntary and involuntary processes, nor between psychological versus biological uniqueness. From a functional perspective, the concept of uniqueness extends to our physiological/biochemical life as much as it does to our psychological life. Biochemical individuality means that your way of digesting food is different than my way of digesting food; the bile synthesized in your liver is different than the bile synthesized in my liver; the food that nourishes you may not be the same food that nourishes me. The following examples illustrate how biochemically diverse we are.

In 1993, a study was published showing the levels of vitamins B12, B6, and folic acid in 64 healthy older adults (20 male, 44 female; mean age 76).[6] Of these subjects, 94% had "normal" serum levels of vitamin B6, vitamin B12, and folate. Yet, when these researchers measured serum levels of three metabolites known to accumulate in the blood when vitamins B6, B12, and folate are deficient—methylmalonic acid (MMA), 2-methylcitric acid (2-MCA), and homocysteine (HCys)—they found that over 63% of the subjects had elevated serum metabolites, indicating intracellular deficiency of at least one of these vitamins. Even more striking was the interindividual variability in the serum metabolites. Subjects showing normal serum levels of vitamins B6, B12, and folate frequently differed radically in their serum HCys levels (between 10 and 50 μM/L). Subjects differed dramatically in their MMA levels as well. This study gives us just one example of how metabolically different healthy individuals can be, given a strikingly similar and normal snapshot glance at vitamin status. Science is continuing to document that many of these differences relate to the interaction between a person's genetics and environment, and that each of us is "wired" to express a different need for these crucial B-vitamins, depending on our unique biochemistry, which is influenced by lifelong behaviors and exposures.

The B-vitamins are by no means the only examples of our biochemical differences. Vitamin E requirements have been reported to show, at minimum, a five-fold variance in normal, healthy adults, and an even greater interindividual variability when dietary intake of polyunsaturated fatty acids is substantially different.[7] Plasma ascorbate (vitamin C) levels regularly vary in healthy individuals by 25 to 30% but disease states like diabetes, inflammatory conditions, and presence of infections can lead to a substantially increased need for the vitamin. Most organizations now indicate a minimum requirement and a maximum amount as the levels to consider (between 100 and 1000 milligrams per day).[8] Levine and colleagues have reported that the level of vitamin C within the neutrophil increases by as much as 10-fold over normal levels depending upon the activation state of the cell.[9] This means, for example, that a cell in an inflammatory state will accept as much as 10 times the amount of vitamin C as will a cell in a non-inflammatory state. That is, the environment affects how much vitamin C the body's cells need at any one time.

The first and foremost guiding principle of a functional approach, namely the principle of biochemical individuality, tells us that we are as different at the biochemical level (e.g., at the level of our everyday involuntary processes) as we are psychologically. And it tells us that we have to do better than the Recommended Dietary Allowances based on bell-shaped distributions of the "average" person, food pyramids with a "one-size-fits-all" philosophy, and the prepackaged "safety net" generic multivitamin approach to nutrition. Many of the specific ways of doing better by incorporating the idea of biochemical individuality are discussed in detail in the subsequent chapters of this book.

Patient-Centered Nutrition

The functional focus on biochemical individuality may leave you thinking: "If everyone is so different, where do I begin?" Clinical nutrition works hand-in-hand with "patient-centered medicine." Emphasizing patient care rather than disease care, this approach honors Osler's admonition that "It is more important to know what patient has the disease than what disease the patient has." It is important to do more than make the patient a real partner in health care, however; clinicians also must understand how to elicit and analyze the patient's whole story. As developed by Leo Galland, MD, in the mid-1990s, the key components of the patient's story are:

antecedents (what preceded the patient's illness?);
triggers (what factors, given the patient's antecedent history, tipped the patient over the edge into a dysfunctional state?); and
mediators (given the initial disease or condition, what has kept the process going, so that health is still out of reach?).

This kind of analysis explicitly recognizes that each person's path to disease (or health) is unique. We need to understand that path in order to modify it and change the momentum away from disease and toward health. Acquiring the patient's full story is the best place to start.

Even the scientific literature is beginning to embrace the idea of "personalized" medicine.

For instance, the term "personalized nutrition" is beginning to be used in relation to how the information from the human genome project can become directly beneficial to the public.[10] Individualized information, like specific genetic patterns, can be detected as "single nucleotide polymorphisms," or "SNPs." Many SNPs are being actively investigated now to find ways to personalize drug dosages and dietary recommendations.[11,12] One of the best understood SNPs codes for an enzyme necessary in the folate pathway. The majority of the population does not contain this SNP. But 20 to 30% of the population does carry at least one copy of this SNP (called the MTHFR C-T), and it appears that these individuals may need more than the RDA level of 400 μmg/d of folate.

Dynamic Balance and Nutrition

A functional medicine approach to healthcare means examining core clinical imbalances that underlie a disease or condition, not just viewing health from a symptom perspective. In order to identify what is "imbalanced," we must first know what it means to promote balance. During your training as a clinician, you may have been asked to read the seminal 1865 work by Claude Bernard, the contemporary of Pasteur, titled *An Introduction to the Study of Experimental Medicine.*[13] In this work, Bernard developed the concept of "homeostasis" and described the "milieu intérieure," the interior environment whose stability serves as the "primary condition for freedom and independence of existence."

Bernard viewed maintaining constancy in this interior environment as the foremost goal of an organism, toward which all vital mechanisms in the body are oriented.

Modern textbooks of medicine define homeostasis as "the relatively stable physical and chemical composition of the internal environment of the body which results from the actions of compensating regulatory systems." Homeostatic systems, then, are systems that function to keep the physical or chemical internal environment relatively constant. Perhaps the most commonly used example of homeostasis is the body's thermoregulatory system (the reason we humans are referred to as "homeotherms"). This system is designed to maintain our body temperature at around $98.2° \pm 0.6°$. Most people experience convulsions at body temperatures near or above 106° Fahrenheit and cannot survive temperatures much greater than 109°. At the other end of the spectrum, heat-producing mechanisms (including vasoconstriction, increased thyroxine production, increased metabolic rate, and shivering) occur with increasing exposure to cold. Our thermoregulatory system maintains a relatively narrow temperature range throughout healthy life. Only with the loss of vitality (for example, in the loss of health that can accompany aging) does this thermoregulatory function become less sensitive. So, we conclude that body temperature is characterized by homeostasis—a constant, fixed parameter of life.

Body temperature, however, is ***not*** a fixed parameter. When we take a temperature, we get a single, fixed number, but that number is not a constant in the body. Body temperature actually fluctuates within about 3° Fahrenheit (from 97° to 100°) throughout the day. And, it is different at the extremities than at internal sites, where it is a bit higher on average. Body temperature also is lower in the mornings and after rest than it is after exertion or intake of food, when the body is more active metabolically. Therefore, body temperature is not static, but rather dynamic. It is in *dynamic balance*, being maintained "around 98.2° Fahrenheit" not always right on the dot, but constantly fluctuating to adjust to the environment and the needs of the body at each moment in time.

This same argument could be applied to the subtle control of blood pH (which is maintained between 7.35 and 7.45), or the subtle differences between alveolar and atmospheric pressure of 760 and 758 mm Hg. The metabolic pathways in our bodies are the same, fluctuating up and down in activity around an average point. Too often, we tend to focus on the average number and not on the range, but it's the ability to adjust that keeps us connected and interacting in a healthy way with the world around us.

One way in which this discussion relates to nutrition, and more importantly to functional medicine, is how we view a single number from a laboratory or physical test. Is that number telling the whole story? Or, is that number just one point that needs to be put into context for the whole individual? Identifying imbalance means understanding that

we are not looking at fixed points, but at a dynamic process that fluctuates, and the range of fluctuation needs our attention in looking at the whole person within the context of his or her own environment.

Web-like Interconnections and Nutrition

Dynamic balance helps us think more completely about the range of changes a person's body goes through every single day, realizing that nothing is entirely "fixed." Web-like interconnections move us out of the "single-agent—single-outcome" way of thinking. Instead, we see the body as a fully interconnected organism, within which everything affects everything else and nothing is truly isolated. For example, a natural, simple, everyday experience like relaxing can have profound effects on nutrition and health. Contraction of the lower esophageal sphincter (the muscle that separates the esophagus from the stomach) and spasm of the intestine (which occurs in nutrition-related gastrointestinal disorders like irritable bowel syndrome) can both be normalized by simple relaxation.[14] From another perspective, we know a fair amount now about the diverse effects that stress has on health (it increases cortisol levels, for example). But that connection goes both ways—not only does stress increase your need for certain nutrients, but the use of certain nutrients can palliate not only the physical symptoms (blood pressure and cortisol) but the subjective response to acute psychological stress as well.[15] The whole system is interconnected and multidirectional, from the mind to the body and back again.

Restoring balance to underlying metabolic patterns is a process that makes demands upon the body. The classical macro- and micronutrients that act to restore and maintain balance must be accompanied by other necessary food factors that also have important parts to play in this orchestration of life. An objective of nutritional therapy is to make sure the appropriate companionships are in place. For example, the companion presence of different molecules has a dramatic effect on nutrient absorption. Certain forms of minerals in an inorganic delivery form require adequate secretion of hydrochloric acid (HCl) by the stomach for proper digestion and absorption. Many nutrients must attach to organic acids or amino acids for proper absorption. The presence of flavonoids along with vitamin C alters and enhances vitamin C absorption. These are examples of how nutrients and other food factors work in concert and synergistically. The functional approach to nutrition looks not just at providing all the basic nutrients, but at supporting these critical relationships as part of nutritional therapy.

Another example of this web-like interconnection is seen with Wilson's disease, a disorder of excess copper absorption and deposition. In this progressive disorder, which leads to cirrhosis of the liver and degeneration of brain tissue, zinc therapy can lower excessively high levels of copper in the blood.[16] This approach recognizes the natural balance (and antagonism) that can occur in the body between copper and zinc. In other words,

what's important is not just what's there that shouldn't be, or what's not there that should be, but also the balance and connection of these different factors with each other.

The body's web is very complex. For example, let's look at the issue of maintaining healthy bone. Historically, when nutrition researchers observed resorption of bone calcium, they perceived absolute quantitative calcium deficiency and recommended calcium supplements. However, "calcium deficiency" is not an isolated deficiency but a problem of balance among nutritional and other parameters. We can't achieve bone remineralization with supplemental calcium alone. Other nutrients—such as magnesium, manganese, zinc, copper, boron, and phosphorus—are equally important for formation of hydroxyapatite and a healthy bone matrix. And, these other nutrients must be present in certain ratios.

Bone restoration involves more than just the presence of the right nutrients in the right amounts. In space, when astronauts are in a zero-gravity environment, minerals leach from their bones because load-bearing movement is difficult without gravity. Similarly, the bones of people who are bedridden lose minerals because those individuals are not upright, engaging in load-bearing activity. From much other research, we now know that building and maintaining healthy bone requires load-bearing on a regular basis. That is to say, adequate nutrients are necessary, but physical activity is also required for the nutrition to "work" and the bones to mineralize properly.

The web is even more complex than just minerals and physical exercise. We also know that many other factors affect bones. Systemic inflammation, such as seen with rheumatoid arthritis, can cause bone resorption; hormonal changes influence bone resorption; and certain drugs also influence bone resorption.[17,18] In addition, bone health can influence other body functions. For example, lead is a toxic metal that, in its ionic form, as it occurs in things like lead pipe found in old plumbing fixtures, can mimic calcium in the body. Small amounts of lead can even affect gene expression by its ability to replace calcium in key regulatory control proteins.[19] A person with a significant exposure to lead will have bones in which some of the calcium has been replaced by lead. Lead can stay in the body for a long time—years, or even decades—sequestered in the bones.[20] Studies suggest that the majority of the body's lead burden resides in the bone and during times of increased bone turnover, such as seen with calcium deficiency, osteoporosis, repair of broken bones, and pregnancy and lactation, this lead will be released.[21,22] If a person has a history of high lead exposure, the newly liberated lead can create functional brain problems that don't seem directly related to the bone, such as learning disabilities, seizures, and even comas.

The subsequent chapters of this book unravel some of this web with respect to nutrition, and provide more examples of these important connections. The final chapters look at some key functionalities (e.g., energy production, environmental interactions with toxicants, and gastrointestinal function) that underlie many different conditions and show how nutrition can support them.

How Nutrition Supports Health as a Positive Vitality

The historical focus on deficiency and negative outcomes is still apparent in many clinical nutrition textbooks where problem avoidance is the exclusive intervention. Examples of this type of intervention include: elimination of high oxalate foods to avoid recurrence of calcium oxalate nephrolithiasis; reduction of dietary fat to avoid exacerbation of intestinal malabsorption; decreased simple sugar intake in the management of dysglycemia. While the problem-avoidance intervention might be critical in symptomatic management of a health condition, it does not address functionality, or reestablishment of a positive balance in underlying metabolic patterns.

Negative outcomes like vitamin deficiency have been the traditional focus of clinical nutrition. Therefore, most nutritional interventions have been designed to remedy deficiency states. The formula has been fairly simple, involving three basic steps: First, the presence of clinical deficiency symptoms is determined—usually by examining some visible, morphological change occurring at an end-stage clinical level. Examples of such observations include rachitic rosary (vitamin D), angular stomatitis or cheilosis (vitamin B2), koilonychias (iron), glossitis (folate), and gingival enlargement or gingivitis (vitamin C). Second, a dietary or laboratory confirmation (or both) is obtained. For example, a diet diary could be entered into a computer software program and could confirm a deficiency in vitamin D intake, or a laboratory panel could help verify an iron-deficiency anemia. Third, the necessary nutrient(s) are provided (often through supplementation) to treat the deficiency.

A functional perspective certainly acknowledges the importance of this basic approach to nutrient deficiency and recognizes such deficiencies as a reason for intervention. However, a functional approach also seeks to enhance the effectiveness of clinical nutrition by bringing "function" more directly into the intervention process. The integration of functional thinking occurs at each step of the process, and might radically alter the final components of the intervention by bringing different considerations into the process at an earlier stage.

What would happen if we could go back in time prior to the appearance of the end-stage, morphological change or frank deficiency? We would likely find that many "invisible" biochemical and physiological changes were occurring for some time prior to the appearance of the deficiency or disease. In other words, subclinical changes were going on long before the patient arrived in our office. Using such knowledge to prevent or treat disease has been called "upstream medicine"—which is what functional medicine at its best can deliver.

A clear example of this issue of "subclinical" effects can be seen in the development of metabolic syndrome, a condition that has been linked to further development of Type II diabetes mellitus, and one that is prevalent in our current society. Metabolic syndrome is called the "deadly quartet" and is characterized by high triglycerides, insulin resistance, low HDL cholesterol, and high blood pressure.[23,24] Much research has now shown that metabolic syndrome does not occur overnight, but involves many changes in how the body handles glucose and insulin, and is influenced by many other factors over time. We can look at fasting glucose and insulin in an individual and find healthy levels, but if we do a challenge test (i.e., give a glucose dose, and then look at blood glucose and insulin in a 2-hr postprandial assessment), we may see something quite different. A much elevated insulin level may indicate that the body is starting to have problems in adjusting to a glucose challenge. Having this information, we can intervene before things become worse, giving us a much better opportunity to fully restore normal function.

As clinicians, we become versed in the signs and symptoms that signal the presence of a disease or condition. However, do we become versed in observing—or noting the absence of—the signs of optimal balance in our patients? Do we know how to evaluate "positive vitality," not just diagnose disease? Understanding key subclinical imbalances and their potential effects on an individual is one way to begin seeing health as the presence of positive vitality not just the absence of disease. Several examples of how determining a patient's nurture status can help identify subclinical imbalances and provide clues to promoting positive vitality are provided in subsequent chapters of this book. In particular, the areas of energy metabolism, gastrointestinal function, and environmental influences on health, including nutrition, are provided specific focus in the latter part of this text.

Promotion of Organ Reserve with Nutrition and Conditionally Essential Nutrients

Underlying all balance is proper nutriture. Moreover, optimal health is more than the ability of the body to operate adequately in a particular moment; it also means the ability of the body to withstand the challenges of everyday life. These challenges may arise from communicable diseases (like flus and colds), increased stress, increased physical activity, a more toxic environment, or dietary changes. A functional approach to health means supporting the body in such a way that it can thrive despite the challenges of living, not just survive. The body, therefore, needs reserves, some storehouse upon which it can draw when it is challenged. And, functional medicine looks at these reserves as part of overall health.

Conventional approaches to nutriture have placed all nutrients within one of two categories: essential or nonessential. Essential nutrients have been defined as nutrients that the body cannot synthesize and that must, therefore, be supplied through the diet. Nonessential nutrients have been defined as nutrients that the body can synthesize and, therefore, need not be obtained through dietary intake. A functional perspective argues that many nutrients cannot be placed accurately within a single category. In many cases, nutrients that have been conventionally described as "nonessential" may be required in the diet, at specific times or in a specific individual. Therefore, a functional understanding of clinical nutrition involves a new classifica-

tion for nutrients within a category called "conditionally essential."

Nutrients can become conditionally essential for a variety of reasons. A human body may have a constitutive genetic "defect" which prevents an ordinary level of synthesis of the nutrient. In other cases, the body may have an induced defect, in which the nutrient-synthesizing enzyme has been inhibited by a toxic substance, resulting in a lower production of the nutrient. The body might have an atypically high need for the nutrient and, although the body synthesizes the nutrient in an amount considered adequate for a typical human body, the nutrient needs would still not be met. In each of these cases, the nutrient in question would conventionally be classified as "nonessential" but would, in fact, need to be supplied exogenously through the diet or through supplementation.

To avoid the dilemma of a "nonessential" nutrient needing to be supplied exogenously, the functional perspective has adopted the term "conditionally essential" to apply to nutrients that can be synthesized by the body but need to be obtained from the diet or supplementation in a specific person at a specific time. Whether the average human body *can* synthesize a nutrient and whether a specific human body *is* actually synthesizing a nutrient are two distinctly different issues. Only the latter issue relates directly to what is going on in a unique individual at a particular moment.

This textbook provides a novel look at nutrients, from macronutrients to micronutrients, from the functional perspective. In addition, this book includes many categories of nutrients that are considered "nonessential" in the conventional sense, but may be essential to some individuals—that is, conditionally essential nutrients—in order to promote, restore, and maintain optimal health for a patient.

SUMMARY

A functional approach to nutrition means analyzing the multiple roles of various nutrients and other necessary food factors (the so-called "non-nutrients"). A functional approach to nutrition means knowing what these key life-sustaining substances are really doing in the body and asking the question: Are they truly supporting health in this particular person's body they way they should be? In the chapters of this text, you will be taken through the conventional naming of

nutrients, and, in addition, this book focuses on the function of those nutrients in supporting health throughout the different systems of the body, as well as a broader perspective on deficiency symptoms (insufficiencies) and how to ameliorate them.

We are excited to accompany you on your journey toward achieving a more effective use of clinical nutrition in your practice. We welcome comments and suggestions for correcting any errors, and for making the book more useful when next we update it. Please do remember that no book can substitute for an individualized, thoughtful decision process by patients and providers. Clinically-related material is not presented as a prescription for care, but rather as an indicator of the kind of information clinicians may want to consider in making treatment decisions for their patients.

CHAPTER 1 REFERENCES

1. Gruber CJ, Tschugguel W, Schneeberger C, Huber JC. Production and actions of estrogens. N Eng J Med. 2002;346:340–350.
2. Bray GA. The underlying basis for obesity: relationship to cancer. J Nutr. 2002;132(11 Suppl): 3451S–3455S.
3. Zhu BT, Conney AH. Functional role of estrogen metabolism in target cells: review and perspectives. Carcinogenesis. 1998;19:1–27.
4. Liehr JG. Is estradiol a genotoxic mutagenic carcinogen? Endocrine Rev. 2000;21(1):40–54.
5. Lord RS, Bongiovanni B, Bralley JA. Estrogen metabolism and the diet-cancer connection: rationale for assessing the ratio of urinary hydrox-

ylated estrogen metabolites. Altern Med Rev. 2002;7:112–129.
6. Joosten E, van den Berg A, Riezler R, et al. Metabolic evidence that deficiencies of vitamin B12 (cobalamin), folate, and vitamin B6 occur commonly in older people. Am J Clin Nutr. 1992;58:468–76.
7. Blumberg JB. Dietary reference intakes for vitamin E. Nutrition. 1999;15:797–798.
8. Levine M, Rumsey SC, Daruwala R, Park JB, Wang Y. Criteria and recommendations for vitamin C intake. JAMA. 1999;281:1415–1423.
9. Washko PW, Wang Y, Levine M. Ascorbic acid recycling in human neutrophils. J Biol Chem. 1993;268:15531–15535.

10. Grimaldi K, Gill-Garrison R, Roberts G. Personalized nutrition: an early win from the human genome project. Integrative Med. 2003;2:34–45.

11. Collins FS, Guttmacher AE. Genetics moves into the medical mainstream. JAMA. 2001; 286:2322–2323.

12. Ames, BN, Elson-Schwab I, Silver EA. High-dose vitamin therapy stimulates variant enzymes with decreased coenzyme binding affinity (increased Km): relevance to genetic disease and polymorphisms. Am J Clin Nutr 2002;75: 616–658.

13. Bernard C. An introduction to the study of experimental medicine. Henry Copley Greene, trans. New York; The MacMillan Co; 1865.

14. Shuster MM. Biofeedback control of gastrointestinal motility. In: Masmajilan JV, ed. Biofeedback—Principles and practice for clinicians. New York;NY: Williams and Wilkins; 1979.

15. Brody S, Preut R, Schommer K, Schurmeyer TH. A randomized controlled trial of high dose ascorbic acid for reduction of blood pressure, cortisol, and subjective responses to psychological stress. Psychopharmacology 2002;159:319–324.

16. Chandra RK. Zinc and immunity. Nutrition. 1994;10:79–80.

17. Richette P, Corvol M, Bardin. Estrogens, cartilage, and osteoarthritis. J Bone Spine. 2003;70: 257–262.

18. Haugeberg G, Orstavik R, Kvien T. Effects of rheumatoid arthritis on bone. Curr Opin Rheumatol. 2003;15:469–475.

19. Bouton CM, Pevsner J. Effects of lead on gene expression. Neurotoxicology. 2000;21:1045–1055.

20. Olmstead MJ. Heavy metal sources, effects, and detoxification. Altern Complementary Med. 2000;Dec:347–354.

21. Vig EK, Hu H. Lead toxicity in older adults. J Am Geriatr Soc. 2000;48:1501–1506.

22. Sowers MR, Scholl TO, Hall G, et al. Lead in breast milk and maternal bone turnover. Am J Obstet Gynecol. 2002;187:770–776.

23. Kelley DE. Overview: what is insulin resistance? Nutr Rev. 2000;58:(II)S2–S3.

24. Ford ES, Giles WH, Dietz WH. Prevalence of the metabolic syndrome among US adults. JAMA. 2002;287:356–359.

2

Carbohydrates

CARBOHYDRATE DEFINES MANY CLASSES of compounds. Among these classes are the simple, monomer sugar molecules like fructose and glucose, as well as large, polymeric, complex chains that constitute fiber. While carbohydrates are best known as valuable energy sources and structural elements in living cells, they are also a diverse group of compounds that perform a number of other vital tasks.

Several epidemiological studies suggest that chronic disease inversely correlates with consumption of whole, natural plant foods and one of the key components that accounts for this health benefit is fiber. In plant foods, carbohydrates may reach 90 to 95% of total caloric content.[1] Carbohydrates account for only 45% of total caloric intake in the United States, and carbohydrates have been labeled by some as unhealthy components of the diet.

One reason for the confusion in whether carbohydrates are healthy or unhealthy is the unfamiliarity with the different types of carbohydrates and their various effects on the body. The digestibility and physiological effects of a carbohydrate-rich meal depend upon the composition and type of carbohydrate. However, most public health guidelines for carbohydrate consumption do not distinguish among the varieties of carbohydrates. For example, the U.S. Department of Agriculture's Food Guide Pyramid recommends that individuals consume 6 to 11 portions of high-carbohydrate food per day but does not distinguish carbohydrate type or content, such as simple sugar or fiber.[2] Likewise, the American Diabetes Association

Exchange Lists do not account for fiber content or degree of processing in their carbohydrate recommendations.[3] Such simplistic approaches fail to recognize carbohydrate complexity and diversity. Moreover, food labeling lumps the different carbohydrates together as one substance, so for processed foods it can be difficult to really know what type of carbohydrate is really being consumed.

Carbohydrates also have received inconsistent clinical attention. For example, high-carbohydrate diets have been treated as "be-all-and-end-all" approaches to macronutrient balance. Pritikin-type diets suggest a carbohydrate intake as high as 75 to 80% of total calories.[4] High-carbohydrate intake has also been recommended for prevention and/or treatment of conditions such as cardiovascular disease, gastrointestinal disease, and diabetes. Other health advisors endorse very-low-carbohydrate diets that take advantage of the dehydration effects of ketosis.

This chapter addresses the need to consider the complexities of carbohydrates as well as their greater roles in the metabolic processes of living organisms. Carbohydrates are not just an important source of rapid energy production. They are critical links to health and disease. Specifically, this chapter outlines the different types of carbohydrates found in food, describes their diverse physiological structures, and discusses the roles of carbohydrates in functional medicine.

CLASSES OF CARBOHYDRATES

Carbohydrates are molecules that contain carbon, hydrogen, and oxygen in the general elemental composition of $C_x(H_2O)_y$ (Figure 2.1). The simple carbohydrates glucose, fructose, and galactose are the most common carbohydrates found in food (Figure 2.1). These simple carbohydrates and their derivatives are the major building blocks from which most other biological material is derived.

Plants begin constructing carbohydrates through photosynthesis—transforming energy

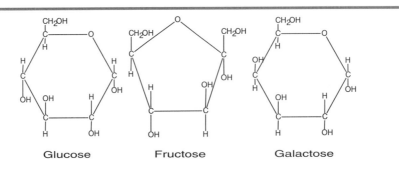

Glucose   Fructose   Galactose

FIGURE 2.1   *Structure of three major monosaccharides*

from sunlight into sugars. Animals then convert the plant sugars they eat into polymers or other noncarbohydrate components such as proteins, fats, and lignins. Animals also use the sugars in plants to create energy. Photosynthesis produces about 200×10^9 tons of biomass each year.[5]

Carbohydrates have traditionally been classified into the oversimplified and misleading categories of "simple" and "complex." Simple refers to molecules of one or two simple sugar units (monosaccharides and disaccharides), and complex refers to polysaccharides (10 or more units). However, most carbohydrates in food are not simple sugars but multimers of these carbohydrate units as either oligosaccharides (2 to 10 monosaccharides) or polysaccharides (more than 10 monosaccharides).

From a functional perspective, neither classification is helpful. On the one hand, "simple" monosaccharides can have extremely complex metabolic roles. Even structurally, they can have far-reaching health consequences. The deposition of galactose in the neuronal myelin sheath and the glycosylation of proteins—now understood as a co-translational event—are examples of highly complex and far-reaching roles for monosaccharides. On the other hand, "complex" carbohydrates like plant cellulose may remain relatively inert metabolically.

Not only are the terms simple and complex misleading, they also exclude the intermediate category: carbohydrates that are neither simple nor complex—*oligosaccharides* ("few-sugar" carbohydrates). Oligosaccharides contain between 2 and 10 monosaccharides, and include such molecules as fructooligosaccharides (Figure 2.2), which are "prebiotic" carbohydrates. That is, they escape degradation in the upper digestive tract and travel to the large intestine where they become fuel for the friendly intestinal flora.

Carbohydrates can be classified according to their physical characteristics (Table 2.1). This type of classification allows for more differentiation of their effects than does the "simple" and "complex" classification system. However, a functional understanding of carbohydrates must consider their biological effects as well as their physical properties. For example, a fiber might be soluble or insoluble, might resist digestion and act as a prebiotic, and might also affect blood sugar control. Since individual carbohydrates can have such differing functional effects, several major carbohydrates from different physical categories are reviewed below.

Fructose

Fructose is the sweetest of the simple sugars and is highly concentrated in honey, fruits, and some vegetables. Fructose metabolism is an active area of research. Studies have shown that liver cells use fructose without the mediating effects of insulin. For this reason, fructose has been suggested as less problematic than glucose for dysglycemic individuals.[6]

Clinical studies have supported this observation. For example, fructose has been shown to attenuate the glycemic rise in blood after a

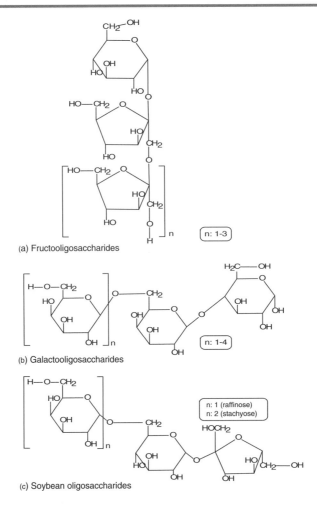

(a) Fructooligosaccharides

(b) Galactooligosaccharides

(c) Soybean oligosaccharides

FIGURE 2.2   *Oligosaccharides having physiological activity include fructooligosaccharides (a), galactooligosaccharides (b), and soybean oligosaccharides (c)*

glucose load.[7] Data continue to support that modest amounts of fructose may be the beneficial choice of sweetener for most people. Consuming large amounts (greater than 50 g) of fructose, however, has been reported to cause an increase in serum triglycerides in some non-insulin-dependent diabetics, particularly those with hypertriglyceridemia.[6] And, large amounts of fructose have also been reported to cause hyperuricemia in gout pa-

TABLE 2.1   *Physiologically Important Classes of Carbohydrates*

Simple Sugars
Monosaccharides and disaccharides Including: glucose, fructose, galactose, maltose, lactose, sucrose
Oligosaccharides
Apolymeric carbohydrates that contain 2 to 10 monosaccharides Including: galactooligosaccharides, fructooligosaccharides, soy oligosaccharides
Starch
Large-chain glucose polymers Including: amylose—straight-chain polymers of glucose; amylopectin—branched-chain   polymers of glucose
Nonstarch Polysaccharides
Large-chain nonstarch carbohydrate polymers Including: cellulose, pectin, hemicellulose, gums

tients.[6] Therefore, as with any sugar, fructose intake should be modest.

Studies illustrate that fructose malabsorption can occur, especially in health-compromised patients. For instance, patients with functional bowel disorders, like irritable bowel syndrome, have been reported to have sugar malabsorption and, in those patients, fructose may provoke symptoms.[8] Some studies suggest fructose malabsorption and consequential symptoms can be decreased or even eliminated when fructose is consumed with glucose. This result is possibly caused by glucose activating the fructose transporter.[6]

High Fructose Corn Syrup (HFCS)

According to studies reported in the 1990s, the average American adult consumes about 40 grams per day of fructose, the majority (~70%) of which comes from a non-natural source of fructose: high fructose corn syrup. HFCS is the main sweetener used in many processed foods, and is a primary sweetener used by the soft drink industry. HFCS is not fructose, but instead is a combination of glucose and fructose, which is produced by conversion of dextrose to fructose. Preparations of HFCS range in composition, but many are about 50% fructose and 50% glucose. Several studies have compared HFCS to fructose and shown distinct differences. For example, HFCS has been shown to lead to a significant increase in blood glucose and insulin levels as compared to the same amount of fructose in non-insulin-dependent diabetics. Therefore, the intake of HFCS should be considered separately in reviewing a patient's diet.

Inulin and Fructooligosaccharides

The large intestine contains symbiotic microbiota that play an important role in health. At least 50 different genera of bacteria exist in the human colon. For fuel, the colonic microbiota use undigested carbohydrates, such as soluble fibers and resistant starch. These symbiotic bacteria support health by producing short-chain fatty acids (SCFAs) from fermentation of carbohydrates. Propionate, acetate, and butyrate are SCFAs that supply up to 70% of the energy used by colonic epithelial cells.

Of those bacteria important to health, bifidobacteria and lactobacilli genera are the most extensively researched. Some carbohydrates selectively promote the growth of these beneficial or "friendly" bacteria. Selective support of bifidobacteria and lactobacilli may cause them to compete for and outgrow other harmful bacteria. As a result, they may act as a targeted, natural approach to antibiotic therapy. A carbohydrate that selectively supports the growth and/or activity of one or both of these species of bacteria and improves host health is called a *prebiotic*.[10] (Table 2.2 indicates which carbohydrates function as prebiotics and which function as colonic food. Figure 2.3 shows many of the activities of bifidobacteria.)

Prebiotics include fructooligosaccharides, inulin, and galactooligosaccharides. Inulin is a member of the fructan family of storage carbohydrates that occur in various flowering plants, especially chicory, onions, asparagus, and Jerusalem artichokes. Food sources of inulin are shown in Table 2.3. Inulin is a polysaccharide composed of repeating fructose units with a terminal glucose unit.[11] Prebiotics, along with a balance of soluble and insoluble dietary fibers, provide substrate for

TABLE 2.2   *Classification of Certain Carbohydrates as Colonic Food and Prebiotics*

Carbohydrate	Colonic Food	Prebiotic
Resistant Starch	Yes	Possibly
Nonstarch polysaccharides		
Plant cell wall polysaccharides	Yes	No
Hemicellulose	Yes	No
Pectins	Yes	No
Gums	Yes	No
Nondigestible oligosaccharides		
Fructooligosaccharides	Yes	Yes
Galactooligosaccharides	Yes	Probably
Soybean oligosaccharides	Yes	Probably
Glucooligosaccharides	Possibly	No

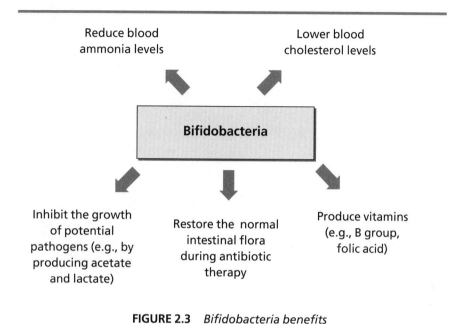

FIGURE 2.3 *Bifidobacteria benefits*

microflora to produce these beneficial SCFAs. When a diet includes prebiotics, intraluminal concentrations of SCFAs increase.

Oligosaccharides resulting from inulin breakdown are called fructooligosaccharides. In dietary research, fructooligosaccharides (oligosaccharides containing between 2 and 10 molecules of the monosaccharide fructose with a terminal glucose unit) are an active area of study. Fructooligosaccharides are the preferential substrate for most bifidobacteria and are ineffective as a substrate for the potentially pathogenic bacterium *Clostridium perfringens*. Supplementing these nutrients in doses of 1–8 g per day favorably affects human microflora balance.[11] Examples of common fructooligo-saccharide molecules are shown in Figure 2.4; food sources are shown in Table 2.4.

TABLE 2.3 *Inulin in Food*

Plant	Inulin Level (%)
Wheat	1–4
Onion	2–6
Murnong	8–13
Leek	10–15
Asparagus	10–15
Chicory root	13–20
Yacon	15–20
Salsify	15–20
Jerusalem artichoke	15–20
Dahlia tuber	15–20
Garlic	15–25

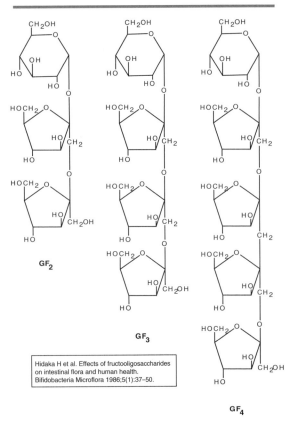

GF$_2$

GF$_3$

Hidaka H et al. Effects of fructooligosaccharides on intestinal flora and human health. Bifidobacteria Microflora 1986;5(1):37–50.

GF$_4$

FIGURE 2.4   *Some fructooligosaccharides*

Nondigestible or "Resistant" Starch

Although starch and nonstarch polysaccharides are both polymers of monomeric sugars, the unique nutritional and physical properties of starch set it apart. Starch is the predominant food reserve in plants, and starch and starch breakdown products, along with sucrose and lactose, are also the predominant carbohydrates digested by humans.[13] Two types of starch polymers exist:

amylose, a straight-chain polymer of glucose, and amylopectin, a branched-chain polymer of glucose (Figure 2.5). The D-glucose units in amylose, an essentially linear molecule, are linked by α-(1→4) glycosidic bonds. Amylopectin consists of glucose linked by α-(1→4)-D-glucan bonds with an occasional α-(1→6) bond. Amylopectin is a large molecule with a molecular weight in excess of 10^7 daltons and has a complex "bush-like" structure.

Starch digestion begins in the mouth, where amylase enzymes start the hydrolysis process, and continues in the small intestine. The enzyme β-amylase cleaves the penultimate glycosidic link from the reducing end of the starch to release maltose. Digestion by β-amylase is often incomplete, and starch must be completely depolymerized to glucose before it can be absorbed in the small intestine. Therefore, many enzymes are involved in starch digestion. In humans, depolymerization is effected by several digestive enzymes that cleave the α-(1→4) and α-(1→6) glucosidic bonds, mainly by the action of α-amylases.

Starch is packaged as granules in plants. Starch granules differ in their composition and ability to be broken down in the digestive tracts of humans. Formation of complexes with fatty acids and guar gum also reduce the digestibility of starch. In addition, the amylose starch complexes are less susceptible to digestion than the amylopectin complexes due to their tight physical structure. These factors (physical inaccessibility, food particle size, cell wall or protein encapsulation, and composition of starch complexes) result in different

TABLE 2.4 *Fructooligosaccharides and Food*

Oligosaccharides		Distribution
GF₂	1-kestone	onion, edible burdock, rye, asparagus, Chinese chive, Jerusalem artichoke
	6-kestone	Gramineae plants
	neokestone	onion, banana, asparagus, sugar maple, Gramineae plants
GF₃	nystose	onion, edible burdock, asparagus
	bifurcose	rye
	neobifurcose	oat
GF₄	fructosylnsystose	onion, edible burdock, asparagus
	bifurcose	rye

Source of data: Mitsuoka T, Hidaka H, Eida T. Effect of fructo-oligosaccharides on intestinal microflora. Die Nahrung 1987;5–6:427–436.

starch digestion rates with some starch being "resistant" to digestion (Table 2.5).

Carbohydrate chemists have defined three categories of starch to describe these phenomena: rapidly digestible starch (RDS), slowly digestible starch (SDS), and resistant starch (RS).[14] The concept of resistant starch is just beginning to receive widespread attention in the literature, and it may eventually have extremely important clinical implications,

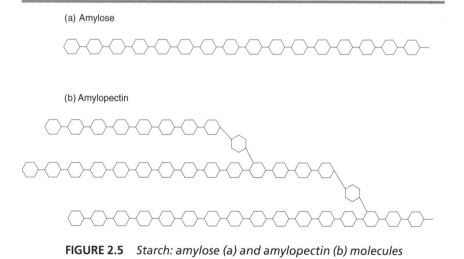

FIGURE 2.5 *Starch: amylose (a) and amylopectin (b) molecules*

TABLE 2.5   *Differential Digestion of Starch Complexes*

Type of Starch	Example of Occurrence	Probable Digestion in the Small Intestine
Rapidly digestible starch (RDS)	Freshly cooked starchy foods	Rapid
Slowly digestible starch (SDS)	Many raw cereals	Slow but complete
Resistant starch (RS)		
1. Physically indigestible starch	Partly milled grains and seeds	Resistant
2. Resistant starch granules	Raw potato and banana	Resistant
3. Retrograded starch	Cooled, cooked potato, bread, and cornflakes	Resistant

particularly in the management of blood sugar and diabetes. For example, the range of digestibility of different starch complexes may account for the variable blood glucose results obtained with various high starch meals (discussed in greater depth in the glycemic index and carbohydrate composition sections). Moreover, starch resistant to digestion may become fermentable substrate or "food" for bacteria in the lower intestinal tract.

Dietary Fibers

Fiber is generally considered the sum of polysaccharides not digested by the endogenous secretions (digestive enzymes) of the human gastrointestinal tract. The polysaccharides in fiber may include nonstarch polysaccharides, such as cellulose, hemicellulose, and pectin, or the nondigestible fraction of starch called resistant starch.

Fiber is also categorized as soluble or insoluble based on its general physiological effects. Insoluble fibers do not form colloidal suspensions in water. These fibers are typically referred to as "bulking agents," and they usually help intestinal flow. Insoluble fibers include celluloses, some hemicelluloses (pentosans), and insoluble pectins. Insoluble fiber adds weight, volume (fecal bulk), and "softness" to the stools, thereby enhancing intraluminal transport (decreasing transit time) and facilitating regular elimination.

Soluble fibers form colloidal suspensions in water. These fibers typically pass through the intestinal tract more slowly than insoluble fibers. Soluble fibers include soluble gums (including beta-glucans), some hemicelluloses, soluble pectins, and other soluble polysaccharides not susceptible to enzymatic degradation. Soluble fiber adds some bulk and "softness" to the stools by its property of water absorption and facilitates ("normalizes") intraluminal stool transit and elimination. However, it is more often associated with certain therapeutic effects—decreasing cholesterol absorption and moderating or delaying the absorption of glucose in the small in-

TABLE 2.6   *Dietary Fibers*

Plant cell walls are composed of fiber and non-fiber components. **Non-fiber components** include: Proteins Cutin Wax Silice Suberin Lignin
Insoluble fibers (insoluble in water, but can swell and absorb up to 20 times their weight in water): Celluloses Lignins Some hemicelluloses
Soluble fibers (soluble in water and form a smooth gel or thickened network): Pectins Gums Mucilages Alginates Carrageenans Some hemicelluloses
Note: Cereal fibers are generally insoluble in water, whereas fruits, vegetables, and nuts contain a higher proportion of soluble fiber.

Reference: Thebaudin JY, Lefebvre AC, Harrington M, Bourgeois CM. Dietary fibres: nutritional and technological interest. Trends Food Sci Tech 1997;8:41–48

testines. Soluble fibers can also delay gastric emptying and increase the satiety value of a meal. A more comprehensive look at the physiological effects of different types of fiber is provided in Table 2.7.

From a functional medicine perspective, estimating dietary fiber may be one of the best "shortcuts" of evaluating a patient's dietary quality, because lack of fiber content takes a greater toll on diet quality than any other component of food. In the United States, average adult fiber intake is below 10 g per day.[15] Worldwide, the average fiber intake is in the 50 to 75-gram range. High rates of intake of processed and animal foods (which universally contain little to no fiber) account for this difference. Fiber intake has been shown to be cardioprotective,[16] glucose regulating,[17] and cancer protective.[18]

Analyzing an individual's diet diary can help determine the quantity and quality of fiber in the overall diet. While the National Cancer Institute recommends 25 to 30 g of fiber per day, observational studies in diabetes research and epidemiological studies in countries where daily fiber consumption reaches a level of 75–100 g, suggest higher levels may be helpful.

EVALUATING FIBER INTAKE

A practitioner can evaluate an individual's fiber consumption in several ways. An individual health history should include questions that assess stool frequency, quality, quantity, and the ease or difficulty with which stools are passed, as well as questions regarding amount of regular fluid intake, laxative use, and exercise. Estimating transit time is also helpful.* If

---

*One of the most common health hazards and problems in Western Civilization is chronic constipation and diseases of the colon, e.g., hemorrhoids, diverticulitis, colitis, and cancer of the colon. Studies of other cultures have consistently shown a correlation between healthy colons, large stools and normal colon transit time. Colon transit time can be measured by asking the patient to eat either a moderate serving of corn or beets (1/2 to 3/4 cup) or take 4 charcoal capsules, and note the time of first and last appearance in the stool.

TABLE 2.7   *Physiological Effects of Soluble/Insoluble Fibers*

Physiological Response	Dietary Fiber		Resistant Starch
	Soluble	*Insoluble*	
Upper GI Tract			
Digestive enzyme activity	Decrease	Decrease	No effect
Rate of mineral & vitamin absorption	Delayed	No effect	No effect
Amount of mineral & vitamin absorption	No effect	No effect	No effect
Blood cholesterol	Decrease	No effect	No effect
Blood glucose	Decrease	No effect	Insufficient data
Blood insulin	Decrease	No effect	Insufficient data
Sterol absorption	Decrease	Small decrease	No effect
Lumen particle size	None	Variable	None
Lumen viscosity	Variable	None	None
Lower GI Tract			
Bacterial growth–biomass	Significant increase	Medium increase	Significant increase
Attachment sites for biomass	None	Variable	None
Gases: CO_2, H_2, CH_4 (methane)	Significant increase	Small increase	Significant increase
Colon pH	Significant decrease	Small decrease	Significant decrease
Colon and fecal:			
SCFAs	Increase	Increase	Increase
Acetate	Increase	Small increase	Increase
Propionate	Increase	Small increase	Increase
Butyrate	Increase	Small increase	Significant increase
Ammonia	Decrease	Small decrease	Significant decrease
Fecal anaerobic bacteria	Change	Small change	Change
Epithelial cell physiology and cell biology:			
DNA repair	Increase	Small increase	Increase
Gene expression	Reduction	Reduction	Insufficient data
Proliferation	Reduction	Reduction	Insufficient data
Apoptosis	Unknown	Unknown	Unknown
Laxative Effects	Weak	Strong	Strong
Fecal bulk; water-holding capacity	Weak	Strong	Strong
Bile acid changes in colon	Positive	Positive	Insufficient data
Intestinal Transit Time	No change	Strong decrease	Decrease

bowel movements are difficult and/or painful, infrequent, small, hard, and dry, and/or transit time is prolonged, additional fiber may be needed. Some laboratory stool analyses provide information regarding total and/or individual short-chain fatty acid content. More information on laboratory testing is provided in Chapter 10.

Increasing Fiber in the Diet

Commonly used and known dietary fiber sources include wheat bran, psyllium, and oat fiber. Unfortunately, many individuals experience reactions to wheat (gluten) and/or psyllium-containing foods and supplements. Less commonly known and yet beneficial food fibers include soy fiber, beet fiber, pea fiber, oat gum, rice bran, apple pectin, apple fiber, cellulose and xanthan gums, and gum arabic.

Consider the following when adding fiber to the diet:

Tolerability: Since many fibers come from gluten-containing products (wheat, rye, and barley), the source of the fiber(s) should be considered within the context of the individual's tolerance or antigenic sensitivities.

Solubility properties: The type and/or proportion of insoluble to soluble fibers may be determined in part by the known physiologic effects of the individual fibers and the desired physiologic changes in a given individual.

Daily fluid intake: As the amount of fiber in the diet increases, increasing fluid (water) intake is generally advised. (Failure to increase fluid intake along with increasing fiber, especially in the elderly and other cases of physiologic compromise can result in stool impaction and bowel obstruction.) Especially with the carbohydrate fibers, drinking water is clinically important. Increasing a patient's fiber amount without simultaneously increasing water may produce constipation, while excessive increases in fiber together with water may produce diarrhea.

Gradual increase: Incrementally increasing fiber in the daily diet is important. *Gradually* increasing the amount over days to weeks, as individually indicated and tolerated, will generally improve tolerance/adaptation while minimizing side effects. For many individuals, as little as 1 teaspoon of additional fiber per day may be the initial limit that will not cause problems.

A FUNCTIONAL APPROACH TO CARBOHYDRATES

Carbohydrate Metabolism and Maldigestion

Gas and bloating are the two most common effects that people experience after eating, and both can be related to carbohydrate intake. Everyone produces gas as a byproduct of digestion. Some amount of gas and bloating throughout the day is normal. Producing some intestinal gas is usually a sign of a good high-fiber diet and good health, and any inconvenience it may cause is social and not medical. The gases humans produce in the process of digestion include hydrogen, methane, hydrogen sulfide, carbon dioxide, nitrogen, and ammonia. Hydrogen sulfide is the gas that causes offensive odor. The average individual produces approximately $1^1/_2$ quarts of gas daily in the course of normal digestion. The number of times a person passes gas in a day varies from as few as 3 times to nearly 40.

It takes 15 minutes to 2 hours for the first part of a meal to pass through the stomach and small intestine to the colon. An entire meal takes much longer. It can take as little as a few hours, to as long as a few days, for meals to pass from the beginning of the digestive tract, the stomach, to the end, the colon. Individuals with a fast transit time send more undigested starch to the colon along with fiber. Most digestion occurs in the small intestine, and is assisted by enzymes produced in the pancreas and bile produced in the liver. Some foods, especially soluble fiber and the prebiotic carbohydrates, result in a large amount of gas as a byproduct of fermentation by colonic bacteria.

Although modest gas production is normal, some individuals experience excessive gas and bloating. Clinical experience suggests that a number of conditions may lead to gas and bloating, including (1) a high-fat diet; (2) hypochlorhydria or inadequate digestive enzymes; and (3) food sensitivity. Foods commonly associated with symptoms of gas and bloating include high-fat foods, fruits and juices containing sorbitol or mannitol (apple juice, pear juice, grapes, prunes, cherries), cabbage and other cruciferous vegetables,

beans, and unripe fruit (which contains a high percentage of pectin). Soy oligosaccharides or legume oligosaccharides have also been implicated in excessive gas and bloating.

Fat and protein are slower to digest than carbohydrate. Therefore, when a high-fat meal is consumed, it remains in the stomach a longer time than a high carbohydrate meal. The carbohydrates associated with the fat and protein in the high-fat diet are presumed to be broken down and possibly fermented earlier in the digestive tract than the lower intestine. Some older people find it more difficult to digest high-protein, high-fat meals than younger individuals. This may be due to the decreased secretion of stomach acid that is sometimes associated with aging. (The high fat content of the standard American diet places a heavy burden on both the pancreas and the gallbladder for the proper digestion and assimilation of fats and may help explain why gallbladder surgery is so common.)

In all chronic cases of gas and bloating, it is essential to consider hypochlorhydria as a prime cause, and to review any medications a patient may be taking to *reduce* stomach acid secretion. Reducing stomach acid secretions can result not only in gas and bloating but also in the malabsorption of a number of important nutrients and other gastrointestinal dysfunctions.

Several cooking techniques can help minimize those symptoms of gas and bloating that are related to carbohydrate consumption. These techniques include soaking beans overnight; draining, rinsing, and adding $^1/_2$ teaspoon of mustard seed to the cooking water of legumes; and cooking cruciferous vegetables like cabbage more quickly—for example, stir-frying instead of boiling or steaming.

Carbohydrate Metabolism and Blood Sugar Regulation

Over eighteen million people in the United States live with diabetes mellitus.[19] Although the 2002 figures represented only 6.3% of the population in that year, the Centers for Disease Control estimated the lifetime risk for Americans born in 2000 to be one in three![20] That makes diabetes the nation's #1 chronic disease prevention and treatment challenge.

The two major types of diabetes, type 1 (insulin-dependent diabetes mellitus or IDDM) and type 2 (non-insulin-dependent diabetes mellitus or NIDDM) are treated differently. In IDDM, a lack of insulin causes elevated levels of blood glucose. In NIDDM, a lack of insulin *sensitivity* is the cause of elevated levels of blood glucose.[21] Ninety percent of all diabetics have NIDDM.[22] The insulin resistance that characterizes NIDDM is often further complicated by the fact that many NIDDM individuals are also obese, which can exacerbate the insulin resistance.[23]

Long-term complications of diabetes, including problems with eyes, kidneys, cardiovascular and nervous systems, can be prevented or delayed by dietary control.[24] Type I diabetics try to maintain proper blood glucose balance with a combination of diet and insulin injections. Type II diabetics are usually treated initially with diet and exercise, which can improve insulin sensitivity.[25,26]

Many individuals with NIDDM are less conscious than they should be of the dangers associated with complications from the disease. Raising their consciousness about the risks enables clinicians to identify and implement preventive strategies that may avoid, or at least delay, the onset of complications such as cardiovascular disease, nephropathies, and neuropathies.[27] Individuals who already have hypertension or hyperlipidemia are at high risk of developing serious cardiovascular complications if they do not attend to their diet and exercise. The 1996 recommendation for "near-normal" glycemia (a glycohemoglobin level no higher than 1.0% above the upper normal limit), published by the American College of Physicians, advises aggressive means to prevent cardiovascular disease, nephropathy, and neuropathy, and suggests that even a small decrease in glycohemoglobin is beneficial.[28,29]

Glycemic index

Carbohydrate metabolism plays an important role in the treatment of both types of diabetes.[30] Much of the research has focused on ways to identify high-risk foods for diabetics, but assessing the amount of glucose entering the bloodstream after a meal and describing the foods to avoid or include in a diet for diabetics can be difficult. The concept of "glycemic index" has been developed to help compare different foods based on their ability to induce a rise in blood glucose. Glycemic index is often abbreviated as GI, and is the calculated value of the blood glucose response to a food as compared to a standard food (usually glucose or white bread).

To determine the GI, the glycemic response of ingesting a portion of food containing 50 g of carbohydrate is compared to the glycemic response of a 50-gram portion of glucose or white bread (Figure 2.6). Most commonly, researchers use white bread instead of glucose as the standard response since GI data from white bread appear to be more reliable.[31,32] The GI of a specific food is typically measured after an overnight fast.

In 1995, researchers compiled the International Table of Glycemic Index to summarize the data obtained from studies about the GI of specific individual foods.[33] GI values were consistent for most foods. However, some foods varied widely, which is difficult to explain. The authors suggested that amylose content of starch and methods of cooking and processing could explain the variations in GI. In addition, the variety, species, or strain of the food source may be different and may result in different responses (e.g., russet potato vs. new potato, basmati rice vs. short-grain rice, ripe banana vs. aged banana). Table 2.8 lists the glycemic index for some commonly eaten foods.

Because the amount of carbohydrate can differ in a typical serving of a food, a new measure termed "glycemic load" (GL) has been introduced. The dietary glycemic load is defined as the product of a food's glycemic index and its carbohydrate content.[34] GL takes into account the idea that foods rated solely on the basis of their GI do not quantify common or customary servings that are eaten. For instance, while carrots have a high GI (92 vs. glucose), a usual serving of carrots has a low total carbohydrate content (6-8 g), and thus would realistically only produce a low glycemic response. Using the GL therefore allows for the assessment of the quantity as well as the quality of the carbohydrate intake in the diet. However, the question of whether the GI of foods, or the GL of a diet, has significance to human health continues to be controversial, and no consensus on its use has been reached in the United States. Recent research in this area, both epidemiological and case controlled, strongly suggests that high GI foods and high GL diets produce increased serum glucose levels and increased insulin demand. These events have been shown,

$$\frac{\text{Glycemic response of a portion of food with 50 g carbohydrate}}{\text{Glycemic response of a 50 g portion of white bread}} \times 100$$

FIGURE 2.6   *Calculation of glycemic index (GI)*

TABLE 2.8 *Glycemic Index Table of Commonly Eaten Foods*

Food	GI—glucose standard	GI—white bread standard
rye bread	63	90
white bread	69	100
whole wheat bread	72	99
white rice	72	81
parboiled 5 min		54
parboiled 25 min		6
brown rice	66	81; 76
high amylose		66
potato (new), boiled	70	80
(russet), baked	56	128; 80
mashed	70	98
sweet potato	48	70
shredded wheat	67	97
milk (skim)	32	46
corn flakes	80	109
sweet corn	59	80
oatmeal	49	93
green peas, frozen	51	65
kidney beans	29	43
lentils	29	38
pearl barley	25	36
spaghetti	50	
boiled 5 min		45
boiled 15 min		61
apple	39	53
banana	62	84
underripe	30	59; 43
orange	40	59
orange juice	46	67
fructose	20	31
glucose	100	138
sucrose	59	89

in predisposed individuals, to increase insulin resistance and the risk for type 2 diabetes. Additionally, epidemiological evidence in the past three years supports the concept that low GL diets are associated with higher HDL-cholesterol and lower triglyceride concentrations, and overall a low GL diet decreases risk for coronary heart disease.[35-39]

Factors affecting glycemic response

Several factors affect the GI of a food, including type of carbohydrate, starch accessibility (e.g., resistant starch), nutrient composition, presence of protein and fat, processing and preparation, and total sucrose and fructose content.[40,41] The same food may produce a different GI based on how it is cooked or what food accompanies it in a meal. In addition, while many tables of general GI values for foods exist, researchers are still unclear about long-term benefits of diets based on low GI foods.[42]

In addition to the debate over these GIs for individual foods, the reliability of GI in predicting glycemic response to a mixed meal is also controversial: does the response to a meal depend only on the GI of the individual foods in that meal? While the literature presents both sides of this issue, several studies with both healthy and diabetic subjects report reliability in predicting glycemic response based on the GI of individual foods contained in a meal.[43,44] However, glycemic response for NIDDM patients may be an exception.[45,46]

As discussed earlier, the starch amylose is digested more slowly than amylopectin, due in part to the ability of amylose to form resistant starch. This observation may help explain why carbohydrates higher in amylose have a lower GI.[47] Starch in raw foods, or in foods with a high moisture content cooked at low temperatures, is less digestible.[48,49] Brand et al. studied the effects of processed vs. unprocessed foods and concluded that food processing also correlates with a higher GI. Sweeteners or other components that may be augmented in processed foods may contribute to this finding.[50] Conversely, high temperatures used in canning can increase starch hydrolysis, rendering it more digestible.

Adding fiber to the diet improves glycemic control compared to the predicted values for foods without added fiber.[51,52] In early studies on fiber supplementation in diabetics, Anderson and Chen reported discontinuing insulin in a group of 8 men who had been taking 16 units of insulin daily.[53] Subjects' diets consisted of 10% protein and 70% carbohydrate, including 60 to 80 g of plant fiber. The authors attributed the decreased insulin needs to the different plant fibers used in the diet. They suggested that the significantly lower glycemic and insulin response produced by barley and oatmeal was created by the high amounts of the soluble fiber β-glucan in the respective grains.[54,55]

Fiber may influence GI in several ways. First, soluble fiber causes a delay in gastric emptying, which could slow absorption of glucose. Second, fiber causes a viscous solution to form in the intestine, which may block enzymatic breakdown.[56] In addition to a high fiber content, legumes also contain phytate and lectins, which can inhibit digestion and absorption.[57] An inverse relationship has been found between the amount of phytate in foods and GI, suggesting that phytate affects starch digestibility.[58]

Second meal effect

The second meal effect is the ability of one meal to improve glucose tolerance of the next meal. Studies using healthy subjects illustrate that a slow and prolonged absorption of carbohydrate at breakfast results in a slower rise in blood sugar levels, a reduced insulin response, and a lessened glycemic response after lunch.[59,60] A low GI dinner meal has been shown to produce the same type of glycemic response after breakfast.[61] Clinically, this "second meal" phenomenon underscores the importance of dietary interventions that evaluate the entire dietary pattern—not simply individual food selections.

The concept of "second meal effect" may also help explain why meal frequency throughout the whole day is important. Carbohydrate and endocrine metabolism and serum lipid levels are affected by the rate at which starches are digested and absorbed.[62] Carbohydrates are absorbed more slowly with increased meal frequency, often resulting in a reduction of insulin response, postprandial blood glucose, and serum cholesterol levels.

Clinical conclusions about carbohydrates and glycemic index

Historically, maintaining optimum blood sugar control has been the most important goal in dietary management of diabetes mellitus.[63,64] Researchers have typically recom-

mended a diet with few refined carbohydrates for diabetics to help reduce long-term complications such as neuropathy, nephropathy, and cardiovascular disease.[65,66] Before diabetes was treated with insulin, diabetics were advised to consume only 20% of their total calories as carbohydrate.[67,68]

In 1997, The American Diabetes Association (ADA) recommended more frequent meals to improve both glucose and lipid control.[69] Consistent with its 1996 position, ADA did not mention GI, nor did it consider fiber to be important. Fiber specifications reflected the 1996 position of 20 to 35 g per day—the same level recommended for healthy individuals.[70] Moreover, a study published in the New England Journal of Medicine in 2000 comparing the ADA guidelines for fiber with a high fiber diet (50 g of fiber with 50% soluble, 50% insoluble) in type 2 diabetic patients reported improved glycemic control and decreased hyperinsulinemia and lipids with the high fiber diet.[71] This again points out the need to look at more than overall carbohydrate, to focus on the variety and amount of key carbohydrates, such as soluble fiber intake in specific health-compromised individuals.

The Exchange List for Meal Planning, developed in 1950 by the Committee on Diabetic Diet Calculations of the ADA, guided meal planning to improve diabetes management.[72] It offered measurements of the available carbohydrate content of foods. Starchy foods were grouped together, and measured amounts were treated as interchangeable. According to Truswell, "Available carbohydrates were assumed to be all digested and absorbed at the same rate and to have the same effect on postprandial blood glucose, except for sugar, or sucrose, which was absorbed more rapidly."[73] Our current understanding about the varying glucose response to different types of carbohydrates suggests that this concept is outdated and is even counterproductive in many regards.

While using the GI of foods as a dietary guide has merit, it also has problems. Patients planning meals with an emphasis on improving blood sugar, serum insulin, or serum lipids have no way of knowing the amylose content of the food they are eating, nor can they know how many times a food has been reheated in a restaurant before it is served, nor what its age may be. The ripeness of fruit, for example, can change its GI (banana is one such example). Different varieties of foods grown and sold in packages give no clue to the consumer about possible differences in GI. It is often difficult to convince individuals with diabetes that it is very important to eat fresh, whole, unprocessed foods. Nonetheless, basic principles used in understanding glycemic response can and should be explained to patients. Moreover, practitioners should encourage patients to incorporate these ideas into their meal planning.

CARBOHYDRATE RESEARCH: FUTURE DIRECTIONS

Although most nutrition-related discussions about carbohydrates focus on their role in metabolism and energy production, carbohydrates and their derivatives are essential in several other biological processes, including cell adhesion, cell development and differentiation, cell signaling events, infection, and metastasis.[74] Intensive study in a new field of carbohydrate research called "glycobiology" focuses on these activities of carbohydrates, which result from the attachment or "decoration" of specific proteins with carbohydrate moieties, a process called glycosylation. The Golgi apparatus inside the cell appears to be the most important site for intracellular glycosylation. The cell is actually able to synthesize the glycan (protein-carbohydrate) molecules without having to code this information into the DNA.[75] Glycosylated proteins appear to play a critical role in cell recognition[76] and the miscommunications that lead to cellular dysfunction, including autoimmune dysfunction and metastases.

SUMMARY

Contrary to the historical idea that carbohydrates are easily defined as "simple" or "complex" compounds with specific, well-defined roles in metabolism, the term actually encompasses a diverse group of compounds that perform multiple important functions in the body. The right selection of carbohydrates supports healthy blood glucose control and gastrointestinal function, helps prevent several diseases and dysfunctional conditions, and provides important nutrients to the body. Because of the many beneficial physiologic functions of different types of carbohydrates, a more sophisticated approach to using carbohydrates to support patient health in a variety of ways is integral to the functional medicine model.

CHAPTER 2 REFERENCES

1. Hegarty V. Nutrition: Food and the Environment. St. Paul, Minn: Eagan Press; 1995:143–168.

2. USDA website, March 2004: <http://www.nal.usda.gov/finic/Fpyr/pyramid.html>

3. American Diabetes Association. Nutrition recommendations and principles for people with diabetes mellitus. Diabetes Care. 1997;20 (Suppl 1):S14–S17.

4. Pritikin N. The Pritikin Permanent Weight-Loss Manual. New York, NY: Bantam Books; 1981.

5. Whistler RL, BeMiller JN. Carbohydrate Chemistry for Food Scientists. St. Paul, Minn: Eagan Press; 1997:1–17.

6. Henry RR, Crapo PA, Thorburn AW. Current issues in fructose metabolism. Ann Rev Nutr. 1991;11:21–39.

7. Moore MC, Mann SL, Davis SN, et al. Acute fructose administration improves oral glucose tolerance in adults with type 2 diabetes. Diabetes Care 2001;24(11):1882–1887.

8. Goldstein R, Braverman D, Stankiewicz H. Carbohydrate malabsorption and the effect of dietary restriction on symptoms of irritable bowel syndrome and functional bowel complaints. Isr Med Assoc J 2000;2:583–587.

9. Elliott SS, Keim NL, Stern JS, Teff K, Havel PJ. Fructose, weight gain, and the insulin resistance syndrome. Am J Clin Nutr. 2002;76:911–922

10. Gibson GR, Roberroid MB. Dietary modulation of the human colonic microbiota: introducing the concept of prebiotics. J Nutr. 1995;125(6):1401–1412.

11. Silva RF. Use of inulin as a natural texture modifier. Cereal Chemistry. 1996;41:792–794.

12. Hidaka H, Hirayama M, Tokunaga T, et al. The effects of undigestible fructo-oligosaccharides on intestinal microflora and various physiological functions on human health. In: Furda I and Brine CJ, eds. New Developments in Dietary Fiber. New York, NY: Plenum Press;1990:105–117.

13. Hidaka H, Hirayama M, Tokunaga T, et al. The effects of undigestible fructo-oligosaccharides on intestinal microflora and various physiological functions on human health. In: Furda I and Brine CJ, eds. New Developments in Dietary Fiber. New York, NY: Plenum Press;1990:117–151.

14. Annison G, Topping DL. Nutritional role of resistant starch: chemical structure vs physiological function. Annu Rev Nutr. 1994;14:297–320.

15. Norris J, Harnack L, Carmichael S, et al. US trends in nutrient intake: the 1987 and 1992 national health interview surveys. Am J Publ Health. 1997;87(5):740–746.

16. Glore SR, Van Treeck D, Knehans AW, et al. Soluble fiber and serum lipids: a literature review. J Amer Diet Assoc. 1994;94:425–436.

17. Nuttal FQ. Dietary fiber in the management of diabetes. Diabetes. 1993;42:503.

18. Ausman LM. Fiber and colon cancer: does the current evidence justify a preventive policy? Nutr Rev. 1993;51:57–63.

19. National Institute of Diabetes and Digestive and Kidney Diseases. National Diabetes Statistics fact sheet: general information and national estimates on diabetes in the United States, 2003. Bethesda, MD: US Dept of Health and Human Services, NIH, 2003.

20. Narayan KMV, Boyle JP, Thompson TJ, Sorensen SW, Williamson DF. Lifetime risk for diabetes mellitus in the United States. JAMA 2003;290(14):1884–1890.

21. Schiltz B. Carbohydrate Metabolism in the Regulation of Glycemic Index. Seattle, WA:1997 Thesis. Bastyr University.

22. Bidlack WR. Interrelationships of food, nutrition, diet and health: The National Association of State Universities and Land Grant Colleges White Paper. J Am Coll Nutr. 1996;15:422–433.

23. Wolever TM. Diet and the role of altered carbohydrate absorption in the treatment of noninsulin-dependent diabetes mellitus. Can J Gastroenterol. 1996;10(1):29–36.

24. Schiltz B. Carbohydrate Metabolism in the Regulation of Glycemic Index. Seattle, WA:1997 Thesis. Bastyr University.

25. Henry RR, Genuth S. Forum one: current recommendations about intensification of metabolic control in non-insulin-dependent diabetes mellitus. Ann Intern Med. 1996;124(1 pt 2): 175–177.

26. Clark CM Jr. The future of NIDDM care: where do we go from here? Ann Intern Med. 1996; 124(1 pt 2):184–186.

27. American Diabetes Association. Nutrition recommendations and principles for people with diabetes mellitus. Diabetes Care. 1997;20 (Suppl1):S14–17.

28. Wolever TM. Diet and the role of altered carbohydrate absorption in the treatment of noninsulin-dependent diabetes mellitus. Can J Gastroenterol. 1996;10(1):29–36.

29. Reaven G. Pathophysiology of insulin resistance in human disease. Physiol Rev. 1995;75:473–486.

30. Bidlack WR. Interrelationships of food, nutrition, diet and health: The National Association of State Universities and Land Grant Colleges White Paper. J Am Coll Nutr 1996;15:422–433.

31. Crapo PA, Reaven G, Olefsky J. Postprandial plasma-glucose and -insulin responses to different complex carbohydrates. Diabetes. 1977;26: 1178–1183.

32. Wolever TM, Jenkins DJ, Jenkins AL, Josse RJ. The glycemic index: methodology and clinical implications. Am J Clin Nutr. 1991;54:846–854.

33. Foster-Powell K, Brand Miller J. International Tables of Glycemic Index. Am J Clin Nutr. 1995; 62(Suppl):871S–893S.

34. Foster-Powell K, Holt SH & Brand-Miller JC. International table of glycemic index and glycemic load values. Am J Clin Nutr 2002; 76(1): p. 5–56.

35. Leeds AR. Glycemic index and heart disease. Am J Clin Nutr 2002;76(1): 286S–9S.

36. Liu S, Manson JE et al. Relation between a diet with a high glycemic load and plasma concentrations of high-sensitivity C-reactive protein in middle-aged women. Am J Clin Nutr 2002;75(3): 492–8.

37. Liu S, Manson JE et al.. Dietary glycemic load assessed by food-frequency questionnaire in relation to plasma high-density-lipoprotein cholesterol and fasting plasma triacylglycerols in postmenopausal women. Am J Clin Nutr 2001; 73(3): 560–6.

38. Liu S, Willett WC. Dietary glycemic load and atherothrombotic risk. Curr Atheroscler Rep 2002;4(6): 454–61.

39. Liu S, Willett WC et al. A prospective study of dietary glycemic load, carbohydrate intake, and risk of coronary heart disease in US women. Am J Clin Nutr 2000;71(6): 1455–61.

40. Parillo M, Riccardi G. Dietary carbohydrates and glucose metabolism in diabetic patients. Diabetes Metab. 1995;21(6):391–401.

41. Jenkins DA, Wolever TM, Taylor RH, et al. Glycemic Index of Foods: A Physiological Basis for Carbohydrate Exchange. Am J Clin Nutr. 1981;34:362–366.

42. Schiltz B. Carbohydrate Metabolism in the Regulation of Glycemic Index. Seattle, WA:1997 Thesis. Bastyr University.

43. Jenkins DJ, Wolever TM, Wong GS, et al. Glycemic responses to foods: possible differences between insulin-dependent and noninsulin-dependent diabetics. Am J Clin Nutr. 1984;40:971–981.

44. Wolever TM, Jenkins DA, Ocana AM, Rao VA, Collier GR. Second meal effect: low-glycemic-index foods eaten at dinner improve subsequent breakfast glycemic response. Am J Clin Nutr. 1988; 48:1041–1047.

45. Laine DC, Thomas W, Levitt MD, Bantle JP. Comparison of predictive capabilities of diabetic exchange lists and glycemic index of foods. Diabetes Care. 1987:10:387–394.

46. Coulston AM, Hollenbeck CB, Swislocki AL, Reaven GM. Effect of source of dietary carbohydrate on plasma glucose, insulin responses to mixed meals in subjects with NIDDM. Diabetes Care. 1987;10(4):395–400.

47. Parillo M, Riccardi G. Dietary carbohydrates and glucose metabolism in diabetic patients. Diabetes Metab. 1995;21(6):391–401.

48. Bjorck I, Granfeldt Y, Liljeberg H, Tovar J, Asp NG. Food properties affecting the digestion and absorption of carbohydrates. Am J Clin Nutr. 1994;59 (Suppl):699S-705S.

49. Parillo M, Riccardi G. Dietary carbohydrates and glucose metabolism in diabetic patients. Diabetes Metab. 1995;21(6):391-401.

50. Brand JC, Nicholson PL, Thorburn AW, Truswell AS. Food processing and the glycemic index. Am J Clin Nutr. 1985; 42:1192–1196.

51. Bjorck I, Granfeldt Y, Liljeberg H, Tovar J, Asp NG. Food properties affecting the digestion and absorption of carbohydrates. Am J Clin Nutr. 1994;59 (Suppl): 699S–705S.

52. Jenkins DA, Jenkins AL, Wolever TM, et al. Low glycemic index: lente carbohydrates and physiological effects of altered food frequency. Am J Clin Nutr. 1994;59(suppl):706S–709S.

53. Anderson JW, Chen WJ. Plant fiber. Carbohydrate and lipid metabolism. Am J Clin Nutr. 1979;32:346–363.

54. Liljeberg HG, Granfeldt YE, Bjorck IM. Products based on a high fiber barley genotype, but not on common barley or oats, lower postprandial glucose and insulin responses in healthy humans. J Nutr. 1996;126:458–466.

55. Truswell AS. Glycaemic index of foods. Eur J Clin Nutr. 1992;46(Suppl 2):S91–S101.

56. Parillo M, Riccardi G. Dietary carbohydrates and glucose metabolism in diabetic patients. Diabetes Metab. 1995;21(6):391–401.

57. Rea RL, Thompson LU, Jenkins DJ. Lectins in foods and their relation to starch digestibility. Nutr Res. 1985;5:919–929.

58. Yoon JH, Thompson LU, Jenkins DJ. The effect of phytic acid on in vitro rate of starch digestibility and blood glucose response. Am J Clin Nutr. 1983;38:835–842.

59. Jenkins DJ, Wolever TM, Taylor RH, Griffiths C, Krzeminska K, Lawrie JA. Slow release dietary carbohydrate improves second meal tolerance. Am J Clin Nutr. 1982; 35:1339–1346.

60. Shaheen SM, Fleming SE. High-fiber foods at breakfast: influence on plasma glucose and insulin responses to lunch. Am J Clin Nutr. 1987; 46:804–811.

61. Wolever TM, Jenkins DA, Ocana AM, Rao VA, Collier GR. Second meal effect: low-glycemic-index foods eaten at dinner improve subsequent breakfast glycemic response. Am J Clin Nutr. 1988; 48:1041–1047.

62. Jenkins DA, Jenkins AL, Wolever TM, et al. Low glycemic index: lente carbohydrates and physiological effects of altered food frequency. Am J Clin Nutr. 1994;59 (Suppl):706S–709S.

63. American Diabetes Association. Principles of nutrition and dietary recommendations for individuals with diabetes mellitus. Diabetes. 1979;28: 1027–1029.

64. Margolis S, Saudek CD. Diabetes. Baltimore, MD: The Johns Hopkins White Papers, 1997.

65. American Diabetes Association. Implications of the diabetes control and complications trial. Diabetes Care. 1993;16:1517–1520.

66. Reaven GM. Parma symposium: current controversies in nutrition. Am J Clin Nutr. 1988;47: 1078–1082.

67. American Diabetes Association. Nutrition recommendations and principles for people with diabetes mellitus. Diabetes Care. 1997;20 (Suppl 1):S14–S17.

68. Parillo M, Riccardi G. Dietary carbohydrates and glucose metabolism in diabetic patients. Diabetes Metab. 1995;21(6):391–401.

69. Schafer RG, Bohannon B, Franz M, Freeman J, Holmes A, McLaughlin S. Translation of the diabetes nutrition recommendations for health care institutions: technical review. J Am Diet Assoc. 1997;20:96–105.

70. American Diabetes Association. Nutrition recommendations and principles for people with diabetes mellitus. Diabetes Care. 1997;20 (Suppl 1):S14-S17.

71. Chandalia M, Garg A, Lutjohann D, von Bergmann K, Grundy SM, Brinkley LJ. Beneficial effects of high dietary fiber intake in patients with type 2 diabetes mellitus. N Engl J Med. 2000;342:1392–1398.

72. Caso EK. Calculation of diabetic diets. J Am Diet Assoc. 1950; 26:575–583.

73. Truswell AS. Glycaemic Index of Foods. Eur J Clin Nutr. 1992;46(Suppl 2):S91–S101.

74. Borman S. Carbohydrates' complexities. Chem Engineering News. 1996:36–38.

75. Axford J. Glycobiology and medicine: an introduction. J Roy Soc Med. 1997;90:260–264.

76. Sharon N, Lis H. Carbohydrates in cell recognition. Sci Am. 1993;268(1):82–89.

3

Proteins and Amino Acids

THE AVERAGE US ADULT CONSUMES over 100 grams of dietary protein per day—nearly twice as much as the Recommended Dietary Allowances (RDAs) range of 46–53 grams.[1,2] Given such information, one is likely to assume that the diet is complete in protein and that the potential for (protein) deficiency is lower than for most nutrients. However, such an assumption would not necessarily be correct. The conventional reasoning grossly misrepresents the metabolic role of protein. It is not protein in its macromolecular form that operates at a functional level, but rather the building blocks of protein—amino acids.

When digested, protein is broken into amino acids and peptides. These smaller molecular components give protein its nutritional impact. Since proteins from different

sources have different amino acid compositions, individuals may consume adequate amounts of total protein but still be deficient in specific amino acids because of the *quality* of the protein. The protein source may have a low amount of a particular amino acid, or the individual may require a higher amount of that amino acid based on unique metabolic needs. Thus, while assessing the diet in terms of total protein intake rather than specific amino acid intake is convenient, it likely misses the most important aspect of protein quality—amino acid composition.

Other problems also arise from a limited perspective on total protein intake. For example, such an approach does not account for the type of protein and its relationship to food allergies and sensitivities and their effects on the immune system. This chapter reorients the

41

protein discussion to include information about amino acid support in clinical nutrition, and emphasizes the importance of studying protein at a metabolic level. Understanding the structure and purposes of macromolecules can help explain how they function in a broader context.

Specifically, this chapter investigates the nutritional role of proteins and amino acids by classifying amino acids, outlining bioactive peptides, exploring the role of proteins in food-allergy-related conditions, and discussing how functional medicine helps manage those conditions.

AMINO ACIDS

Amino acids are the molecules that constitute the building blocks of proteins. The simplest definitions of protein, "molecules composed of amino acids in peptide linkage," "high polymers," and "polyamides," recognize that the alpha-amino carboxylic acid building blocks, or amino acids, give proteins their primary structure. Most amino acids consist of an asymmetric carbon bonded to four different covalent partners. The amino acids that make up proteins differ only by what is attached to the fourth bond of the carbon, known as the *side chain*. Biochemists identify amino acids by these side chains.

The major classes of amino acids include those with acid, base, aliphatic, or aromatic side chains (Figure 3.1). When amino acids are synthesized chemically, two stereoisomers, called the D- and L-forms, result. Biological synthesis produces only the L-form.

This form is used in the synthesis of protein. The only D-form amino acids that humans can use are methionine and phenylalanine. Both amino acids can be converted to their respective L-forms by a transamination reaction in the body.[3]

Most biochemistry texts identify only 20 amino acids as the building blocks of proteins. However, several other amino acids and derivatives of amino acids generally not associated with protein are also important in metabolism. They include creatine, carnitine, betaine, taurine, ornithine, and citrulline.

Essential and Nonessential Amino Acids

Nutrition has traditionally divided amino acids into two categories, *essential* and *nonessential*. Most people can synthesize about half of these amino acids, or *nonessential* amino acids, as long as their diet includes organic nitrogen. Conventional medicine has designated the remaining amino acids as *essential*. It teaches that the body is unable to synthesize these amino acids and thus must obtain them from food in prefabricated form. These essential amino acids include leucine, isoleucine, valine, lysine, phenylalanine, tryptophan, threonine, and methionine. Most clinical intervention has been limited to these "essential" amino acids.

Whether the average human body *can* synthesize a nutrient is a simpler issue than whether it *is* synthesizing that nutrient. Only the latter relates directly to function—what is actually going on in an individual at a given moment. In this sense, all amino acids play a critical role in

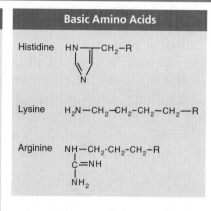
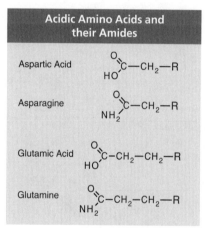
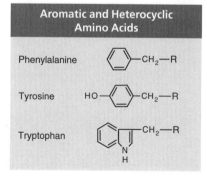
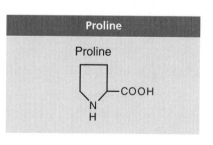

Aliphatic Amino Acids

Glycine H—R

Alanine CH_3—R

Valine CH_3—CH—R (CH_3)

Leucine CH_3—CH—CH_2—R (CH_3)

Isoleucine CH_3—CH_2—CH—R (CH_3)

Serine HO-CH_2—R

Threonine HO—CH—R (CH_3)

Cysteine HS-CH_2—R

Methionine CH_3—S—CH_2—CH_2—R

Basic Amino Acids

Histidine HN—CH_2—R

Lysine H_2N—CH_2—CH_2—CH_2—CH_2—R

Arginine NH—CH_2·CH_2-CH_2—R, C=NH, NH_2

Acidic Amino Acids and their Amides

Aspartic Acid O=C(HO)—CH_2—R

Asparagine O=C(NH_2)—CH_2—R

Glutamic Acid O=C(HO)—CH_2—CH_2—R

Glutamine O=C(NH_2)—CH_2—CH_2—R

General Formula for all Amino Acids except Proline

H_2N—C—C(=O)(OH) with H and X attached

The figure directly above is an R group. The full structure for each amino acid is shown by connecting the X point shown above to each of the R points shown in the figures to the left. Only the elements shown at left change; the R group stays constant. This general formula applies to all amino acids except proline.

Aromatic and Heterocyclic Amino Acids

Phenylalanine ⬡—CH_2—R

Tyrosine HO—⬡—CH_2—R

Tryptophan (indole)—CH_2—R

Proline

Proline (ring)—COOH

FIGURE 3.1 *Formulas of the 20 common amino acids*

human metabolism and are essential at some level. At least eight amino acids have been used clinically but have not been classified as essential since the body has metabolic pathways for their synthesis. These amino acids include cysteine, taurine, glycine, arginine, citrulline, ornithine, tyrosine, and glutamine.

The little attention given to "nonessential" amino acids has created problems since nonessential amino acids play many unique, *non*interchangeable roles in metabolism. For example, the sulfur-containing amino acid cysteine serves anti-inflammatory and antioxidant roles, activities that the essential sulfur-containing amino acid, methionine, cannot provide. The "nonessential" amino acid arginine is unique in its ability to serve as a nitric oxide generator and in the urea cycle. The

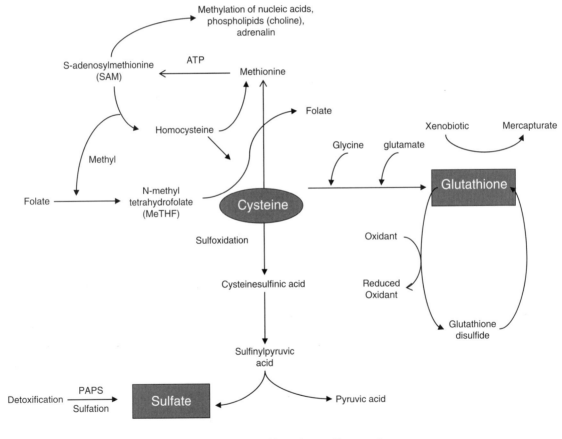

FIGURE 3.2 *Trans sulfuration-sulfate pathways*

"nonessential" amino acids taurine and glycine help the body detoxify. In each example, the metabolic roles are unique to specific, "nonessential" amino acids. Furthermore, if the body is actively using these amino acids for anti-inflammation, for detoxification, or as antioxidants, the body must replace what it uses. Therefore, these "nonessential" amino acids are only "nonessential" if the body can synthesize these amino acids as quickly as it uses them. When need becomes greater than the ability to synthesize an amino acid, it moves from the category of non-essential to "conditionally essential."

Amino Acids and Amino Acid Derivatives: Examples

The sulfation cycle: cysteine, methionine, and betaine

The sulfur amino acids, methionine and cysteine, play several roles in metabolism. Cysteine is a methyl donor in many biochemical pathways, including the conversion of homocysteine to methionine (Figure 3.2). Cysteine is also a sulfur donor for one of the Phase II detoxification pathways, sulfation, in which non-water-soluble substances are converted to water-soluble substances by the addition of a sulfate moiety prior to excretion in the urine. Cysteine also helps synthesize glutathione, an important element in antioxidant defense and detoxification. Sulfation also helps control intercellular communication and signal transduction by producing membrane-active sulfated glycoproteins.

Methionine can be converted to s-adenosylmethionine (SAM) and used by many biochemical pathways as a methyl donor. Betaine is a methyl donor for the conversion of homocysteine to methionine. Only recently have theories developed about undermethylation and its relationship to health. Methylation of DNA is one of the mechanisms the body uses to control DNA expression. The role of undermethylation of DNA in promoting conditions like cancer is only beginning to be explored.[4] The conversion of methionine to homocysteine, and the contribution of homocysteine to atherogenesis, is also gaining more medical attention (Figure 3.3).[5]

Individuals may overproduce homocysteine because of metabolic imbalances in cobalamin or folate status or because of an inborn deficiency of cystathionine beta-synthase or methylenetetrahydrofolate reductase (MTHFR).[6] Recent research links high plasma homocysteine to an increased risk of cardiovascular disease.[7,8] Supplementing the diet with cofactors vitamin B6, vitamin B12, folate, and betaine has been successful in decreasing plasma homocysteine levels and rebalancing the methylation pathway.[9]

Amino acid conjugation: taurine and glycine

Detoxification removes exogenous and endogenous toxins from the body. Detoxification consists of a set of reactions designed to convert a lipophilic substance (how most toxic molecules exist) into a water-soluble substance that can be excreted. Most toxins

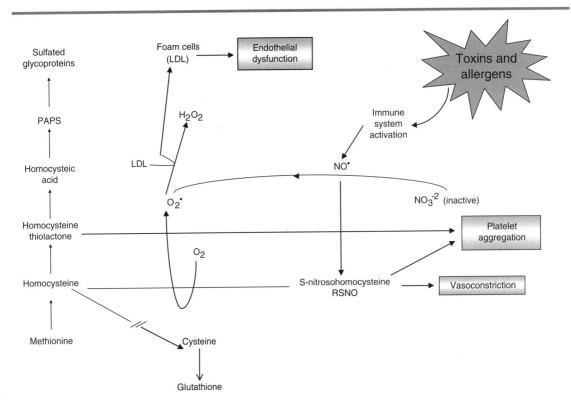

FIGURE 3.3   *Atherogenic mechanisms of homocysteine and their modulation by nitrogen oxides*

require a two-step detoxification process: Phase I activation, which uses oxygen to produce an active site on the toxin; and Phase II conjugation, which adds a water-soluble substance to the active site on the molecule (Figure 3.4). Many Phase II conjugation reactions require amino acids, including sulfation, glutathione conjugation, and amino acid conjugation.

The first identified detoxification pathway involving amino acids was the conjugation of benzoic acid with glycine to form hippuric acid.[10] Although many amino acids are used in Phase II conjugation, a commonly observed amino acid conjugate is glycine.[11] Glycine biotransformation is important for carboxylic acids and heterocyclic amines, including salicylates (e.g., aspirin) and phenylacetic acid. Glycine is also one of the amino acids used for biosynthesis of the tripeptide glutathione.

The end product of sulfur metabolism in mammals is the amino acid taurine. But tau-

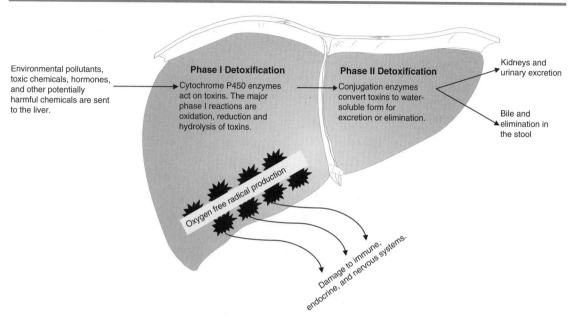

FIGURE 3.4 *Detoxification in the liver*

rine does not exist in protein. Instead, it is the most abundant free amino acid in many animal tissues, including muscle, platelets, and the central nervous system. While all of taurine's roles are not yet clear, research indicates that taurine is required for some Phase II detoxification and bile acid conjugation reactions. Taurine helps regulate calcium availability in heart muscle, platelets, and, possibly, the developing nervous system. It may even act as an antioxidant and component in some low molecular weight biologically active peptides such as the neurotransmitter glutaurine (gamma-L-glutamyl-taurine).[12]

Although most requirements for taurine are met through its endogenous synthesis, many nutritionists consider taurine to be a "conditionally essential" amino acid in infants, individuals on enteral nutrition, or individuals deficient in vitamin B6, methionine, or cysteine.[13] It also helps in states of hypernatremic dehydration or trauma.[14,15] Taurine is most abundant in animal products and does not exist in commonly consumed plants.[16]

The urea cycle and signal transduction: arginine, ornithine, and citrulline

The body disposes of nitrogen from amino acids during amino acid degradation through the urea cycle. Nitrogen balance studies have suggested that the amino acids in the urea cycle, primarily arginine, are dispensable (i.e., they can be removed from the diet without any apparent effect). However, this view has been challenged on two accounts. First, when the intake of amino acids is relatively high, arginine is indispensable. Its removal from the diet may result in hyperammonemia.[17] Second, the amino acids in the urea cycle are also involved in the nitric oxide signal transduction pathway (Figure 3.5).

Nitric oxide is synthesized from arginine by nitric oxide synthase (NOS). Two distinct types of NOS exist in the body: 1) a constitutive NOS which is calcium-dependent and present in endothelium, neural tissues, and platelets, and 2) an inducible NOS which is calcium-independent and present in immune cells, vascular smooth muscle cells, endothelial cells, and myocytes.[18] Nitric oxide is a mediator of immune, nervous, and cardiovascular systems (Figure 3.6). It is linked to pathophysiological states such as shock, hypertension, stroke, and neurodegenerative diseases.[19]

Recent studies have explored potential methods for modulating nitric oxide production and thereby influencing the inflammatory process or vascular biology. For example, corticosteroids prevent the production of inducible NOS without affecting the constitutive activity. This may account for their anti-inflammation activity.[20] Some re-

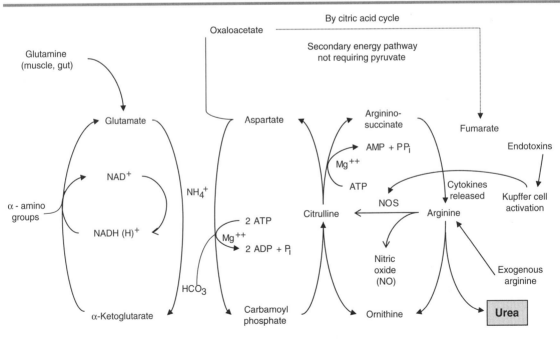

FIGURE 3.5 *Hepatic urea cycle — nitric oxide synthase relationship*

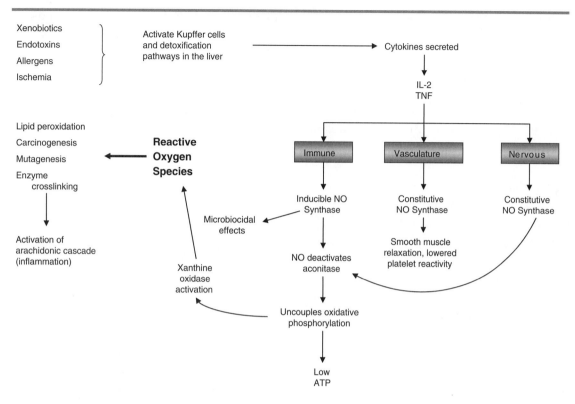

Xenobiotics
Endotoxins
Allergens
Ischemia

Activate Kupffer cells and detoxification pathways in the liver → Cytokines secreted

IL-2
TNF

Lipid peroxidation
Carcinogenesis
Mutagenesis
Enzyme crosslinking

Reactive Oxygen Species

Activation of arachidonic cascade (inflammation)

Immune   Vasculature   Nervous

Inducible NO Synthase   Constitutive NO Synthase   Constitutive NO Synthase

Microbiocidal effects

Xanthine oxidase activation

NO deactivates aconitase

Smooth muscle relaxation, lowered platelet reactivity

Uncouples oxidative phosphorylation

Low ATP

FIGURE 3.6 *The multiple influences of nitric oxide on immune, vascular, and nervous systems*

search indicates that supplemental arginine may promote enhanced nitric oxide production, which may benefit immune deficiency and cardiovascular endothelial function mediated through endothelial relaxing factor (NO).[21] However, research is still tentative. While some studies show that supplemental arginine increases host immune functions, others do not.[22,23] Citrulline may also be useful in preventing hyperammonemia and modulating nitric oxide-mediated functions. Watermelon contains a relatively large quantity of citrulline (around 100 mg of citrulline per 100 gram serving).[24]

The branched-chain amino acids: leucine, isoleucine, and valine

Compared to other amino acids, the branched-chain amino acids (BCAAs) differ metabolically. BCAAs, and leucine in particular, directly stimulate protein synthesis; are able to be oxidized completely in mitochondria to provide energy; and, within the liver, can act as precursors for lipids or ketone bodies.

Because the mitochondria preferentially transport BCAAs across their membranes for use as substrates in aerobic energy production, these amino acids provide nutritional support primarily for energy-related disorders, stress, and muscle building. Research strongly indicates that BCAAs play a key role in maintaining muscle protein reserves.[25]

For brain entry, BCAAs share a transport mechanism with the aromatic amino acids tryptophan, phenylalanine, and tyrosine. Tryptophan is a precursor for serotonin; high serotonin levels seem to play a role in pathogenesis of cancer anorexia. Recent research on cancer anorexia suggests that BCAAs may safely improve caloric intake in cancer patients with anorexia by competitively decreasing the amount of tryptophan transported to the brain.[26] The BCAAs are particularly concentrated in the germs of grains, in fish, and in dairy products. However, they are especially deficient in most grain flours and in most nuts and seeds.

Mitochondrial metabolism: creatine and carnitine

Creatine and carnitine play key roles in energy metabolism and are discussed in greater depth in Chapter 8. Briefly, creatine is synthesized from arginine and glycine in the liver and kidneys. The majority of creatine is transported to skeletal muscle cells where it is phosphorylated to phosphocreatine, an important energy storage molecule. Lean meat is one of the richest sources of creatine; a 1 kilogram steak contains approximately 4 grams of creatine.[27] The estimated dietary requirement for creatine is 2 grams per day and can be obtained from other meat sources such as fish. However, humans generally obtain less than half this amount. Creatine is converted to creatinine for excretion. Since creatinine is neither reabsorbed nor produced by the kidneys, its excretion rate is used to measure kidney function.[28]

The amino acid derivative carnitine is receiving a well-deserved and growing reputation as a valued nutrient. Aerobic energy produced by mitochondria begins when a substrate is successfully transported into the mitochondrial matrix. In this process, carnitine not only transports fatty acids and pyruvate into the mitochondrial space, it also transports mitochondrial "waste" out of the mitochondria and into the cytoplasm.[29] Carnitine also helps detoxify certain organic acids (Table 3.1).[30] Alternative practitioners are beginning to use ratios of acyl-to-free carnitine in diagnosing energy-related disorders.

Carnitine is synthesized in the body by carboxylation and methylation of lysine. This process requires vitamin C, vitamin B3, vitamin B6, and iron as enzymatic cofactors. Carnitine can also be obtained from the diet, where it exists in high levels in animal protein (Table 3.2). Although adults with average diets usually meet carnitine requirements, carnitine is considered a conditionally essential nutrient since it is depleted in many conditions. Therefore, dietary carnitine may be necessary to maintain adequate levels for support of mitochondrial energy production (see Chapter 8). For example, individuals who cannot synthesize carnitine well, have low ac-

TABLE 3.1 *Carnitine in Detoxification*

Acids Excreted as Carnitine Esters	Conditions Under Which Organic Acid Accumulates
CH_3CH_2COOH Propionic acid	Propionyl-CoA carboxylase and methylmalonyl-CoA mutase deficiencies
$(CH_3)_2CHCH_2COOH$ Isovaleric acid	Isovaleric acidemia
$HOOCCH_2CH(CH_3)CH_2COOH$ 3-methylglutaric acid	3-Hydroxy-3-methylglutaryl-CoA lyase deficiency
$CH_3(CH_2)_6COOH$ Octanoic acid	Medium-chain acyl-CoA dehydrogenase deficiency
$(CH_3)_3CCOOH$ Pivalic acid	Pivampicillin treatment
$(CH_3CH_2CH_2CH_2)_2CHCOOH$ Valproic acid	Valproic acid therapy

tivity of the mitochondrial carnitine transport enzyme(s), or experience excessive loss of carnitine from hemodialysis, enteral feeding, organic acidemias or increased xenobiotic excretion, require supplemental carnitine.[31]

Glutamine

Glutamine contains two nitrogen moieties and is the most abundant amino acid in whole blood.[32] Combined with alanine, it transports more than half of circulating amino acid nitrogen. It is also the principal carrier of nitrogen from the periphery to visceral organs. For these reasons, glutamine has been called the "nitrogen shuttle" for interorgan amino acid exchange. It is avidly consumed by replicating cells, including intestinal epithelial cells and fibroblasts. The gastrointestinal tract mucosal cells (enterocytes), lymphocytes and macrophages use glutamine as a preferred respiratory fuel. The uptake of glutamine by the mucosal cells from both the intestinal lumen and arteriolar circulation increases in catabolic states and glucocorticoid (anti-inflammatory steroid) therapy.[33]

Glutamine is involved in regulation of acid/base balance since it is the precursor for urinary ammonia. It is also an important precursor of nucleic acids, amino sugars, and proteins and acts as a "conditionally essential" amino acid during stress states associated with injury, sepsis, and inflammation. Adding glutamine to enteral nutrient formulas helps maintain its level in plasma and intracel-

TABLE 3.2 *Carnitine Content of Selected Foods*
Micromole/100g or 100 mL

Dairy Products		Bread and Cereal	
Whole milk	20.4	Whole-wheat bread	2.26
Butter	3.1	White bread	0.912
American cheese	23.2	Rice (cooked)	0.090
Cottage cheese	7.0	Macaroni	0.780
Ice cream	23.0	Corn flakes	0. 078
Vegetables		**Non-Dairy Beverages**	
Green beans (cooked)	0.019	Coffee	0.009
Green peas (cooked)	0.037	Orange juice	0.012
Asparagus (cooked)	1.210	Tomato juice	0.030
Beets (cooked)	0.020	Grape juice	0.093
Broccoli (fresh)	0.023	Grapefruit juice	Not detected
(cooked)	0.011	Cola	Not detected
Carrots (fresh)	0.041	**Miscellaneous**	
(cooked)	0.039		
Potato (baked)	0.080	Eggs	0.075
Lettuce	0.007	Peanut butter	0.516
Fruits		**Meat Products**	
Apples	0.0002	Beef steak	592
Bananas	0.0056	Ground beef	582
Strawberries	Not detected	Chicken breast	24.3
Peaches	0.0060	Cod fish	34.6
Pineapple	0.0063	Pork	172
Pears	0.107	Bacon	145

lular pools. This addition improves nitrogen balance and augmentation of cell proliferation.[34] Since glutamine breaks down fairly rapidly in solution, any glutamine-containing powdered product should be consumed as soon as possible after it is mixed with liquid.

Excitatory amino acid: glutamate

Researchers have identified more than 30 different signaling molecules in the central nervous system, including the amino acids aspartate, glutamate, glycine, and gamma-aminobutyric acid. Of these, glutamate is the principal excitatory amino acid in the brain. Its interactions with specific membrane receptors are responsible for many neurological functions including cognition, memory, movement, and sensation.[35] Although several different membrane-bound receptors are involved in the neuronal response to glutamate, mobilization of calcium is the major mechanism for the excitatory signal from glutamate (Figure 3.7).

PROTEINS AND PEPTIDES

The human body contains tens of thousands of different kinds of proteins, each performing a specific function and possessing a unique structure. Proteins function in structural support, storage, substance transport, signaling, movement, defense, and, as enzymes, selective acceleration of cellular chemical reactions.

Biologically Active Peptides

When consumed, protein is broken down by acid hydrolysis in the stomach with the help of intestinal proteases, resulting primarily in amino acids. However, many small peptides, primarily dipeptides and tripeptides, are not totally broken down (digested) into amino acids. Instead, these di- and tripeptides escape full digestion and are carried across the brush border membrane.[36] Measurable amounts of peptides exist in peripheral blood or urine after a protein-rich meal.[37] Studies show faster absorption rates for di- and tripeptides than for individual amino acids, suggesting that peptide-based formulas may be more efficacious in individuals with markedly impaired absorptive capacity.

Studies illustrate that many small peptides have specific biological activity.[38] These peptides are called biogenic or bioactive amines. Research is still investigating the amount and type of bioactive amines produced from most

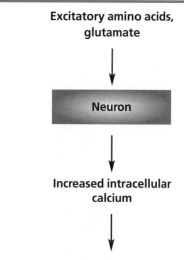

Excitatory amino acids, glutamate

Neuron

Increased intracellular calcium

- Protein kinase C
- Calcium/calmodulin-dependent protein kinase II
- Phospholipases
- Proteases
- Phosphatases
- Nitric oxide synthase
- Endonucleases
- Ornithine decarboxylase
- Xanthine oxidase

FIGURE 3.7
Pathophysiologic consequences of the activation of cellular enzyme systems by excitatory amino acid-evoked increases in intracellular calcium

protein preparations. The ability of some peptides to escape digestion and carry out specific biological functions may explain the association between enhanced immune function and lactalbumin consumption, lower blood pressure after vegetable protein consumption, and increased transit time after soy protein consumption.[39,40]

The best-researched bioactive amine is glutathione (Figure 3.8). The tripeptide glutathione (L-γ-glutamyl-L-cysteinylglycine, or GSH) plays an important role in detoxifying xenobiotic compounds. It also acts as an antioxidant of reactive oxygen species and free radicals.[41] The influence of GSH on cellular metabolism seems to expand, almost exponentially, as research increases. GSH is involved in regulation of redox balance, free radical scavenging, regulation of prostaglandin metabo-

lism, deoxyribonucleotide synthesis, cell proliferation, and immune messaging.[42] Glutathione reductase and glutathione peroxidase enzymes shuffle glutathione between its reduced (GSH) and oxidized (glutathione disulfide, or GSSG) forms. The reductase also requires vitamin B2 and the reducing factor NADPH (generated by the hexose monophosphate shunt, or HMS metabolic pathway). Glutathione peroxidase (GPO) is a selenium-requiring enzyme.

In both animals and humans, exercise appears to induce the activity of the enzymes superoxide dismutase (SOD), glutathione

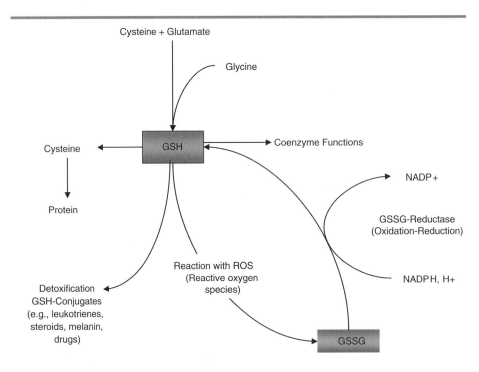

FIGURE 3.8   *Overview of glutathione function and metabolism*

peroxidase (GPO), and catalase (CAT).[43] Although results have been mixed, the ratio of reduced-to-oxidized glutathione (GSH:GSSG) appears to decrease in many tissues in response to strenuous activity. This decrease is dependent upon dietary intake, nutritional supplementation, and endocrine balance.[44,45,46]

Glycoproteins and Proteoglycans

Many classes of proteins exist in the body. Amino acid composition and protein conformation help determine a protein's potential to bind to a cell membrane or to be soluble in aqueous media. Some proteins are synthesized with sugar moieties covalently bound to selected amino acids. These proteins are called glycoproteins and may contain a short oligosaccharide chain or an extensive, sophisticated polysaccharide. The specific sugar moieties attached to glycoproteins are important in cell recognition and anchoring to other cells. Glycoproteins usually contain between 1 and 60 percent carbohydrate by weight and many short polysaccharide units (15 or fewer sugars per polysaccharide moiety). A sialic acid residue exists at the end of each polysaccharide.[47]

Proteoglycans are another class of proteins to which polysaccharides attach. Proteoglycans help hold tissues together, as they are a part of the connective tissue, or extracellular matrix (ECM), to which cells attach. Proteoglycans differ from glycoproteins since proteoglycans contain between 90 to 95 percent carbohydrate by weight, all of which is in the form of glycosaminoglycan chains.[48] Glucosaminoglycans (GAGs) are polysaccharides that contain at least one amino sugar (N-acetylglucosamine or N-acetylgalactosamine) and no sialic acid residues.

In addition to their structural role in connective tissue, GAGs play important metabolic roles. Ion transport, diffusion of nutrients, water retention, collagen fibrogenesis, growth factor binding, cell signaling, and other aspects of cell regulation depend upon proper GAG functioning.[49] Growth factors such as platelet-derived endothelial cell growth factor (PDGF), transforming growth factor beta (TGF-b), and basic fibroblast growth factor (bf GF) have been widely studied in molecular medicine. They mediate cell signaling, angiogenesis, and carcinogenesis and are found attached to the GAG-containing extracellular matrix.[50] In addition, specific GAGs are produced during the early stages of wound healing.[51]

Many hexosamines, uronic acids, and GAGs are available as oral supplements and have been widely used to nutritionally support damaged connective tissue. Examples include glucosamine sulfate, galactosamine sulfate, d-glucuronic acid, and chondroitin sulfates. Numerous studies indicate that oral glucosamine sulfate has helped individuals with osteoarthritis, and other chronic degenerative articular disorders. In a double-blind study comparing glucosamine sulfate to ibuprofen in treatment of osteoarthritis of the knees, glucosamine sulfate was found to be slower in alleviating symptoms but more effective over an eight-week period.[52] A large, multi-center trial in Portugal involving 252 physicians and 1,208 subjects found oral supplementation to be more effective than all previous treatments (except glucosamine injection) in reducing pain from exercise and decreasing limitations on active and passive movement after 6 to 12 weeks.[53] Availability of glucosamine appears to be the rate-limiting step in the synthesis of many GAGs.[54,55]

Soy Protein

The amino acid profile of the soybean is unusually complete for a plant protein.[56] Soy protein contains adequate quantities of the essential amino acids histidine, isoleucine, leucine, lysine, tryptophan, valine, phenylalanine, and tyrosine. Initial research in rats to determine the protein efficiency ratio (PER) suggested that the protein quality of adequately processed soybean protein was 62 to 92 percent that of casein. However, several researchers have found that rat bioassays, such as PER, generally underestimate the protein quality of soy protein for humans. This is because rats have higher relative amino acid requirements for the sulfur amino acids methionine and cysteine, and soy protein contains a lower amount of methionine than casein.[57]

In human health, the protein quality of a food is determined by both the pattern of essential amino acids and digestibility. How well the human body utilizes protein from food is determined by monitoring the nitrogen balance after consumption of a specific protein. Several studies indicate that humans use soy protein at a higher rate than the rat PER bioassays suggest.[58,59,60] The past 15 years of research on the quality of soy protein suggest that soy protein has the highest nutritive value of any plant protein source.[2] The digestibility of commercial soy foods such as tofu, soy protein isolates, and soy flour ranges from 85 to 90 percent.[61] Furthermore, the level of soy protein consumption *without* methionine supplementation needed to maintain nitrogen balance in humans is similar to animal source protein like egg, milk, and meat.[6]

Bioavailability of minerals such as zinc and iron from soy is influenced by the form of soy product and presence of fiber and/or phytic acid. Phytic acid (inositol hexaphosphate), generally found in high-fiber foods, can bind minerals in the gastrointestinal tract to decrease their absorption during digestion. The relatively high level of minerals in soy partially overcomes this effect. And most soy products are processed in ways that decrease or remove phytic acid. When mineral content is of concern, supplementing minerals can increase the nutritive value of soy products.

Raw soybeans contain a family of proteins called protease inhibitors. Inhibitors bind with proteolytic digestive enzymes such as trypsin and inhibit their action. Although no direct evidence indicates that low-level intake of these inhibitors is harmful to humans, some researchers have suggested that consumption of these inhibitors may be of concern. Trypsin inhibitors are ubiquitous in food. For example, raw potato contains twice the trypsin inhibitor activity of raw soy flour; raw egg contains an amount comparable to soy. Heat treatment can destroy protease inhibitors. Cooking soybeans or processing of soy, such as the heat treatment used in preparation of soy protein isolates, partially denatures the proteins, decreasing the activity of these protease inhibitors. The heat processing of soy protein also increases its digestibility.[62]

The hypocholesterolemic effect of soy protein has been extensively studied. A meta-analysis of 38 controlled clinical trials concluded that consumption of soy protein rather than animal protein significantly decreased serum concentrations of total cholesterol, LDL cholesterol, and triglycerides in hypercholesterolemic individuals.[63] The changes in serum cholesterol and LDL cholesterol concentrations directly related to initial serum cholesterol concentrations. In other words, soy protein consumption did not affect the concentration of serum cholesterol in normolipidemic individuals. Instead, it led to decreased total cholesterol, LDL cholesterol, and triglyceride levels in individuals with elevated serum lipids. Although the mechanism(s) of this hypocholesterolemic effect is(are) unknown, the two best-supported theories suggest that the type and/or amino acid composition of the soy protein and the isoflavones are key in lowering cholesterol.[64]

The connection between soy protein consumption and maintaining or promoting healthy blood cholesterol levels is so strong that in 1999 the US Food and Drug Administration granted a food claim stating that "diets low in saturated fat and cholesterol that include 25 grams per day of soy protein may reduce the risk of heart disease."

Soy-derived phytosterols, such as beta-sitosterol, support prostate health.[65] The iso-flavone genistein, abundant in soybeans, inhibits tyrosine kinase activity and angiogenesis *in vitro*.[66] Human clinical trials investigating the effect of soy protein on estrogenic-dependent conditions are only beginning, but researchers at the University of Illinois report that adding soy protein with isoflavones (also called phytoestrogens) to a low-fat, low-cholesterol diet increases bone density in post-menopausal women.[67] In a placebo-controlled trial, Burke and coworkers at the Bowman Grey School of Medicine in Winston-Salem, NC, observed that women who consumed soy protein that contained isoflavones reported less intense menopausal symptoms compared to women who received the placebo.

The most common substitutes for cow's milk are soy-based formulas, which are nutritionally similar to cow's milk formulas. Soy-based formulas have the advantage of being lactose-free. Between 1 and 3 percent of children appear to have an allergic response to cow's milk, and 30 percent of atopic children show evidence of allergy to cow's milk.[68] Allergies to soy are far less prevalent. However, children with food sensitivities should be evaluated for soy protein allergy prior to use of soy-based formulas: approximately 25 percent of children allergic to cow's milk appear also to be allergic to soy.

Rice Protein

Rice, a major source of nutrition for much of the world's population, is widely considered by nutritionists to be one of the least sensitizing and most easily digestible protein sources available. Rice has historically been perceived as hypoallergenic and is the only grain allowed on an extensive elimination diet for allergy testing.[69] Rice is gluten-free and often recommended to replace wheat or corn. In the United States and populations consuming a Western diet, rice allergy is rare. However, this is not the case in Japan, where some statistics show that rice-associated allergy is increasing, with rice ranking second only to egg white as the most common potential allergen in the Japanese diet.[70]

Recent technological advances in food processing have led to the production of a low-allergy-potential rice protein extract.[71] Therefore, rice protein extract is ideal to build a diet for nutritional management of food allergies and chemical and environmental sensitivities. High-quality proteins supply all essential amino acids. Like other cereal grains, rice protein is rich in sulfur-containing amino acids cysteine and methionine but low in threonine and lysine. These two limiting amino acids in rice should be augmented in rice protein-based diets.

A FUNCTIONAL APPROACH TO AMINO ACIDS, PROTEINS, AND PEPTIDES

For at least 20 years, information on amino acid requirements for children and adults has been available to clinicians. These recommendations are based on the work of Hamish Munro and his colleagues at MIT, and are determined primarily from results of nitrogen balance studies.[72] In nitrogen balance studies, all amino acids are assumed equal in terms of their ability to contribute to both nitrogen losses (through feces, urine, sweat, hair, sloughed epithelial cells, exhaled ammonia, nasal secretions, seminal fluid, and menstrual blood) and nitrogen intake from the diet. From a functional perspective, treating all amino acids as equal overlooks the unique role that individual amino acids and amino acid groupings have in supporting health.

Oxidative Stress and N-Acetylcysteine

Researchers have studied the effects of selenium and N-acetylcysteine (NAC) supplementation on oxidative stress. Oral supplementation with NAC helps repair oxidatively damaged tissue in lung disease.[73] Along with severe depletion of liver glutathione, this type of damage frequently occurs in athletes participating in ultramarathon-type events.[74] Doses of NAC in oxidative-stress studies range from 1000 mg to approximately 7000 mg (or 100 mg per kg body weight) per day.[75]

Glutamine and the NMDA Receptor Pathway

Glutamate activation of the N-methyl-D-aspartate (NMDA) receptor pathway is important in functional medicine. NMDA receptor activation results in calcium influx, which leads to stimulation of nitric oxide synthase and subsequent production of nitric oxide (Figure 3.9).[76] Overstimulation of the NMDA receptor can lead to increased levels of nitric oxide production and concomitant produc-

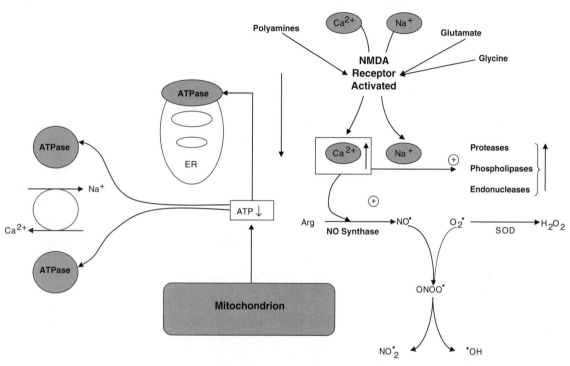

FIGURE 3.9   *Energy failure*
Albers DS, Beal MF. Mitochondrial dysfunction and oxidative stress in aging and neurodegenerative disease. J Neural Transm 2000;59:133–154.

tion of high levels of reactive oxygen species. Many neurologic disorders, such as stroke, dementia, epilepsy, Huntington's, Parkinson's and Alzheimer's diseases, and amyotrophic lateral sclerosis have been associated with injury to neurons, as have both hypoglycemia and trauma. Overstimulation of receptors such as the NMDA receptor may be partially responsible for such damage.[77,78] Agents that inhibit nitric oxide production, such as nitroglycerin, can block neurotransmitter release from NMDA-glutamate excited neurons. An-

tioxidants may provide some protection from production of reactive oxygen species in situations of NMDA overstimulation.

This overstimulation of NMDA receptors may result from high levels of glutamate either transported to the brain or synthesized within the brain itself (Table 3.3). Some controversy exists about whether glutamate from the diet can contribute to high levels of brain glutamate. While glutamate is a normal constituent of protein, monosodium glutamate (MSG), a sodium salt of glutamate, is often

TABLE 3.3   *Chronic Neurodegenerative Diseases thought to be Mediated in Part through Stimulation of Glutamate Receptors*

Good evidence for involvement of glutamate receptors, at least to some extent, in neuronal damage:

Huntington's disease (pathological process mimicked by injection of the endogenous NMDA agonist quinolinate; mitochondrial inhibitors, which make neurons more susceptible to glutamate toxicity, can reproduce this process)

AIDS dementia complex (human immunodeficiency virus-associated cognitive-motor complex) (evidence that neuronal loss is ameliorated by NMDA antagonists in vitro and in animal models)

Neuropathic pain syndromes (e.g., causalgia, or painful peripheral neuropathies with a central component blocked by NMDA-receptor antagonists or inhibitors of nitric oxide synthase)

Suggestive evidence of involvement of glutamate receptors, at least to some extent, in neuronal damage:

Olivopontocerebellar atrophy (some recessive forms associated with glutamate dehydrogenase deficiency)

Parkinsonism (mimicked by impaired mitochondrial metabolism, which renders neurons more susceptible to glutamate-induced toxicity)

Amyotrophic lateral sclerosis (primary defect may be mutation in superoxide dismutase gene, which may render motor neurons more vulnerable to glutamate-induced toxicity; there is also evidence for decreased glutamate reuptake)

Mitochondrial abnormalities and other inherited or acquired biochemical disorders (partial listing)

MELAS syndrome (mitochondrial myopathy, encephalopathy, lactic acidosis, and stroke-like episodes due to point mutation in mitochondrial DNA)

MERRF (myoclonus epilepsy with ragged-red fibers, signifying mitochondrial DNA mutation; also frequently accompanied by ataxia, weakness, dementia, and hearing loss)

Leber's disease (point mutation in mitochondrial DNA, presenting with delayed-onset optic neuropathy and occasionally degeneration of basal ganglia, with dystonia, dysarthria, ataxia, tremors, and decreased vibratory and position sense)

Wernicke's encephalopathy (thiamine deficiency)

Rett syndrome (disease of young girls, presenting with seizures, dementia, autism, stereotypical hand wringing, and GALT disorder)

Homocysteinuria (L-homocysteic acid is an agonist for some glutamate receptors)

Hyperprolinemia (L-proline is a weak NMDA-like agonist)

Nonketotic hyperglycinemia (a case report of some improvement after treatment with an NMDA antagonist)

Hydroxybutyric aminoaciduria

Sulfite oxidase deficiency

Combined systems disease (vitamin B12 deficiency, which may result in accumulation of homocysteine)

Lead encephalopathy

Some or slight evidence for involvement of glutamate receptors in pathophysiology or neuronal damage:

Alzheimer's disease (some data that the vulnerability of neurons to glutamate can be increased by β-amyloid protein)

Hepatic encephalopathy (perhaps a component, although inhibitory neurotransmitters are more clearly involved)

Tourette's syndrome (deficits in basal ganglia have been proposed to be mediated by glutamate or glutamate-like toxins)

Drug addiction, tolerance, and dependency (animal models suggest that NMDA antagonists may be helpful in treatment) added to food in significant amounts to enhance taste. MSG produces a taste sensation, called *umami* taste, which is separate from the taste produced by the sweet, sour, and salty sensations of other food ingredients.[79] Umami taste, produced by MSG, appears to induce cephalic-phase insulin secretion and stimulate pancreatic flow.[80,81] High levels of MSG have even induced asthma and caused shudder-like attacks in children.[82] Researchers do not fully understand how an additive identical to one of the building blocks of protein can create such powerful responses.[83] Perhaps it is not the presence or absence of the substance that is important but rather the absolute amount consumed with respect to other amino acids.

Detoxification, Sulfate Reserves, and Neurodegenerative Diseases

Over the past several years, Steventon and Waring have reported that defects in the metabolism of sulfur amino acids, including cysteine and homocysteine, are associated with motoneuron and neurodegenerative diseases.[84] Elevated excretion of cysteine and a reduced excretion of sulfate have been noted in patients with Parkinson's disease, Alzheimer's disease, and other motoneuron diseases, as compared to controls without neurodegenerative disorders. Not only are a variety of motoneuron diseases associated with poor sulfation and low sulfate reserves, but inflammatory conditions such as rheumatoid arthritis, delayed food sensitivity, multiple chemical sensitivities, and diet-responsive autism have also been associated with poor

sulfation. Approximately 2.5 percent of the general population are currently thought to be "poor sulfoxidizers." In other words, they have the phenotypic uniqueness of poor conversion of cysteine and homocysteine into inorganic sulfate. These conditions may relate to endogenous toxicity associated with poor sulfoxidation and sulfation.

Evidence indicates a single steroid sulfotransferase with broad specificity is involved in the sulfation of steroids, lipids, peptides, neurotransmitters, thyroid hormones, bile acids, and a multitude of xenobiotics.[85] Control of sulfotransferases and, to some extent, cysteine/homocysteine sulfoxidation is related not only to genes, but also to diet, toxins, and other environmental factors. Dietary constituents like red wine, coffee, certain cheeses, and chocolate, are known to be potent inhibitors of sulfotransferases. They can result in inhibited sulfation reactions when individuals consume high levels of these foods on a regular basis. Poor sulfoxidation can also result from heavy metals like lead and mercury, resulting in decreased detoxification ability.

Closely connected to sulfation is the conversion of sulfite to sulfate through the enzyme sulfite oxidase. Sulfite oxidase provides another source of sulfate for PAPS (phospho-adenosine-phosphosulfate), and its activity depends on molybdenum. Molybdenum insufficiencies can cause sulfite to accumulate and increase the risk of sulfite-induced neuromuscular toxicity. Diets with low levels of molybdenum can induce sulfite oxidase insufficiency, which, in conjunction with a high protein diet, may cause sulfite to accumulate and make it difficult for sulfation to occur. As a consequence, controlling PAPS through the availability of inorganic sulfate has an important regulatory effect in both neurological and vascular system function.[86]

Food Intolerance, Allergies, and the Elimination Diet

Food allergies and intolerances cause a variety of clinical symptoms. However, not all adverse responses to food components qualify as food allergies. A food allergy occurs when a food component, most commonly a protein or peptide in the food, elicits an immune response. A food intolerance occurs when an individual responds to a food with symptoms that do not involve an immune response. For example, a lactase deficiency, which underlies lactose intolerance, would not be considered an allergic reaction.

Although the underlying mechanisms that elicit food allergy responses are complex and still somewhat controversial, the clinical management strategy is more universally accepted. Several studies show that avoiding suspected foods, such as with an elimination diet, substantially improves clinical symptoms. Clinical studies suggest that 8 percent of U.S. children younger than 6 years old have evidence of food intolerance, and 2 to 4 percent of them experience reproducible allergic reactions to foods, most often eggs, milk, peanuts, soy, fish, and wheat.[87] Surveys suggest that 1 to 2 percent of adult Americans are sensitive to foods, most commonly nuts, peanuts, fish, and shellfish.[88,89,90]

One dietary approach that has been very helpful in patients who complain of food intolerance or allergy-related symptoms is the modified elimination diet. The primary guidelines are shown in Table 3.4 and include:

1. Eliminate dairy products such as milk, cheese, and ice cream. (Note: varying amounts of natural, unsweetened, live-culture yogurt may be tolerated by some individuals.)

2. Avoid meats such as beef, pork, or veal. Chicken, turkey, lamb, and cold-water fish such as salmon, mackerel, and halibut are acceptable if the individual is not allergic or intolerant to these foods. Select from free-range sources whenever possible.

3. Eliminate gluten and any grains that contain proteins that can exacerbate a gluten sensitivity. Avoid any food that contains wheat, spelt, kamut, rye, barley, amaranth, quinoa, or malts. This is the most important part of the diet but also can be the most difficult. Unfortunately, these grains are contained in many common foods such as bread, crackers, pasta, cereals, and products containing flour made from these grains. Products made from rice, corn, buckwheat, and gluten-free flour, potato, tapioca, and arrowroot may be used as desired by most individuals.

4. Drink at least two quarts of water, preferably filtered, daily.

5. Avoid all alcohol-containing products including beer, wine, liquor, and over the counter products that contain alcohol.

TABLE 3.4 *Modified Elimination Diet Summary*

Foods to Include	Foods to Exclude
Whole fruits and diluted juices; fruit juice concentrates for baking	Citrus: oranges, grapefruit, lime, lemon; grapes
Dairy substitutes: rice and nut milks such as almond milk, coconut milk	Dairy and eggs: milk, cheese, eggs, cottage cheese, cream, yogurt, butter, ice cream, frozen yogurt, non-dairy creamers
Non-gluten grains: brown rice, millet, oats*, quinoa, amaranth, teff, buckwheat	Grains: wheat, corn, barley, spelt, kamut, rye, triticale
Fresh ocean fish, wild game, lamb, duck, organic chicken and turkey	Pork, beef/veal, sausage, cold cuts, canned meats, frankfurters, shellfish
Dried beans, split peas and legumes	Soybean products (soy sauce, soybean oil in processed foods; tempeh, tofu, soymilk, soy yogurt, textured vegetable protein)
Nuts and seeds: walnuts, pumpkin, sesame and sunflower seeds, hazelnuts, pecans, almonds, cashews, nut butters such as almond or tahini	Peanuts and peanut butter, pistachio nuts
All raw, steamed, sautéed, juiced or baked vegetables, except as specifically excluded in the box to the right.	Mushrooms, corn, all nightshades including: tomatoes, any variety of potatoes (sweet potatoes and yams are allowed), eggplant, peppers (green, red, yellow), ground cayenne and paprika
Cold pressed olive and flax seed oils, expeller pressed safflower, sesame, sunflower, walnut, canola, pumpkin, and almond oils	Butter, margarine, shortening, processed oils, salad dressings, mayonnaise, and spreads
Drink at least 6-8 cups of filtered water per day. Herbal teas acceptable.	Alcohol, coffee and other caffeinated beverages, soda pop
Brown rice syrup, fruit sweeteners (see page 8), molasses, stevia	Refined sugar, white/brown sugars, succanat, honey, maple syrup, corn syrup, high fructose corn syrup, evaporated cane juice

Things to Watch For

- Corn starch in baking powder and any processed foods
- Corn syrup in beverages and processed foods
- Vinegar in ketchup, mayonnaise & mustard is usually from wheat or corn
- Breads advertised as gluten-free which contain oats, spelt, kamut, rye
- Many amaranth and millet flake cereals have oats or corn
- Many canned tunas contain textured vegetable protein which is from soy; look for low-salt versions which tend to be pure tuna, with no fillers
- Multi-grain rice cakes are not just rice. Purchase plain rice cakes.

*While oats do not contain gluten and should not exacerbate celiac or food intolerance symptoms, it has been shown that cross-contamination with wheat is common in oat-containing, processed products. Therefore, if intolerance to wheat is suspected, care should be taken in selection of oat-containing products (or they should be avoided).

6. Avoid all caffeine-containing beverages including coffee, caffeine-containing tea, and soda pop. Coffee substitutes from gluten-containing grains should also be avoided, along with decaffeinated coffee.

SUMMARY

This chapter provides the groundwork for more innovative nutritional research by exploring the role of amino acids from a functional medicine perspective. Research investigating the connections among nutrition and bioactive peptides, glycoproteins, and proteoglycans is still in its infancy but will surely bring protein to the forefront of nutrition research once again. It may seem strange at first to suggest that the micromolecular form of protein, the amino acids, plays a key role in food allergy and related conditions, because we have been reading about trends in protein research on a macromolecular level. However, recent studies clearly indicate that many food-related symptoms result from the interplay of nutrition and amino acids, many of which have previously been considered *non*essential.

CHAPTER 3 REFERENCES

1. Crim MC, Munro HN. Proteins and amino acids. In: Shils ME, Olson JA, Shike M, eds. Modern nutrition in health and disease, 8th ed. Philadelphia, Pa: Lea & Febiger. 1994;Vol.1:3–35.
2. Subcommittee on the tenth edition of the RDAs, Food and Nutrition Board, Commission of Life Sciences, National Research Council. Recommended Dietary Allowances. 10th ed. Washington, D.C.: National Academy Press; 1989:52–77.
3. Crim MC, Munro HN. Proteins and amino acids. In: Shils ME, Olson JA, Shike M, ed. Modern nutrition in health and disease. 8th ed. Philadelphia, Pa: Lea & Febiger. 1994; Vol. 1:3–35.
4. Feinberg AP, Rainer S, DeBaun MR. Genomic imprinting, DNA methylation, and cancer. JNIC. 1995;17:21–26.
5. Stamler JS, Slivka A. Biological chemistry of thiols in the vasculature and in vascular-related disease. Nutr Rev. 1996;1:1–30.
6. Nygard O, Vollset SE, Refsum H, et al. Total plasma homocysteine and cardiovascular risk profile. JAMA. 1995;274:1526–1533.
7. Boushey CJ, Beresford SAA, Omenn GS, Motulsky AG. A quantitative assessment of plasma homocysteine as a risk factor for vascular disease. JAMA. 1995;274:1049–1057.
8. Verhoef P, Stampfer MJ. Prospective studies of homocysteine and cardiovascular disease. Nutr Rev. 1995;53:283–288.
9. Wilcken DEL, Wilcken B, Dudman NPB, Tyrrell PA. Homocystinuria—The effects of betaine in the treatment of patients not responsive to pyridoxine. N Engl J Med. 1983;309:448–453.
10. Smith RL, Williams RT. In: Fishman WH, ed. Metabolic conjugation and metabolic hydrolysis. Vol 1. London: Academic Press; 1970:1–19.
11. Hutt AJ, Caldwell J. Amino acid conjugation. In: Mulder G, eds. Conjugation reactions in drug metabolism. New York: Taylor & Francis; 1990:273–305.
12. Hayes KC, Trautwein EA. Taurine. In: Shils ME, Olson JA, Shike M, ed. Modern nutrition in health and disease. 8th ed. Philadelphia, Pa: Lea & Febiger. 1994; Vol. 1: 477–485.
13. Laidlaw SA, Grosvenor M, Kopple JD. The taurine content of common foodstuffs. J Parent Enteral Nutr. 1990;14:183--88.
14. Mallinckrodt E, Hauhart RE, Dirgo JA. Taurine: A role in osmotic regulation of mammalian

brain and possible clinical significance. Life Sci. 1980;26:1561–1568.

15. Paauw JD, David AT. Taurine supplementation at three different dosages and its effect on trauma patients. Am J Clin Nutr. 1994;60:203–206.

16. Laidlaw SA, Grosvenor M, Kopple JD. The taurine content of common foodstuffs. J Parent Enteral Nutr. 1990;14:183–188.

17. Laidlaw SA, Kopple JD. Newer concepts of the indispensable amino acids. Am J Clin Nutr. 1987;46:593–605.

18. Masters BSS. Nitric oxide synthases: why so complex? Annu Rev Nutr. 1994;14:131–145.

19. Bredt DS, Snyder SH. Nitric oxide: A physiological messenger molecule. Annu Rev Biochem. 1994;63:175–195.

20. McCall T, Vallance P. Nitric oxide takes centre-stage with newly defined roles. TIPS. 1992;13:1–6.

21. Preli, RB et al. Review: Vascular effects of dietary L-arginine supplementation. Atherosclerosis 2002;162:1–15.

22. Barbul A. Arginine: Biochemistry, physiology, and therapeutic implications. J Parent Enteral Nutr. 1986;10:227–238.

23. Larrick JW. Metabolism of arginine to nitric oxide: An area for nutritional manipulation of human disease. J Opt Nutr. 1994;3:22–31.

24. Larrick JW. Metabolism of arginine to nitric oxide: An area for nutritional manipulation of human disease. J Opt Nutr. 1994;3:22–31.

25. Smith R, Elia M. Branched-chain amino acids in catabolic states. Proc Nutr Soc. 1983;42:473–487.

26. Cangiano C, Laviano A, Meguid MM, et al. Effects of administration of oral branched-chain amino acids on anorexia and caloric intake in cancer patients. JNCI 1996;88:550–552.

27. Harris RC, Soderlund K, Hultman E. Elevation of creatine in resting and exercised muscle of normal subjects by creatine supplementation. Clinical Science. 1992;83:367–374.

28. Greenhaff PL. Creatine and its application as an ergogenic aid. Int J Sport Nutrition. 1995;5: S100–S110.

29. Tanphaichitr V, Leelahagul P. Carnitine metabolism and carnitine deficiency. Nutr 1993; 9: 246–254.

30. Broquist HP. Carnitine. In: Shils ME, Olson JA, Shike M, eds. Modern Nutrition in health and Disease. 8th ed. Philadelphia, Pa: Lea & Febiger. 1994; Vol. 1:459–65.

31. Feller AG, Rudman D. Role of carnitine in human nutrition. J Nutr. 1988;118:541–547.

32. Teran JC, Mullen KD, McCullough AJ. Glutamine—a conditionally essential amino acid in cirrhosis? Am J Clin Nutr. 1995;62:897–900.

33. Smith RJ, Wilmore DW. Glutamine nutrition and requirements. J Parent Enteral Nutr. 1990; 14: 94S–99S.

34. Ziegler TR, Benfell K, Smith RJ, et al. Safety and metabolic effects of L-glutamine administration in humans. J Parent Enteral Nutr. 1990;14: 137S–146S.

35. Lipton SA, Rosenberg PA. Excitatory amino acids as a final common pathway for neurologic disorders. N Engl J Med. 1994;330:613–622.

36. Steele RD, Harper AE. Proteins and amino acids. In: Brown ML, ed. Present Knowledge in Nutrition. 6th ed.. Washington, D.C.: International Life Sciences Institute Nutrition Foundation. 1990:67–79.

37. Grimble GK. The significance of peptides in clinical nutrition. Annu Rev Nutr. 1994;14: 419–447.

38. Roberts PR, Zaloga GP. Dietary bioactive peptides. New Horizons. 1994;2:237–243.

39. Grimble GK, Keohane PP, Higgins BE, Kaminski MV Jr, Silk DBA. Effect of peptide chain length on amino acid and nitrogen absorption from two lactalbumin hydrolysates in normal human jejunum. Clin Sci. 1986;71:65–69.

40. Roberts PR, Zaloga GP. Dietary bioactive peptides. New Horizons. 1994;2:237–243.

41. Bray TM, Taylor CG. Tissue glutathione, nutrition, and oxidative stress. Can J Physiol Pharmacol. 1993;71:746–751.

42. Bray TM, Taylor CG. Tissue glutathione, nutrition, and oxidative stress. Can J Physiol Pharmacol. 1993;71:746–751.

43. Reddy VK, Kumar CT, Prasad M, et al. Exercise-induced oxidant stress in the lung tissue: role of dietary supplementation of vitamin E and selenium. Biochem Int. 1992;26(5):863–871.

44. Reddy VK, Kumar CT, Prasad M, et al. Exercise-induced oxidant stress in the lung tissue: role of dietary supplementation of vitamin E and selenium. Biochem Int. 1992;26(5):863–871.

45. Rokitzki L, Logemann E, Sagredos AN, et al. Lipid peroxidation and antioxidative vitamins under extreme endurance stress. Acta Physiol Scand. 1994;151(2):149–158.

46. Sen CK, Atalay M, Hanninen O. Exercise-induced oxidative stress: glutathione supplementation and deficiency. J Appl Physiol. 1994;77(5): 2177–2187.

47. Alberts B, Bray D, Lewis J, et al. Molecular Biology of the Cell. New York: Garland Publ, Inc; 1983:50–53.

48. Alberts B, Bray D, Lewis J, et al. Molecular Biology of the Cell. New York: Garland Publ, Inc; 1983:692–707.

49. Leadbetter WB. Cell matrix response in tendon injury. Clin Sports Med. 1992;July 11(3):533–578.

50. Shyjan AM, Heldin P, Butcher EC, et al. Functional cloning of the cDNA for a human hyaluronan synthase. J Biol Chem. 1996;271 (38):23395–23399.

51. McCarty MF. Glucosamine for wound healing. Med Hypoth. 1996;47:273–275.

52. Vaz AL. Double-blind clinical evaluation of the relative efficacy of ibuprofen and glucosamine sulfate in the management of osteoarthrosis of the knee in out-patients. Curr Med Res Opin. 1982;8(3):145–149.

53. Tapadinhas MJ, Rivera IC, Bigamini AA. Oral glucosamine sulphate in the management of arthrosis: report on a multi-centre open investigation in Portugal. Pharmatherapeutica. 1982; 3(3):157–168.

54. Saleh M, LoBuglio A. Platelets in rheumatic diseases. In: McCarty DJ and Koopman WJ. (eds.). v Arthritis and applied conditions. A textbook of rheumatology. Vol 1. Philadelphia. Pa: Lea & Fibiger;1993.

55. Karzel K, Domenjoz R. Effects of hexosamine derivatives and uronic acid derivatives on glycosaminoglycan metabolism of fibroblast cultures. Pharm. 1971;5:337.

56. Erdman JW, Fordyce EJ. Soy products and the human diet. Am J Clin Nutr. 1989;49:725–737.

57. Torun B, Viteri FE, Young VR. Nutritional role of soya protein for humans. JAOC. 1981; 58:4 00–406.

58. Kies C, Fox HM. Comparison of the protein nutritional value of TVP, methionine-enriched TVP, and beef at two levels of intake for human adults. J Food Sci. 1971; 36:841–845.

59. Zezulka AY, Calloway DH. Nitrogen retention in men fed varying levels of amino acid from soy protein with or without added L-methionine. J Nutr. 1976; 106:212–221.

60. Young VR, Puig M. Queiroz E, Scrimshaw N, Rand WM. Evaluation of the protein quality of an isolated soy protein in young men: relative nitrogen requirements and effect of methionine supplementation. Am J Clin Nutr. 1984;39:1 6–24.

61. Messina M, Messina V, Setchell K. The Simple Soybean and Your Health. Garden City Park, New York: Avery Publishing Group; 1994:19–33.

62. Erdman JW, Fordyce EJ. Soy products and the human diet. Am J Clin Nutr. 1989;49:725–737.

63. Anderson JW, Johnstone BM, Cook-Newell ME. Meta-analysis of the effects of soy protein intake on serum lipids. N Engl J Med. 1995; 333: 276–282.

64. Potter SM. Overview of proposed mechanisms for the hypocholesterolemic effect of soy. J Nutr. 1995;125:606S–611S.

65. Berges RR, Windeler J, Trampisch HJ, et al. Randomized, placebo-controlled, double-blind clinical trial of b-sitosterol in patients with benign prostatic hyperplasia. Lancet. 1995; 345: 1529–1532.

66. Messina MJ, Persky V, Setchell KDR, Barnes S. Soy intake and cancer risk: a review of the in vitro and in vivo data. Nutr Cancer. 1994b; 21:113–131.

67. Genetic Engineering News. 1996; November 1:34.

68. Wilson NW, Hamburger RN. Allergy to cow's milk in the first year of life and its prevention. Ann Allergy. 1988;61:323–327.

69. Van Hooser B, Crawford LV. Allergy diets for infants and children. Compr Ther. 1989;15:38–47.

70. Sampson HA. Food hypersensitivity: manifestations, diagnosis, and natural history. Food Tech. 1992;May:141–144.

71. Liska DJ, King M, Peterson B, Medcalf D. Antigenicity of rice protein concentrate and rice flours. Functional Medicine Research Center, Research Report Number 102. 1997;March:1–9.

72. Crim MC, Munro HN. Proteins and amino acids. In: Shils ME, Olson JA, Shike M, eds. Modern Nutrition in Health and Disease. 8th ed. Philadelphia, Pa: Lea & Febiger. 1994; Vol. 1:3–35.

73. Suter PM, Domenghetti G, Schaller, et al. N-acetylcysteine enhances recovery from acute lung injury in man. A randomized, double-blind, placebo-controlled clinical study. Chest. 1994; 105:190–194.

74. Pyke S, Lew H, Quintanilha A. Severe depletion in liver glutathione during physical exercise. Biochem Biophys Res Commun.1986;139(3): 926–931.

75. Sochman J, Vrbska J, Musilova B, et al. Infarct size limitation: acute N-acetylcysteine defense (ISLAND trial): preliminary analysis and report after the first 30 patients. Clin Cardiol. 1996;19: 94–100.

76. Beal MF. Aging, energy, and oxidative stress in neurodegenerative diseases. Ann Neurol. 1995; 38:357–366.

77. Lipton SA, Rosenberg PA. Excitatory amino acids as a final common pathway for neurologic disorders. N Engl J Med. 1994;330:613–622.

78. Masliah E, Alford M, DeTeresa R, Mallory M, Hansen L. Deficient glutamate transport is associated with neurodegeneration in Alzheimer's disease. Ann Neurol. 1996;40:759–766.

79. Baylis LL, Rolls ET. Responses of neurons in the primate taste cortex to glutamate. Physiol Behavior. 1991;49:973–979.

80. Niijima A, Togiyama T, Adachi A. Cephaliphase insulin release induced by taste stimulus of monosodium glutamate (umami taste). Physiol Behavior. 1990;48:905–908.

81. Naim M, Ohara I, Kare M, Levinson M. Interaction of MSG taste with nutrition: perspective in consummatory behavior and digestion. Physiol Behavior. 1991;49:1019–1024.

82. Allen DH, Delohery J, Baker G. Monosodium L-glutamate-induced asthma. J Allergy Clin Immunol. 1987;80:530–537.

83. Barinaga M. Amino acids: how much excitement is too much? Science. 1990;247:20–22.

84. Steventon GB, Waring RH, Heafield MT, et al. Plasma cysteine and sulphate levels in patients with motor neurone, Parkinson's and Alzheimer's disease. Neurosci Letts. 1990;110: 216–220.

85. Comer KA, Falany CN. Immunological characterization of dehydroepiandrosterone sulfotransferase from human liver and adrenal. Molecular Pharmacol. 1992;41:645–651.

86. Coughtrie MW. Sulphation catalysed by the human cytosolic sulphotransferases-chemical defence or molecular terrorism? Human Exp Toxicol. 1996;15:547–555.

87. Sampson HA. Food hypersensitivity: manifestations, diagnosis, and natural history. Food Tech. 1992;May:141–144.

88. Carini C, Brostoff J, Wraith DG. IgE complexes in food allergy. Ann Allergy. 1987;59:110-117.

89. Halpern GM, Scott JR. Non-IgE antibody mediated mechanisms on food allergy. Ann Allergy. 1987;58:14–27.

90. Van Hooser B, Crawford LV. Allergy diets for infants and children. Compr Ther. 1989;15:38-–7.

4

Fats

EW NUTRIENTS HAVE BEEN INCORPORATED into conventional nutritional practice with as little regard for function as dietary fats. As macronutrients, fats have been associated so closely with caloric density, adiposity, and excessive intake that nutritionists have largely ignored the functions of fats. For example, decreased intake of dietary fat has been repeatedly recommended by nearly all U.S. healthcare organizations (e.g., American Dietetic Association, American Diabetes Association, American Heart Association, and National Cancer Institute). Clinically, far too many nutritionists have taken a static, quantitative approach to dietary fat, focusing on reduction of total intake. Simultaneously, low-fat and nonfat foods have been the fastest growing segment of the food industry. According to a 1997 national survey, one out of

every five non-college-educated U.S. adults believes that fat should be totally eliminated from his or her diet.[1] The exception to this viewpoint has been the equally imbalanced view expounded for the low carb diet made popular by Dr. Atkins. However, in his later writings he did begin to make distinctions between good fats and riskier saturated fats. These evolving ideas were further elaborated in the South Beach Diet popularized by Dr. Arthur Agaston.

Moreover, when the issue of fat *quality* has been addressed by mainstream healthcare organizations, it has largely been relegated to the question of saturated fat. By and large, these organizations have treated saturated fat as a negative risk factor for cardiovascular disease and recommended reduced dietary intake. From the perspective of function, however, all saturated fat is not the same, especially because short-chain fatty acids (like butyric acid, which is highly concentrated in butter) play such a critical role in supporting the health of the intestinal cell lining.

Many mainstream recommendations are not clinically effective from a functional medicine point of view, because they do not fully consider the purpose of fats within the body. In terms of function, the best way to make clinical decisions about dietary fat intake is to focus on the *purpose* of the fats in a specific health condition, and to understand how fat fits within the design of the body and works with its metabolic processes. This chapter explores fatty acid metabolism, dietary modification of fat intake, and individualized fatty acid supplementation by taking a functional approach to fats. It investigates the mechanisms underlying the structure, physiological function, and relationships among fats and other dietary constituents to better address the issue of fat quality.

FATS AND CELL MEMBRANES

Cell membranes illustrate well the importance of fats in physiological systems. The fat composition of cell membranes varies dramatically throughout the body's different tissues and structures, and these differences in fat composition directly influence membrane function. Fatty acid shape physically regulates membrane function, and membrane permeability is often directly altered by fatty acid composition.

For example, in much of the body, cell membrane phospholipids (which each contain two fatty acids) rarely contain the omega 3 fatty acid DHA (docosahexaenoic acid). However, in the brain 35 percent of all phospholipids contain DHA. In the eye, photoreceptor phospholipids may contain up to 60 percent DHA. Especially in developing infants, changes in DHA composition in nervous system tissue have been suggested as contributive to such conditions as attention deficit and hyperactivity disorder[2] and may influence visual capacity.[3]

Tissue structures that are highly fat-dense appear to be influenced by both the amount and quality of fat. The myelin sheath insulating nerve cells, for example, is almost 80 percent fat. Changes in fatty acid composition of this sheath have been linked to dysfunction in a variety of myelinated nerves, including the sciatic and optic nerves.

Fat Classification

Although many healthcare providers have focused primarily on fatty acids in their clinical practice, the category of nutritional fats includes more than fatty acids. In biochemical terms, fats are classified as *lipids* and defined as substances that are insoluble in water, soluble in organic solvents like ether or chloroform, and able to be used by the body. It is important to note that this definition of lipids is based on function rather than structure. Because of this functional definition, lipids actually include a wide variety of substances that are also commonly classified in other ways. Many vitamins and hormones, for example, are lipid-derived molecules (Chapter 5). So are phospholipids, sphingolipids, and glycosphingolipids, as well as many of the body's universal regulatory substances like prostaglandins, prostacyclins, leukotrienes, and thromboxanes.

Lipid-derived substances also include fat transport molecules like lipoproteins, which make fats water-soluble to allow for blood transport, and sterols—like cholesterol—which are not only found in cell membranes but also serve as the starting point for synthesis of bile, vitamins, and steroid hormones. Unlike fatty acids, the basic building blocks for many types of fats, many of the above substances are not available from food and

the influence of diet and lifestyle in their synthesis is not fully understood. Research in these areas is advancing rapidly, however, and it is only a matter of time until these lesser-known lipid-derived substances are widely used in clinical practice.

FATTY ACID CLASSIFICATION

Fatty acids, the best known components of the lipid classification system, have a consistent and fairly simple chemical identity (Figure 4.1). All fatty acids are carbon chains

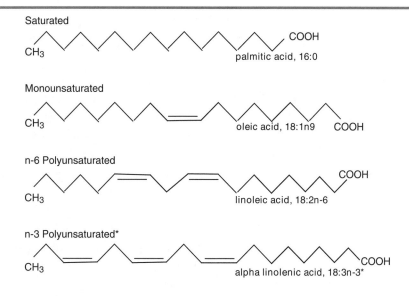

FIGURE 4.1 *Types of fatty acids*

with a carboxyl group at one end and a methyl group at the other. For chain lengths six carbons and longer, even numbers of carbon atoms predominate.

The carbon atoms in a fatty acid may or may not be connected by double bonds. If one or more double bonds do occur, the fatty acid is described as *unsaturated*. If only one double bond occurs, the category is further specified as *monounsaturated*. If more than one double bond occurs, the designation becomes *polyunsaturated*.

Saturated fatty acids, which contain no double bonds, vary in the body in carbon chain length. Very-short-chain fatty acids (VSCFA) contain 2–3 carbons (e.g., acetic, propionic), short-chain fatty acids (SCFA) contain 4–6 carbons (e.g., butyric, valeric, caproic), medium-chain fatty acids (MCFA) contain 8–14 carbons (e.g., caprylic, capric, lauric, myristic), and long-chain fatty acids (LCFA) contain 16 or more (e.g., palmitic) carbon atoms. Some well-known long-chain fatty acids with 20 or more carbon atoms include arachidonic acid (20 carbons), behenic acid (22 carbons), tricosanoic acid (23 carbons), lignoceric acid (24 carbons), and cerotic acid (26 carbons). All of these fatty acids have research-proven functions in the body, and most are available in food or supplements. Table 4.1 provides examples of SCFAs, MCFAs, and LCFAs.

When naming unsaturated fatty acids, researchers sometimes count from the methyl end and at other times from the carboxyl end. Fatty acids that are named using the methyl end procedure are classified in terms of an omega number, which is defined as the carbon atom initiating the first double bond when counting from the methyl end of the molecule. In humans, three omega families of unsaturated fatty acids predominate: the omega 3, omega 6, and omega 9 families.

Desaturase enzymes that can insert a double bond into these specific positions on fatty acid carbon chains appear to be differentially distributed in the animal world. Humans and other mammals do not appear to synthesize desaturase enzymes that can insert a double bond closer than 7 carbon atoms away from the methyl end of the carbon chain. For this reason, humans cannot convert omega 9 family fatty acids into omega 6s, or omega 6s into omega 3s.

However, within each of these families, further elongation of the carbon chain and desaturation of the molecules is possible. For example, the omega 6 fatty acid *linoleic acid* (an 18-carbon unsaturated fatty acid with two double bonds, the first of which occurs at carbon 6) can be desaturated by the enzyme delta 6 desaturase into gamma linolenic acid (an 18-carbon unsaturated fatty acid with three double bonds, the first of which still begins at carbon 6) but not into alpha linolenic acid (an 18-carbon unsaturated fatty acid with three double bonds, the first of which begins at carbon 3). In contrast, the omega 9 fatty acid *oleic acid* containing 18 carbon atoms and one double bond can be synthesized in the body from the saturated fatty acid *stearic acid* (an 18-carbon fatty acid). Clinically, these principles translate into a dietary requirement for at least two un-

TABLE 4.1 *Examples of Short-, Medium-, and Long-Chain Fatty Acids*

No. Carbon Atoms		Systematic Name	Common Name	Abbreviation*
		Saturated fatty acids		
SCFA	1	Methanoic	Formic	
	2	Ethanoic	Acetic	
	3	Propanoic	Propionic	
	4	Butanoic	Butyric	4:0
MCFA	12	Dodecanoic	Lauric	12:0
	14	Tetradecanoic	Myristic	14:0
LCFA	16	Hexadecanoic	Palmitic	16:0
	18	Octadecanoic	Stearic	18:0
	20	Eicosanoic	Arachidic	20:0
	22	Docosanoic	Behenic	22:0
	24	Tetracosanoic	Lignoceric	24:0
		Unsaturated fatty acids		
SCFA	4		Crotonic	4:1(2t)
LCFA	16		Palmitoleic	16:1(9c)
	18		Oleic	18:1(9c)
	18		Vaccenic	18:1(11c)
	18		Linoleic	18:2(9c,12c)
	18		Linolenic	18:3(9c,12c,15c)
	20		Arachidonic	20:4(5c,8c,11c,14c)

* The number of carbon atoms appears first, followed by the number of double bonds. The positions of the lowest numbered carbon of each double bond, and whether the configuration is *cis* (c) or *trans* (t), are indicated in parentheses.

saturated fatty acids (linoleic, an omega 6, and alpha linolenic, an omega 3), which are known as essential fatty acids (EFAs).

Fatty Acids in the Laboratory

Several dozen fatty acids can be measured readily in the plasma using capillary gas chromatography. From these measurements, ratios and patterns can be analyzed to help determine dietary needs and to monitor the efficacy of intervention. Unique patterns of fatty acid composition have been found for such diverse health conditions as eczema[4] and prostate cancer.[5]

A common measure of EFA deficiency is the **triene** (20:3ω9) to **tetraene** (20:4ω6) ratio, or the T/T ratio. A T/T ratio > 0.2 is stated in most textbooks as a marker of essential fatty acid deficiency (EFAD). Using improved capillary GLC methods, Siguel lowered the upper normal limit of T/T to 0.025,[6] a 10x increase in sensitivity allowing the identification of patients with an early biochemical deficiency.

EFA deficiency was proposed as an important factor in the etiology of coronary artery disease (CAD) in the 1950s,[7] but could not be proved. Before 1980, studies had not found many of the biochemical changes associated with EFAD and the proposed link between heart disease and EFAs was abandoned. Siguel proposed that EFAD was found rarely because previously used measures of EFAs lacked adequate sensitivity. Using an improved fatty acid assay,[1] Siguel and Lerman reported a strong association between insufficient levels of EFAs and CAD.[8] The authors stated that insufficient EFA levels appear to be one of the most significant nutritional factors in the etiology of cardiovascular disease. Similarly, they reported a relationship between elevated plasma *trans* fatty acids (TFAs) and CAD.[9]

EFA deficiency is likely to be far more prevalent than previously suspected. Using highly sensitive assay techniques, biochemical evidence of EFAD was found in more than 25 percent of the US adult population.[10] Therefore, EFA deficiency may be a more important factor in nutrition and chronic disease than hitherto appreciated.

Omega Family Fatty Acid Ratios

Ratios of fatty acids between the different fatty acid families appear to play a critical role in a wide variety of health conditions, including cancer, skin-related disorders, immune-related disorders, endocrine-related disorders,

and cardiovascular disorders. High levels of omega 9 fatty acids, for example, may be indicative of fat-related dysfunction, since the body's production of omega 9 fatty acids appears to be increased primarily when the supply of omega 6 fatty acids is deficient. Similarly, inflammatory events appear to be exacerbated by increased ratios of omega 6 to omega 3 fatty acids. The following sections review fatty acid ratios in more detail and explore the clinical relevance of dietary interventions that can help balance omega fatty acid ratios.

ARACHIDONIC ACID CASCADE

The *arachidonic acid cascade* pathway is familiar to many clinicians. It begins with the release of arachidonic acid (AA) from cell membrane phospholipids through the activity of phospholipase A2. It ends with the production of fatty acid-derived regulatory substances including the pro-inflammatory series 2 prostaglandins (PGE$_2$s) (Figure 4.2).

Arachidonic acid, an omega 6 fatty acid containing 20 carbon atoms and four double bonds, lies at a critical juncture in fatty acid metabolism. When acted upon by the enzyme cyclooxygenase, it can be converted into the series 2 prostaglandins and prostacyclins. When acted upon by the enzyme lipoxygenase, it can be converted into the series 4 leukotrienes. These molecules are referred to as "eicosanoid" molecules because of their 20-carbon length. When synthesized in excess, eicosanoids can promote chronic inflammation and are considered proatherogenic. How-

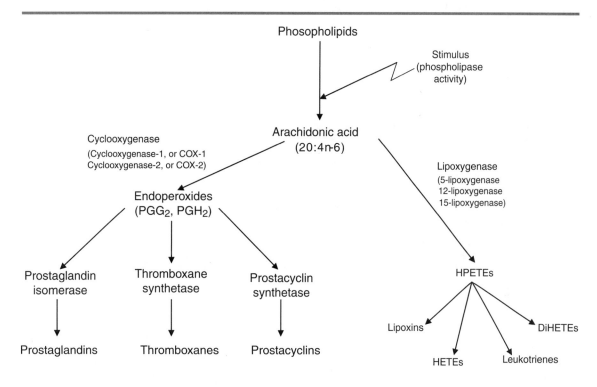

FIGURE 4.2 *Arachidonic acid (AA) cascade*

ever, when they are undersupplied, the body becomes inadequately supported in times of infection and injury. Part of the increased immune-related risk associated with bottle-feeding rather than breastfeeding, for example, involves the generous supply of arachidonic acid in human milk in contrast with the absence of AA in most plant-based formulas.[11]

When simply desaturated and elongated, AA can be converted into adrenic acid and docosapentaenoic acid (DPA). Although DPA has been less investigated than some of the other AA metabolites, research on DPA sup-plementation suggests it can suppress prostacyclin synthesis in a manner similar to EPA (eicosapentaenoic acid) and DHA (docosahexaenoic acid) supplementation. It is also likely to be important in managing inflammatory-related conditions.[12] Because of these diverse metabolic fates, the metabolism and nutritional modulation of AA have been the subject of much research especially related to diet and inflammation.

As Figure 4.3 illustrates, phospholipase A2, located on the cell membrane, is initially responsible for mobilizing arachidonic acid

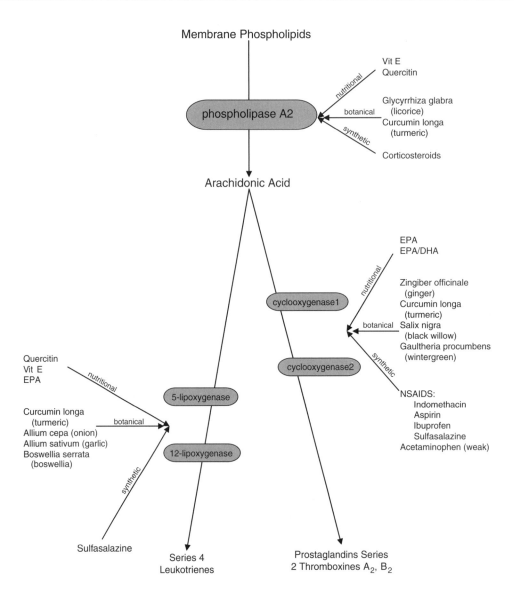

FIGURE 4.3   *Nutritional, botanical, and synthetic inhibitors in the arachidonic acid cascade*

Calder PC. N-3 polyunsaturated fatty acids and inflammation: from molecular biology to the clinic. Lipids 2003;38(4):343-352.

Harbige LS. Fatty acids, the immune response and autoimmunity: a question of n-6 essentiality and the balance between n-6 and n-3. Lipids 2003;38(4):323-341.

(20:4ω6), which is the substrate for eicosanoid synthesis. Activity of this pathway is inhibited by numerous dietary antioxidants, including vitamin E, quercetin, and licorice. The corticosteroid drugs also work as anti inflammatories through inhibition of this pathway.

Synthesis of the series 2 prostaglandins and series 2 thromboxanes requires transformation of arachidonic acid by the cyclooxygenase enzyme. This enzyme is found in at least two isoforms (COX-1 and COX-2). Moreover, because the COX-2 form is highly inducible, its excessive conversion of arachidonic acid into series 2 prostaglandins can be critical to excessive inflammatory response. Production of reactive oxygen species (ROS) is also associated with COX-2 activity. Nonsteroidal antiinflammatory drugs (NSAIDs) primarily inhibit COX-2 and not COX-1, which is why they are called COX-2 specific (or selective) inhibitors.[13] Ginger and turmeric are dietary inhibitors of the enzyme.

Production of leukotrienes from arachidonic acid requires activity of the lipoxygenase enzyme. Activity of this enzyme generates epoxide and peroxide metabolites, which may help regulate leukotriene production but also pose oxidative risk. Dietary inhibitors of the lipoxygenase enzyme include onion, garlic, turmeric, and vitamin E. (See summary in Table 4.2.)

Arachidonic Acid, Omega Ratios, and Inflammation

The ratio of omega 3 to omega 6 fatty acids appears critical to balancing pro-inflammatory eicosanoid synthesis from arachidonic acid.[14] In the United States, omega 3:omega 6

TABLE 4.2 *List of Nutritional, Botanical, and Synthetic Inhibitors in the Arachidonic Acid Cascade*

Enzyme	Nutritional Inhibitors	Botanical Inhibitors	Synthetic Inhibitors
Phospholipase A$_2$	Vitamin E Quercetin	Licorice Turmeric	Corticosteroids
Cyclooxygenase	EPA DHA	Ginger Turmeric Black willow Wintergreen	NSAIDS: Indomethacin Aspirin Ibuprofen Sulfasalazine Acetaminophen
Lipoxygenase	Quercetin Vitamin E EPA	Turmeric Onion Garlic Boswellia	Sulfasalazine

ratios fall in a 1:10 to 1:25 range—compared to a worldwide average of 1:2. Virtually all dietary recommendations from public health agencies have ignored this ratio, either by focusing on intake of omega 9 fatty acids (e.g., recommendations of increased olive oil in the diet) or by encouraging use of plant oils extremely high in omega 6 fatty acids (e.g., safflower, sunflower).

Omega 3 fatty acids are difficult to obtain from animal products, where they are essentially limited to cold-water fish like salmon and halibut. They are more abundant in plant sources but still limited. Especially rich sources include seeds (and their oils) like flax and black currant. Ability of the body to convert omega 3 fatty acids into antiinflammatory regulatory molecules like series 3 prostaglandins and thromboxanes depends upon enzyme activity. Because omega 6 fatty acids use the same elongase and desaturase enzymes for conversion into their prostaglandin and thromboxane equivalents, excessive intake of omega 6:omega 3 fatty acids can saturate enzyme activity and prevent manufacture of antiinflammatory substances even when omega 3 fatty acids are available. Figure 4.4 lists dietary sources of the fatty acids in the AA cascade. Table 4.3 summarizes food sources of these fatty acids.

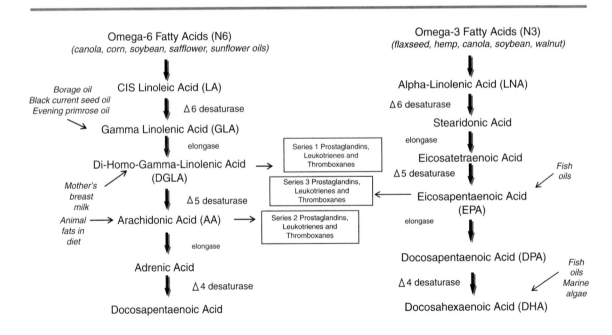

FIGURE 4.4   *Dietary sources and the arachidonic acid (AA) cascade*

TABLE 4.3 *Fatty Acids in Certain Oils*

	Saturated Fats	Oleic Acid	Linoleic Acid	Gamma-linolenic Acid (Omega 6)	Alpha-linolenic Acid (Omega 3)
Cooking Oils					
Canola	7	54	30	0	7
Olive	16	76	8	0	0
Soy	15	26	50	0	9
Corn	17	24	59	0	0
Safflower	7	10	80	0	0
Medicinal Oils					
Evening Primrose	10	9	72	9	0
Black Currant Seed	7	9	47	17	13
Borage	14	16	35	22	0
Flaxseed	9	19	14	0	58

Plant Oil Supplementation and the Arachidonic Acid Cascade

The enzymes that elongate and desaturate omega 6 fatty acids are the same enzymes that elongate and desaturate omega 3 fatty acids. Therefore, it is reasonable to expect that simple modification of the 3:6 ratio can inhibit inflammatory response. However, supplementation with omega 6 oils can also help inhibit inflammation, if those oils move omega 6 fatty acids away from arachidonic acid formation. Borage oil, black currant seed oil, and evening primrose oil (EPO) are three such oils. Because these three oils are rich in gamma linolenic acid (GLA), they are able to act as direct precursors for di-homo gamma linolenic acid (DGLA), which preferentially promotes formation of antiinflammatory series 1 prostaglandins. Black currant seed oil has the double advantage of being rich in stearidonic acid (SDA), a precursor to eicosapentaenoic acid

(EPA) in the omega 3 pathway, which can inhibit further arachidonic acid formation and also serve as a precursor for antiinflammatory series 3 prostaglandins.

Trans Fatty Acids

For more than two decades, the food industry has increased the solidification of plant oils by adding a nickel catalyst to them, heating them, passing hydrogen through them, rebleaching them, and then removing the nickel catalyst by filtration. This process, called hydrogenation, has no health benefit and has been promoted by the food industry as a harmless means of increasing the stability of oils, allowing for convenience and availability of products. During the process of hydrogenation, however, the structure of many fat components is altered. In chemical terms, the fatty acid configuration is switched from *cis* to *trans*. Because oil contains virtually no *trans* fatty acids in its natural state, many nutritionists have questioned its health impact. Since its inception, intake of *trans* fatty acids has been shown to have a negative impact on serum lipid levels and composition,[15] as well as on cell membrane function[16] (Figure 4.5).

Fats and Oxidative Insult

Polyunsaturated fats containing numerous double-bond carbons are highly susceptible to damage by oxygen under conditions of high oxidative stress. Oxidative stress is defined as a physiological condition in which increased concentration of reactive oxygen species (ROS) is not properly counterbalanced by increased presence of oxygen metabolite-processing enzymes and free radical-quenching molecules.

At a molecular level, oxidative stress is related to electrochemical redox potential. Because biological oxidations are electron transfer reactions, the activities of reducing agents (electron donors) and oxidizing agents (electron acceptors) are required to bring about redox reactions. When molecules are left with single, unpaired electrons as a result of electron transfer processes, the molecules become "free radicals"—the most reactive type of ROS. (Table 4.4.)

Lipid Peroxides and Antioxidant Protection of Cell Lipids

The term *lipid peroxides* describes fats that have been chemically damaged by oxygen free radicals. Fats can react with free hydroxy radi-

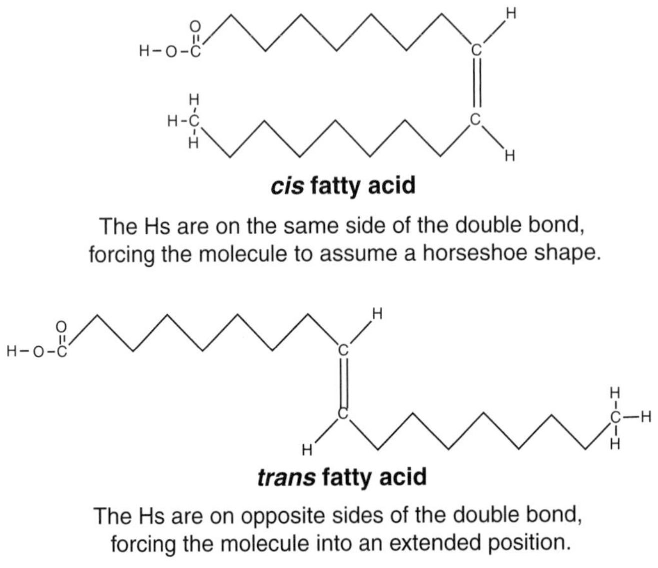

cis fatty acid

The Hs are on the same side of the double bond, forcing the molecule to assume a horseshoe shape.

trans fatty acid

The Hs are on opposite sides of the double bond, forcing the molecule into an extended position.

FIGURE 4.5   *Configuration of* cis *fatty acid and* trans *fatty acid*

TABLE 4.4 *Formation of Certain Free Radicals*

Name	Formula	Comments
Trichloromethyl	$CCl_3^{\bullet}$	A carbon-centered radical (i.e., the unpaired electron resides on carbon). $CCl_3^{\bullet}$ is formed during metabolism of the solvent carbon tetrachloride in liver and contributes to the toxic effects of this solvent. Carbon-centered radicals usually react quickly with O_2 to make peroxyl radical, e.g., $CCl_3^{\bullet} + O_2 \rightarrow CCl_3O_2$.
Superoxide	$O_2^{-\bullet}$	An oxygen-centered radical. Has limited reactivity.
Hydroxyl	$OH^{\bullet}$	A highly reactive oxygen-centered radical. Very reactive indeed: attacks most molecules in the human body.
Peroxyl, alkoxyl	$RO_2^{\bullet}$, $RO^{\bullet}$	Oxygen-centered radicals formed (among other routes) during the breakdown of organic peroxides.
Oxides of nitrogen	$NO^{\bullet}$, $NO_2^{\bullet}$	Nitric oxide ($NO^{\bullet}$) is formed in vivo from the amino acid L-arginine. Nitrogen dioxide ($NO_2^{\bullet}$) is made when $NO^{\bullet}$ reacts with O_2 and is found in polluted air and smoke from burning organic materials (e.g., cigarette smoke).

cals to form lipid carbon-centered radicals, and with molecular oxygen to form lipid carbon-centered radicals and perhydroxy radicals. Lipid carbon-centered radicals can interact further with molecular oxygen to produce lipid peroxyl radicals. Free iron can also generate lipid peroxyl radicals when lipid hydroperoxide or peroxidized fatty acids are present.

A newer test not yet widely available to measure lipid peroxidation involves F_2-isoprostane measurement. The F_2-isoprostanes are prostaglandin-type molecules that are created through the interaction of oxygen radicals with membrane phospholipids (Figure 4.6). For this reason, they may be more sensitive to specific types of free radical damage to the lipid membrane.[17]

The relationship between lipid peroxide levels and risk of atherosclerosis is well documented.[18] Serum lipid peroxides can be measured in the blood by a thiobarbituric acid reactive substance (TBARS) test. Levels of serum lipid peroxides have been correlated with numerous cardiovascular conditions, including atherosclerosis, cardiac ischemia, and cerebral ischemia, as well as with cancers, allergies, respiratory distress syndrome, thermal injury, irradiation, heavy metal toxicity, and other free radical-generating conditions.

Any activities that require substantially increased oxygen intake or result in unexpected low oxygen concentrations can place the body's lipid structures at high oxidative risk. Strenuous exercise, for example, can

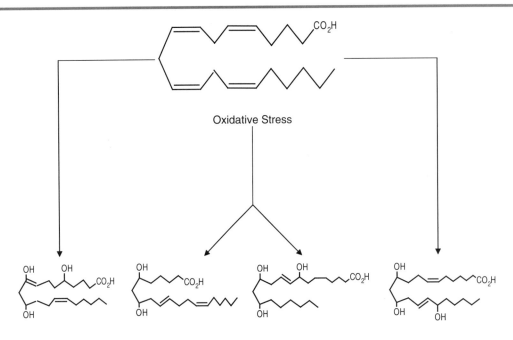

FIGURE 4.6   *The formation of F_2-isoprostanes*

Hansen HS. New biological and clinical roles for the n-6 and n-3 fatty acids. Nutr Rev 1994;52(5):162–167.

increase oxygen consumption as much as 10 to 15 times over resting levels.[19] This increased oxygen uptake occurs at a whole-body level, but it is particularly important in skeletal muscle.

The ability of mitochondria within muscle to regenerate adenosine triphosphate (ATP) for muscular energetics depends upon the availability of oxygen. However, during mitochondrial regeneration of ATP, about 2 to 5 percent of available oxygen becomes converted to ROS, including hydrogen peroxide, superoxide anion radical, and hydroxyl radical.[20] It is the increased presence of ROS that places high demands on the body's capacity to scavenge free radicals with molecular redox agents and maintain proper activity of enzymes, reducing oxidative stress.

Key redox agents studied in oxidative stress literature include ascorbic acid (vitamin C), tocopherol (vitamin E), glutathione (tripeptide consisting of glycine-cysteine-glutamic acid), lipoic acid, and cysteine. Key oxidative enzymes include superoxide dismutase (SOD), which is needed to convert superoxide anion radical into hydrogen peroxide; glutathione peroxidase (GPO), which is able to convert hydrogen peroxide into water; and catalase, which is also able to produce water from hydrogen peroxide in the presence of molecular oxygen. Each oxidative enzyme listed above requires at least one nutrient cofactor. For intracellular SOD, specific ratios of zinc to copper are required; for mitochondrial SOD, the mineral manganese is required; for catalase, enzymatic activity changes are required in relationship to its mineral cofactor, iron (Table 4.5).

Vitamin E and Lipid Protection

Vitamin E supplementation has been shown to reduce oxidative damage to muscle when measured by reduced serum creatine kinase activity.[21] A double-blind, placebo-controlled study of young (22–29 years) and older (55–74 years) adult men doing eccentric treadmill running at 75 percent maximum heart rate after 48 days of supplementation at 800 IU/day of d-alpha-tocopherol indicated numerous protective effects. These indicators included alterations in fatty acid composition, vitamin E concentration, and lipid-conjugated dienes in muscle, together with changes in

urine lipid peroxides. The researchers viewed the changes as consistent with a protective effect of vitamin E against oxidative injury produced by strenuous exercise.

Supplemental doses of vitamin E in clinical studies have ranged widely, from 400 to 1600 IU, but most interventions have targeted a 400-800 IU range. The ability of vitamin E to protect phospholipid bilayers[22] of cell membranes and to scavenge free radicals[23,24] has been clearly demonstrated in medicine. In addition, vitamin E is important in clinical intervention in a wide variety of oxidative stress-related conditions (Chapter 5).

Vitamin C and Lipid Protection

Vitamin C has long been identified as a free radical scavenger and key component in oxidative metabolism. Dietary deficiency of vitamin C has been shown to reduce oxidative capacity, especially during exercise and heightened activity.[25] The vitamin is also involved in carnitine synthesis, which is required for shuffling fatty acid substrate into the mitochondria for aerobic conversion to adenosine triphosphate (ATP).[26]

At Recommended Dietary Allowance levels established by the U.S. Food and Nutrition Board of the National Academy of Sciences, vitamin C may be unable to reduce lipid peroxidation as measured by the TBARS test. However, at the 1 gram per day level, supplementation has been shown to reduce exercise-induced oxidative stress and lipid-related damage as measured by TBARS.[27] (Chapter 5)

TABLE 4.5 *Molecular Redox Agents and Oxidative Enzymes*

Redox Agents	Oxidative Enzymes
Vitamin C	Superoxide dismutase
Vitamin E	Glutathione peroxide
Glutathione	Catalase
Lipoic acid	
Cysteine	

Coenzyme Q10 and Lipid Protection

Research on the clinical use of ubiquinone (commonly referred to as coenzyme Q10 and the benzoquinone with a conjugated iso-prenoid side chain) has produced over 300 indexed journal articles reporting on its use for conditions like arrhythmia, atherosclerosis, cardiomyopathy, and congestive heart failure. The many positive findings should not be surprising, since cardiac muscle is one

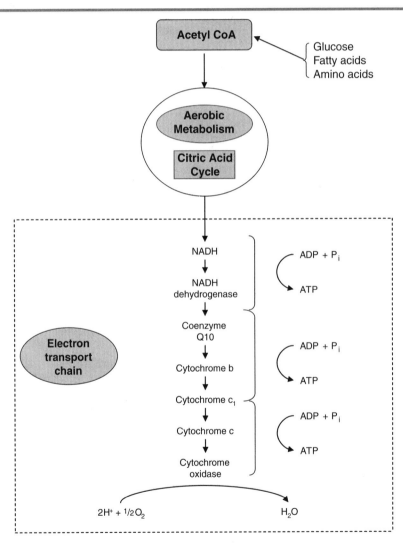

FIGURE 4.7   *Electron transport chain of the mitochondrion*

of the few tissues in the body to be continuously aerobic, and coenzyme Q10 occupies a unique and central spot in aerobic metabolism. Stationed near the center of the mitochondrial electron transport chain (Figure 4.7), it is the only non-protein component of the chain and the only component with the capability of moving two electrons simultaneously along the chain.

While coenzyme Q10 activity may not be directly involved in protection of lipid membrane components, the synergy between coenzyme Q10, vitamin E, and vitamin C is well researched. In its reduced form, coenzyme Q10 helps reduce oxidized forms of vitamin E.[28] Redox potentials of vitamins C and E are interlinked, and the vitamins have been shown to interact synergistically in scavenging free radicals[29] and reducing lipid peroxides in human subjects.[30] Thus, supplementing use of coenzyme Q10 is important to nutritional protection of cell lipids.

STEROLS: THE SECOND MAJOR CATEGORY OF LIPIDS

In addition to the straight carbon chain fatty acids, the lipid family contains a wide variety of ring-like structures, collectively referred to as sterols. The ring structure of the sterols makes them highly hydrophobic and structurally rigid, unlike the highly modifiable long-chain unsaturated fatty acids. Through hydroxylation, sterols are converted in the body into alcohols and then further metabolized into cholanic acids that become bile salts. Other metabolic pathways convert the sterols into vitamins or hormonal messengers (Figure 4.8).

Cholesterol

Despite its bad reputation, cholesterol is a type of lipid (belonging to the category of steroids) that exists in all cell membranes. Cholesterol is vital for such physiological functions as transmission of nerve impulses, formation of vitamin D, synthesis of testosterone and estrogen, and formation of bile. Approximately 80 percent of total body cholesterol is manufactured in the liver, and 20 percent is derived from the diet. As total body cholesterol increases, rate of liver synthesis decreases. Conversely, if dietary intake is low, liver synthesis increases to meet functional needs (provided, of course, that the body and its metabolic function are healthy). When dietary intake is chronically high, however, the ability of the liver to compensate with decreased production may become compromised.

Numerous risk factors have been directly associated with increased risk of high blood cholesterol (hypercholesterolemia). These factors include low fiber intake, high sugar intake,[31] intake of caffeine,[32] stress, lack of exercise,[33] smoking, and high-fat intake when accompanied by nutrient deficiency.

Cholesterol serves as a starting point for sterol-based synthesis of four critical regulatory hormones in the body: cortisol, dehydroepiandrosterone (DHEA), testosterone, and estrogen. Through conversion to pregnenolone and subsequent hydroxylation, cholesterol can be used by the body to form cortisol, the key

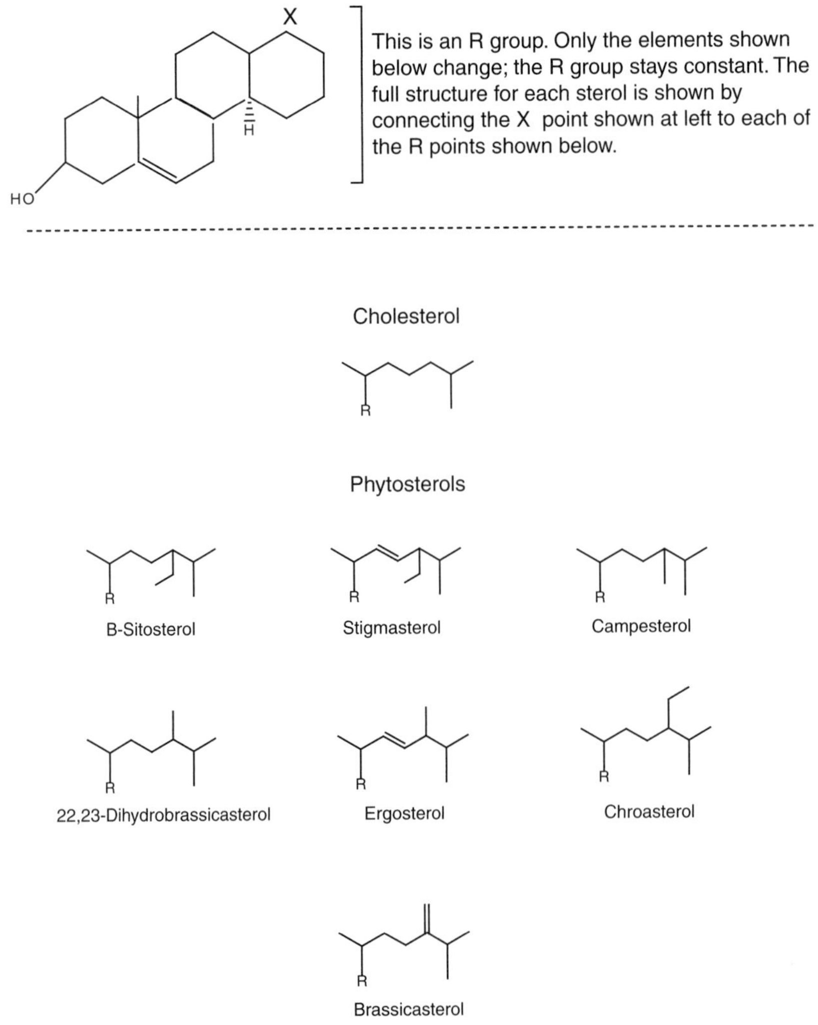

X

This is an R group. Only the elements shown below change; the R group stays constant. The full structure for each sterol is shown by connecting the X point shown at left to each of the R points shown below.

Cholesterol

Phytosterols

B-Sitosterol

Stigmasterol

Campesterol

22,23-Dihydrobrassicasterol

Ergosterol

Chroasterol

Brassicasterol

FIGURE 4.8   *Some sterols*

glucocorticoid "counter-regulatory" hormone. In naturally secreted amounts, cortisol helps provide resistance to exogenous and endogenous stressors.

Cytochrome P450 lyase activity can help transform cholesterol into DHEA (a molecule that, together with its sulfated conjugate, is the most abundant steroid hormone in the body). While DHEA has been shown to have anti-diabetogenic, anti-stress, and weight-loss promoting effects, these effects are still not understood in terms of biological mechanism, and studies have raised important questions about the role of DHEA in metabolic health. Emotional stress, for example, has been shown to cause as much as a 20-fold increase in urinary excretion of DHEA,[34] and serum DHEA levels have been shown to be significantly elevated in postmenopausal women with breast cancer.[35] DHEA itself can be further converted in the body to both estrogens and androgens (Figure 4.9).

Based on this metabolic map, it appears that cholesterol manipulation in the diet (as well as cholesterol levels in the blood) may be a much more complex phenomenon than anyone previously assumed. Furthermore, cholesterol status may be intimately related to immune status as well as reproductive hormone balance. Attempts to regulate cholesterol levels without first considering and addressing these other possible areas of dysfunction may be clinically inappropriate.

Fatty Acids and Thyroid Function

A further hormone-connected issue involving dietary fats is thyroid function. As with all tissues, essential fatty acids are needed to establish and maintain cell membrane integrity and fluidity in the thyroid gland. Moreover, the activity of membrane-dependent enzyme systems and hormone receptors largely depends upon fatty acid composition of the phospholipid membrane.[36] While essential fatty acids affect thyroid architecture, elevated T4 may alter the desaturase enzymes necessary to elongate essential fatty acids. Thus, altered thyroid hormone levels may change the fatty acid constitution of cell membranes in ways that impair membrane structure and function.[37]

Eczema and other skin problems may also be symptoms of poor thyroid function. The skin's integrity depends on the metabolism of certain types of essential fats in the diet. Low thyroid function results in poor utilization of these fats to maintain skin integrity.[38]

SHORT-CHAIN FATTY ACIDS

Largely overlooked in clinical practice have been the short-chain fatty acids (SCFAs). The SCFAs include the 2- (acetic) and 3- (propionic) carbon fatty acids, as well as the 4- (butyric), 5- (valeric), and 6- (caproic) carbon fatty acids. In clinical treatment of intestinal disorders, butyric acid has been especially effective since it is the preferred fuel for the colonocytes, and is even preferred over L-glutamine and D-glucose as a metabolic source of energy. SCFA concentration varies inversely with luminal pH in the intestine, and it increases in direct proportion to increased pancreatic enzyme secretion. As SCFA concentrations increase, sodium and water absorption by the colon also increase. Butyrate administration has also been found to have anti-cancer effects in the colon: it appears to alter cancer cell doubling time, increase

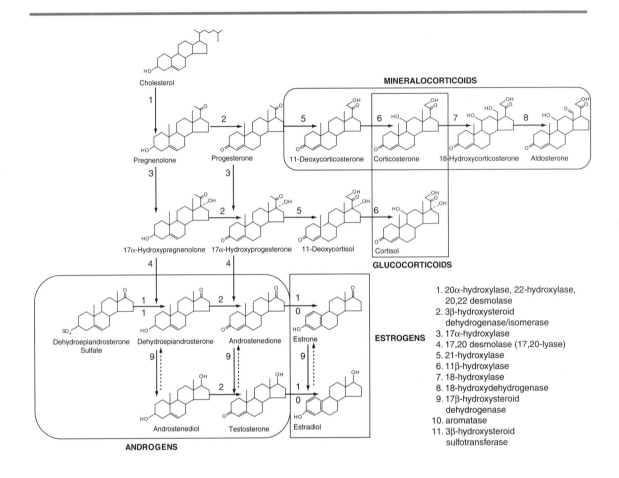

FIGURE 4.9   *Hormone synthesis from cholesterol*

hyperacetylation of histones, and inhibit DNA synthesis.[39,40]

Anaerobic bacteria in the large intestine are themselves capable of producing SCFAs if given an adequate amount of specific substrate. Specifically, approximately 50 to 60 g of dietary carbohydrate rich in fiber can be used to produce over 35 g of SCFAs. Soy polysaccharide, pectin, guar gum, various vegetable fibers, lactulose, and beta-glucan have all been shown to serve as fiber substrate for SCFA production by colonic anaerobes.

In addition to oral supplementation, SCFAs have been administered colonically or enterally to provide more direct support of colonic mucosa. Colonic blood flow can be increased successfully through colonic infusion of SCFAs, and enteral feedings of SCFAs have been shown to increase jejunal and ileal mucosal cell numbers in humans. Clinical use of short-chain fatty acids is discussed further in Chapter 7.

MEDIUM-CHAIN FATTY ACIDS AND MEDIUM-CHAIN TRIGLYCERIDES (MCFAS AND MCTS)

Medium-chain fatty acids (MCFAs) are fatty acids that contain 6 to 24 carbon atoms. These fatty acids include caprylic (8 carbons), capric (10 carbons), lauric (12 carbons) and myristic acid (14 carbons). Triglycerides are molecular compounds that contain three fatty acids attached to a glycerol backbone. They are formed from a monoglyceride and two fatty acids that are attached to the free hydroxyl group on the monoglyceride. (Figure 4.10) When triglycerides contain predominantly MCFAs, they are classified as medium-chain triglycerides (MCTs).

Clinical Use of MCTs

Commercially produced MCT oils have been used since the 1950s to improve the health status of individuals with fat malabsorption problems. There are two reasons for using MCTs. First, MCTs, unlike long-chain fatty acids (LCTs), can be taken up from the intestines into the circulation while bypassing certain physiological steps ordinarily required for fat uptake. For example, chylomicron formation is not required for MCT absorption, nor is a properly working lymphatic system or carnitine shuttle system.[41] Second, MCTs can be metabolized into usable forms of energy as quickly as glucose, a simple sugar that has traditionally been viewed as the body's most readily available form of energy.[42]

Commercial Preparation of MCT Oils

The naturally occurring plant fats referred to as the *lauric fats* have traditionally been used by food chemists as the primary sources for commercial preparation of MCTs. The name itself is derived from the high (nearly 50 percent) concentration of lauric acid (a 12-carbon MCFA) in these fats. Coconut oil and palm kernel oil are the two most widely used starting points for MCT preparation. However, the important goal of MCT preparation is not to produce an oil high in lauric acid (12-carbon), but an oil that is high in the shorter MCFAs, namely caprylic (8-carbon) and capric (10-carbon) acids. MCT oils containing 90 percent or more of these two MCFAs are the only MCT oils that have been shown to be clinically effective in improving the health status of compromised individuals. The MCFA composition of most commercial preparations has resembled the composition of Mead Johnson's best-selling MCT oil Portagen™, which contains 67 percent caprylic and

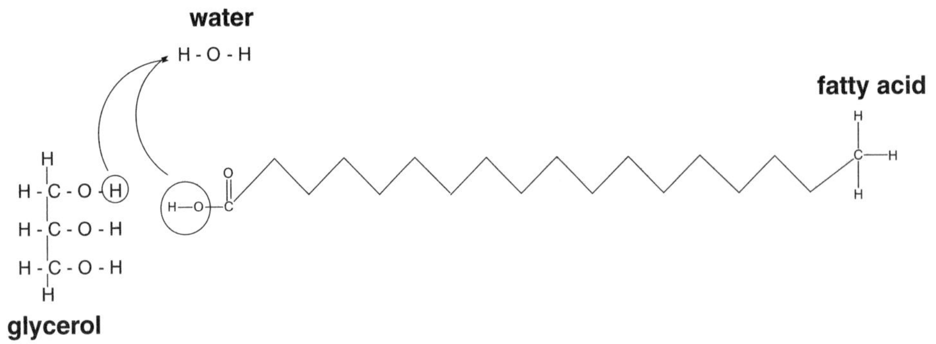

FIGURE 4.10   *The formation of a monoglyceride*

23 percent capric MCFAs. In the process of MCT oil preparation, small amounts of other MCFAs remain within the final product, including lauric acid (12-carbon), which is typically present at 1 to 4 percent in commercial products.

Clinical Effectiveness of 8-Carbon and 10-Carbon MCFAs within MCT Oils

The use of MCT oils containing varying mixtures of MCFAs has consistently improved the course of numerous health problems (perhaps by increasing calories), including pancreatic insufficiency, liver cirrhosis, altered intestinal permeability, lymphatic obstruction, surgical stress, epilepsy, glycogen storage disease, and cystic fibrosis. The results from exclusive use of 8-carbon and 10-carbon MCFAs as the "marker" compounds

within the oils have been equally consistent. Some studies have used the 8-carbon (caprylic) fatty acid exclusively,[43] but most have looked at 8-carbon (caprylic)/10-carbon (capric) mixtures.[44,45,46,47] In each instance, metabolic and physiologic properties of the oils have been shown to depend upon their 8-carbon and 10-carbon constituents.

Hypercholesterolemic Effects of Lauric and Myristic Acids

While traditional arguments against excessive dietary use of coconut and palm oil have focused on their LCFA content, recent research has shown that the lauric/myristic acid component of these oils has a more pronounced hypercholesterolemic effect upon blood lipids than the palmitic acid (LCFA) component.[48] Previous clinical and epidemiological studies have also found lauric acid intake raises LDL and total cholesterol levels.[49]

FATS AND DIETARY MACRONUTRIENT BALANCE

Desirable levels of dietary fat remain a prevalent topic in clinical debate. At one end of the spectrum are Pritikin-type diets, which follow the extremely low-fat recommendations of Nathan Pritikin, providing as little as 10 g of dietary fat per day or less than 5 percent of total calories. At the other end of the spectrum are extremely high-fat, ketogenic recommendations providing as much as 175 g and over 70 percent of total calories of dietary fat per day. Traditional healthcare organizations have typically recommended 30 percent of total calories from fat. On a 2,000-calorie diet, 10 percent of calories would translate into 22 g of total fat, 20 percent of calories into 45 g, and 30 percent of calories into about 67 g.

It is interesting to compare these fat levels to fatty acid supplementation levels commonly used by nutritionally-oriented practitioners. Six g of evening primrose oil is commonly used therapeutically for conditions like atopic skin disorders, premenstrual syndrome, and immune-related disorders. Similar levels of omega 3 oils are used to treat skin conditions like psoriasis. In lipoprotein-fish oil studies, over 100 g of fatty fish two to three times per week have proven helpful. Clearly, it would be difficult for a patient to achieve any of these therapeutic levels while trying to restrict dietary fat intake to 10 percent of total calories.

Consumption of a 25 to 30 percent fat diet may be clinically more appropriate than consumption of a 20 to 25 percent fat diet regimen for specific types of individuals. Gerald Reaven, a medical doctor and researcher at the Stanford University School of Medicine, has described a condition called "Syndrome X," in which insulin resistance and compensatory hyperinsulinemia are accompanied by changes in blood pressure and serum triglyceride and uric acid levels.[50] In Syndrome X individuals (identifiable through two-hour oral glucose and insulin tolerance testing together with measurement of above-mentioned laboratory parameters), high-fat diets (with the right types of fats) may be able to better support eicosanoid synthesis, avoid insulin hypersecretion, and reduce dyslipidemia and insulin resistance.

Because the average U.S. adult consumes more than 66 pounds of pure, added dietary fat per year (including 26 pounds of oil, 22 pounds of shortening, 11 pounds of margarine, 5 pounds of butter, and 2 pounds of lard), together with 183 pounds of meat, 233 pounds of milk, and 26 pounds of eggs, increased intake of dietary fat is not likely to help most patients. For the majority of patients, reducing dietary fat is still likely to help without reducing total consumption to 20 percent or less of total calories level.

However, for most patients, reducing dietary fat may not be the simplest way to support body function and balance fatty acid intake. Neither would the recommendation simply to substitute unsaturated for saturated fats, or worse, substitute monounsaturated for polyunsaturated fatty acids. The single simplest recommendation might be to focus on overall fat quality and derive as much dietary fat as possible from whole, natural food sources—particularly plant sources, beginning with seeds and nuts. However, nutritionally oriented practitioners will go well beyond a single simple recommendation and address the more complex nature of fatty acid balance appropriate for their individual patients.

FOOD FATS AND PLANT OILS

Among consumers, widespread confusion exists about fat concentrations and fat quality in the commercial food supply. Consumers widely recognize fried foods as sources of concentrated fat, but they typically classify as "sweets" many foods that are predominantly fat in content, such as donuts, croissants, and numerous baked goods that taste sweeter and appear more starchy than is expected of high-fat foods. Nuts and seeds are sometimes not recognized as concentrated food sources of fat, nor are many meats that appear "lean" (without much visible white "marbling"). Regardless of fat *concentration*, fat *quality* is largely ignored in these cases. With the exception of saturated fat, which has been traditionally linked to poor health, quality is not generally taken into consideration by consumers in the derivation, processing, handling, cooking, or storage of foods. Practitioners can help advance the health and self-care abilities

of their patients by taking the time to educate their patients about the relationship between fats and foods.

For example, beef fat is the largest single source of arachidonic acid in the U.S. diet, significantly overshadowing all other individual sources. For individuals eating whole-grain foods, germs of grains can provide substantial fat quality and diversity when they are eaten in rotation. But the most undervalued foods in terms of their ability to support fatty acid metabolism and fat-related health processes are nuts, seeds, and their oils.

Nuts, Seeds, and Their Oils

Many cultures still use seeds and nuts as the sole source of cooking fats. These plant reproductive organs can supply highly concentrated amounts of most omega 3 and omega 6 fatty acids. Although most commercial supplements extract oils from nuts and seeds, many cultures sprout, grind into pastes, or boil and press them into nut and seed milks.

Handling of nuts, seeds, and their oils requires extreme care. Polyunsaturated oils, particularly flax seed oil, cannot be stored at room temperature, and must be kept in light protective, opaque containers. Monounsaturated oils, such as olive or canola oil, do not need to be refrigerated. It is also helpful to understand which oils work best in different cooking techniques.

Some oils should be used in high-heat cooking to avoid peroxidation of double bonds, which would occur with use of the less saturated oils. Other oils should be used in medium-heat cooking (200-300 degrees Fahrenheit), while still other oils should only be used under low-heating conditions (for example, in the slow heating of soups or, even better, in salad dressings). (See Table 4.6).

Fat and Physical Performance

In the popular press (and contemporary research to a much lesser extent), a 1990s equivalent to the 1960s carbohydrate-loading practice has emerged, referred to by some researchers as "fat loading."[51] In this practice, a carbohydrate-sparing effect of increased fat intake is proposed, along with increased availability of fatty aids as fuel sources for aerobic metabolism in endurance events. Several researchers have even investigated exercise effects of an 85 percent fat diet for men, revealing a neutral effect upon their performance.[52] Medium-chain triglyceride (MCT) feeding has also failed to elevate serum fatty acids or improve endurance following increased consumption.[53]

Caffeine has been proposed as an ergogenic aid capable of elevating free fatty acid pools before exercise because of its inhibitory effect on the phosphodiesterase enzyme. In fact, several international competitions have even prohibited pre-event consumption of caffeine for this reason. However, research in this area has been mixed. Several studies using caffeine amounts similar to the caffeine contained in two 8-ounce cups of coffee, or approximately 100–150 mg[54] suggested that while caffeine may benefit untrained individuals, training and consumption of high-carbohydrate foods with caffeine may largely negate the effect of caffeine.

SUMMARY

The most important nutrition concept to change may be the understanding that a simple reduction in dietary fat will not necessarily result in improved health status. Recognizing the roles that fats have in structure and physiologic functioning is a vital step toward establishing the appropriate dietary and supplementary fatty acid intake for an individual.

From their important place in the structure of the membranes surrounding the trillions of cells in our bodies to their critical roles in neurologic, hormonal, immune, and cardiovascular functioning, fats are best viewed in

TABLE 4.6 *Preferred Cooking Techniques of Selected Oils*

High-heat cooking	Medium-heat cooking	Low-heat cooking
Coconut	Olive	Almond
Peanut*	Corn	Sesame
High oleic safflower	Hazelnut	Sunflower Butter

* Critical to use organic because of high-pesticide use.

light of their molecular interactions with the other components of human tissue. Simply reducing total fat intake may not address the need to change the type of fat being consumed.

Cellular destruction, unchecked inflammation, and reduced ability to respond to cellular communications may remain problematic even with reduced fat intake.

CHAPTER 4 REFERENCES

1. 1997 Nutrition Trends Survey. Chicago, IL: American Dietetic Association; 1997.
2. Stevens LJ, Zentall SS, Deck JL, et al. Essential fatty acid metabolism in boys with attention-deficit hyperactivity disorder. Am J Clin Nutr. 1995 Oct;62(4):761–768.
3. Hoffman DR, Birch EE, Birch DG, Uauy RD. Effects of supplementation with omega 3 long-chain polyunsaturated fatty acids on retinal and cortical development in premature infants. Am J Clin Nutr. May 1993;57(5 suppl):807S–812S.
4. Oliwiecki S. Levels of essential and other fatty acids in plasma and red cell phospholipids from normal controls in patients with atopic eczema. ACTA Derm Venerol Stockh. 1993;71:224–228.
5. Persad RA, Gillatt DA, Heinemann D, Habib NA, Smith PJ. Erythrocyte to stearic to oleic acid ratio in prostatic carcinoma. Br J Urol. 1990; 65(3):268–270.
6. Siguel EN, Chee, KM, Gong J, Schaefer, EJ. Criteria for essential fatty acid deficiency in plasma as assessed by capillary column gas-liquid chromatography. Clin Chem;33:1869–1873, 1987.
7. Sinclair HM. Essential fatty acids—an historical perspective. Biochem Soc Trans:18:756–761, 1990.
8. Siguel EN, Lerman, RH. Fatty acid patterns in patients with angiographically documented coronary artery disease. Metabolism; 43(8):982–993, 1994.
9. Siguel EN, Lerman, RH. Trans fatty acid metabolism in patients with angiographically documented coronary artery disease. Am J Cardiol;71(11):916–920, 1993.
10. Siguel E. The role of essential fatty acids in health and disease. Nutrition Issue. Contemporary Therapy; 20(9):500-510, 1994.
11. Koletzko B, Decsi T, Demmelmair H. Arachidonic acid supply and metabolism in human infants born at full term. Lipids. 1996;31(1):79–83.
12. Benistant C, Achard F, Ben Slama S, Lagarde M. Docosapentaenoic acid (22:5,n-3): metabolism and effect on prostacyclin production in endothelial cells. Prostaglandins Leukot Essent Fatty Acids. 1996 Oct;55(4):287–292.
13. Masferrer JL, Kulkarni PS. Cyclooxygenase-2 inhibitors: a new approach to the therapy of ocular inflammation. Surv Ophthalmol. 1997 Feb;41(suppl)2:S35–S40.
14. Boudreau MD, Chanmugam PS, Hart SB, Lee SH, Hwang DH. Lack of dose response by dietary n-3 fatty acids at a constant ratio of n-3 to n-6 fatty acids in suppressing eicosanoid biosynthesis from arachidonic acid. Am J Clin Nutr. 1991 July;54(1):111–117.
15. Wood R, Kubena K, O'Brien B, Tseng S, Martin G. Effect of butter, mono- and poly-unsaturated fatty acid-enriched butter, trans fatty acid margarine, and zero trans fatty acid margarine on serum lipids and lipoproteins in healthy men. J Lipid Res. 1993 Jan;34(1):1–11.
16. van den Reek MM, Craig-Schimdt MC, Clark AJ. Use of published analyses of food items to determine dietary trans octadecenoic acid. J Am Diet Assoc. 1986 Oct;86(10):1391–1394.
17. Morrow JD, Frei B, Longmire AW, et al. Increase in circulating products of lipid peroxidation (F2-

isoprostanes) in smokers. Smoking as a cause of oxidative damage. N Engl J Med. 1995 May; 332(18):1198–1203.

18. Ledwozyw A, Michalak J, Stepien A, Kadziolka A. The relationship between plasma triglycerides, cholesterol, total lipids and lipid peroxidation products during human atherosclerosis. Clin Chim Acta. 1986 Mar 28;155(3):275–283.

19. Clarkson PM. Antioxidants and physical performance. Crit Rev Food Sci Nutr. 1995 Jan;35 (1-2):131–141.

20. Chance B, Sies H, Boveris A. Hydroperoxide metabolism in mammalian organs. Physiol Rev. 1979 Jul;59(3):527–605.

21. Rokitzki L, Logemann, Huber G,Keck E, Keul J. Alpha-tocopherol supplementation in racing cyclists during extreme endurance training. Int J Sport Nutr. 1994 Sep;4(3):253–264.

22. Liebler DC, Kling DS, Reed DJ. Antioxidant protection of phospholipid bilayers by alpha-tocopherol. Control of alpha-tocopherol status and lipid peroxidation by ascorbic acid and glutathione. J Biol Chem. 1986 Sep 15;261(26): 12114–12119.

23. Burton GW, Joyce A, Ingold KU. First proof that vitamin E is a major lipid-soluble, chain-breaking antioxidant in human blood plasma. Lancet. 1982 Aug 7;2(8293):327.

24. Kamal-Eldin A, Appelqvist LA. The chemistry and antioxidant properties of tocopherols and tocotrienols. Lipids. 1996 Jul;31(7):671–701.

25. Packer L, Gohil K, deLumen B, Terblanche SE. A comparative study on the effects of ascorbic acid deficiency and supplementation on endurance and mitochondrial oxidative capacities in various tissues of the guinea pig. Comp Biochem Physiol. [B]1986;83:235–240.

26. Johnston CS. Supplemental vitamin C, carnitine, and endurance performance. J Am Coll Nutr. 1993;12(5):615/Abstract 124.

27. Alessio HM, Goldfarb AH, Cao G. Exercise-induced oxidative stress before and after vitamin C supplementation. Int J Sport Nutr. 1997 Mar; 7(1):1–9.

28. Maguire JJ, Kagan V, Ackrell BA, Serbinova E, Packer L. Succinate-ubiquinone reductase linked recycling of alpha-tocopherol in reconstituted systems and mitochondria: requirement for reduced ubiquinone. Arch Biochem Biophys. 1992 Jan;292(1):47–53.

29. Lambelet P, Saucy F, Loliger J. Chemical evidence for interactions between vitamins E and C. Experientia. 1985 Nov 15;41(11):1384–1388.

30. Kunert KJ, Tappel AL. The effect of vitamin C on in vivo lipid peroxidation in guinea pigs as measured by pentane and ethane production. Lipids. 1983 Apr 18;18(4):271–274.

31. Yukin J. Dietary factors in atherosclerosis: sucrose. Lipids. 1978;13(5):370–372.

32. Arnesen E, Forde OH, Thelle DS. Coffee and serum cholesterol. Br Med J. 1984 Jun 30;288 (6435):1960.

33. Danner SA, Wieling W, Havekes L, et al. Effect of physical exercise on blood lipids and adipose tissue composition of young healthy men. Atheroscler. 1984 Oct;53(1):83–90.

34. Ludwig H, Spiteller M, Egger HJ, et al. Correlation of emotional stress and physical exertions with urinary metabolite profiles. J Isr Chem. 1997;16:7–11.

35. Gordon GB, Bush TL, Helzlsouer KJ, Miller SR, Comstock GW. Relationship of serum levels of dehydroepiandrosterone and dehydroepiandrosterone sulfate to the risk of developing postmenopausal breast cancer. Cancer Res. 1990 Jul 1;53(13):3859–3862.

36. Ioannides C, Barnett CR, Irizar A, Flatt, PR. Expression of cytochrome P450 proteins in disease. In: Ioannides C, ed. Cytochromes P450: Metabolic and Toxicological Aspects. Boca Raton, Fla: CRC Press, Inc; 1996:303.

37. Chen YDI, Loch F. Thyroid control over biomembranes. Arch Biochem Biophys. 1977; 181:470–483.

38. Takeuchi H, Matsuo T, Tokuyama K, Suzuki M. Serum triiodothyronine concentration and Na+,K(+)-ATPase activity in liver and skeletal muscle are influenced by dietary fat type in rats. J Nutr. 1995 Sep;125(9):2364–2369.

39. Pouillart P, Cerutti I, Ronco G, Villa P, Chany C. Butyric monosaccharides ester-induced cell differentiation and anti-tumor activity in mice. Importance of their prolonged biological effect for clinical applications in cancer therapy. Int J Cancer. 1991 Aug 19; 49(1):89–95.

40. Berdanier CD, Baltzell JK. Comparative studies of the responses of two strains of rats to an essential fatty acid deficient diet. Comp Biochem Physiol A. 1986;85(4):725–727.

41. Babayan VK. Medium-chain triglycerides and structured lipids. Lipids 1987;22(6):417–420.

42. Babayan VK. Medium-chain triglycerides and structured lipids. Lipids 1987;22(6):417–420.

43. Linscheer WG, Castell DO, Platt RR. A new method for evaluation of portosystemic shunting. The rectal octanoate tolerance test. Gastroenterology. 1969 Oct;57(4):415–423.

44. DeGaetano A, Castagneto M, Mingrone G, et al. Kinetics of medium-chain triglycerides and free fatty acids in healthy volunteers and surgically stressed patients. JPEN. 1994 Mar;18(2):134–140.

45. Gogos CA, Zoumbos N, Makri M, Kalfarentzos F. Medium- and long-chain triglycerides have different effects on the synthesis of tumor necrosis factor by human mononuclear cells in patients under total parenteral nutrition. J Am Coll Nutr. 1994 Feb;13(1):40–44.

46. Johnson RC, Young SK, Cotter R. Medium-chain triglyceride lipid emulsion: metabolism and tissue distribution. Am J Clin Nutr. 1990 Sep;52(3):502–508.

47. Swift LL, Hill JO, Peters JC, Greene HL. Medium-chain fatty acids: evidence for incorporation into chylomicron triglycerides in humans. Am J Clin Nutr. 1990 Nov;52(5):834–836.

48. Sundram K, Siru OH. Dietary palmitic acid results in lower serum cholesterol than does a lauric-myristic acid combination in normolipemic humans. Am J Clin Nutr. 1994 Nov;59:841–846.

49. Denke MA, Grundy SM. Comparison of effects of lauric acid and palmitic acid on plasma lipids and lipoproteins. Am J Clin Nutr. 1992;56(5):895–898.

50. Reaven GM. Pathophysiology of insulin resistance in human disease. Physiol Rev. 1995 Jul; 75(3):473–486.

51. Sherman WM, Leenders N. Fat loading: the next magic bullet? Int J Sport Nutr. 1995 Jun; 5suppl:S1–S12.

52. Phinney SD, Bistrian BR, Wolfe RR, Blackburn GL. The human metabolic response to chronic ketosis without caloric restriction: physical and biochemical adaptation. Metabolism. 1983 Aug;32(8):757–768.

53. Decombaz J, Arnaud MJ, Milon H, et al. Energy metabolism of medium-chain triglycerides versus carbohydrates during exercise. Eur J Appl Physiol. 1983;52(1):9–14.

54. O'Neil FT, Hynak-Hankinson MT, Gorman J. Research and application of current topics in sports nutrition. J Am Diet Assoc. 1986 Aug; 86(8):1007–1015.

5

Vitamins

THE VITAMIN ERA BEGAN IN THE EARLY part of the 1900s when some of the essential nutrients were extracted from natural foods and their chemical compositions were identified. In 1911, Polish biochemist Casimir Funk identified the substances in natural foods that provided protection against beriberi. Funk named these substances "vitamines," a term he derived from the Latin word "vita," meaning "life," and the chemical term "amine," meaning it contained nitrogen. "Vitamines" was later changed to "vitamins" when it was discovered that some of these substances did not contain nitrogen.

When chemical names were originally given to vitamins, many people believed that each name referred to one substance with a specific function. We know now that a number of different molecular forms of a given vitamin have biological activity. The term

"vitamers" now describes these variant forms of a vitamin. For example, vitamin A is typically considered to include the molecular form called retinol. However, retinoic acid and retinal also have biological activity in the body. Since Funk, many people have contributed to our advanced understanding of vitamins by discovering connections between vitamin deficiencies and illness. Early pioneers include Dutch physician Christian Eijkman and his collaborator Gerrit Grijns, who discovered a link between beriberi and rice polish in 1897. Later, Robert R. Williams and his colleagues identified the chemical composition of this rice polish ingredient as thiamin. Other vitamin pioneers included Joseph Goldberg and Conrad Elvehjem (niacin and pellagra), Albert Szent-Gyorgi (vitamin C and scurvy), Roger Williams (pantothenic acid and folic acid), Linus Pauling (vitamin

C), and Dorothy Hodgkin (vitamin B12). This chapter explores and builds upon their understanding of how vitamins can treat the vitamin deficiency diseases by providing an overview of vitamin structure, absorption in humans, physiologic function, food source, therapeutic considerations, and safety. Each discussion concludes by exploring each vitamin's role in physiologic functioning.

VITAMIN STRUCTURE AND FUNCTION

Vitamins are organic compounds required in small amounts by the body for normal metabolic functions. While these compounds are required for life, they cannot be manufactured by the body and are therefore deemed essential. The vitamins cannot themselves be converted into energy by the body, but some of them are required in the process of energy production.[1]

When considering the importance of vitamins to the human body, it is necessary to reflect on the fundamental biochemical interactions that must take place for humans to survive. For instance, pantothenic acid is needed for synthesis of coenzyme A, a crucial component of the Krebs cycle, which is used for energy production. Vitamin B6 is required for the transfer of amino groups, which is critical to amino acid metabolism throughout the body. Riboflavin is needed for activation of the enzyme glutathione reductase, regenerating the vital antioxidant compound glutathione.

The body generally does not use vitamins as they occur in food. Vitamins must first be transformed into their respective coenzyme or cofactor forms. For example, niacin is transformed into nicotinamide adenine dinucleotide (NADH) or nicotinamide adenine dinucleotide phosphate (NADPH)—the active functional forms the vitamin ultimately takes for metabolism. Riboflavin is converted to flavin mononucleotide (FMN) or flavin adenine dinucleotide (FAD) to fulfill its primary role in metabolism.

VITAMIN CLASSIFICATION

Vitamins are classified according to whether or not they are soluble in fat or water. Fat-soluble vitamins include vitamins A, D, E, and K. The water-soluble vitamins include the B vitamins and vitamin C. B vitamins can be further subdivided into a convenient classification system, which includes those influencing energy release, hematopoiesis, and other metabolic action.[2]

B vitamins that influence energy metabolism include thiamin (B1), riboflavin (B2), niacin (B3), pantothenic acid, biotin, and vitamin B6 (pyridoxine, pyridoxal).[3] B vitamins that affect hematopoiesis include folic acid, cobalamin (B12), vitamin B6, and pantothenic acid (B5). B vitamins are also involved in many metabolic activities beyond those already mentioned (see Table 5.1).

VITAMIN INSUFFICIENCY, DEFICIENCY, AND BIOCHEMICAL INDIVIDUALITY

Vitamin insufficiency resulting from poor nutrition has many facets, and evaluating an individual's nutritional status may reveal a

TABLE 5.1 *Classification of B Vitamins by Function*

Energy Metabolism	
Thiamin	B1
Riboflavin	B2
Niacin	B3
Pantothenic acid	B5
Pyridoxine	B6
Biotin	

Hematopoiesis	
Folic acid	
Cobalamin	B12
Pyridoxine	B6
Pantothenic acid	B5

Other Metabolic Actions	
Thiamin	B1
Riboflavin	B2
Niacin	B3
Pyridoxine	B6
Cobalamin	B12
Biotin	
Folic acid	

gradation of deficiency symptoms. Myron Brin, Ph.D., suggests this gradation may start with a preliminary reduction of nutrient stores with no symptomatology, which may lead to a biochemical reduction in enzyme activity through lack of nutrient-derived coenzymes. This may be followed by physiological impairment that evolves as adverse behavioral and personality effects, moves toward classical deficiency syndromes, and finally becomes terminal tissue pathology. In 1979, Brin noted that the first clinical effects in undernutrition with respect to B vitamins are insomnia, adverse Minnesota Multiphasic Personality Inventory scores, irritability, modified appetite, sugar craving, impaired drug metabolism, and reduced immune competency.

Thus, classic signs associated with such "deficiency diseases" may be end-stage manifestations of sustained nutrient inadequacy. Clinicians should carefully monitor patient insufficiency, in which nutrient needs for optimum metabolism have not been met but the insufficiency is not severe enough to cause the overt disease typically associated with that nutrient. One can imagine that single nutrient insufficiency has the potential to influence metabolism adversely and encourage disease. More commonly, however, insufficiencies exist in more than one nutrient.

Roger Williams, pioneer of the concept of biochemical individuality, spent many years studying unique patterns of supposedly similar animals and humans. To his surprise, body chemistry varied widely, often in animals bred to be genetically similar. He wrote:

> Some inbred rats on identical diets excreted 11 times as much urinary phosphate as others; some, when given a chance to exercise at will, ran consistently 20 times as far as others; some voluntarily consumed 16 times as much sugar as others; some drank 20 times as much alcohol; some appeared to need about 40 times as much vitamin A as others; some young guinea pigs required, for good growth, at least 20 times as much vitamin C as others.[4,5,6]

Williams's work suggests that a wide variation exists among individuals and that these variations interact in unique ways to determine who we are biochemically. These biochemical differences express themselves with unique requirements and unique suscepti- bilities. When we add environmental influ- ences to this formula for diversity, we are left with a human who is fundamentally the same, but practically different. The task of clinicians is to recognize that each patient is unique and discover these unique patterns. Therapy then becomes specifically designed, not to the text- book or to epidemiological studies, but to the distinct needs of a particular human being. It is with this understanding that clinical nutrition can evolve within the core of the healing arts.

DIETARY REFERENCE INTAKES (DRIS): RELEVANCE TO CLINICAL THERAPEUTICS

Governmental agencies have tried to develop standards with which to determine necessary nutrient levels for individuals. Initially, the In- stitute of Medicine's Food and Nutrition Board (FNB) was asked to develop guidelines or "Recommended Dietary Allowances" (RDAs) for use in preparing canned foods and meals, such as for troops overseas during the World Wars. The Board published the first set of standards, the RDAs, in 1941. These stan- dards were developed on data using deficiency diseases, and they set intake limits based upon levels necessary to avoid a deficiency in the majority of individuals, and were continued in the same form until the last publication of RDAs in 1989. The RDAs set the standard not just for preparing foods for large popula-

tions, but also for how a food was labeled. Today, we are used to the idea of a food label saying "this food contains XX percent of the RDA" and many consumers use these state- ments as a means to provide adequate nutri- tion to themselves and their families.

Much controversy has arisen around the RDAs, mainly because data since the 1940s have shown that adequate intake of nutrients is related to more than just a deficiency disease, such as scurvy. Inadequate nutrient intake has been associated with many of the chronic dis- eases common today, such as heart disease, diabetes, and inflammatory conditions like arthritis. In addition, unique life circumstances, such as genetic heritage, personal health his- tory, and biochemical individuality of a person may require that specific nutrients be given at levels well beyond those set forth in the RDAs. Because researchers questioned the value of RDAs in working with individuals and not populations, several different approaches were published in the literature, including the con- cepts of using lowest and highest tolerable lev- els of a nutrient, and calculating nutrient needs based upon the average intake in a population (assuming most individuals were healthy) and not the minimum amount needed to ward off deficiency diseases.

In response to these concerns, the FNB was asked to reevaluate the RDA approach and provide a set of guidelines that would be more suited to current knowledge about nutri- tion and that would incorporate these differ- ent standards. The FNB quickly assessed that it could not provide just one level or amount of a nutrient for general groups of people (female, male, different age groups, etc.) because there are too many variables with respect to nutrient needs. The FNB has revised its approach and now sets a standard called the Dietary Reference Intakes (DRIs). The DRIs are based upon four dietary references: the RDA, the Estimated Average Requirement (EAR), the Adequate Intake (AI), and the Tolerable Upper Intake Level (UL). Definitions of these dietary references are shown in Table 5.2.

The DRIs are useful as an approximation, but are still mainly focused on preventing overt disease in a population. A summary of the DRIs for vitamins is shown in Table 5.3. The DRIs are most useful for setting public policy, providing consistent values from company to company for food labeling, and making foods for large populations. A functional

medicine approach requires that a clinician use these as guidelines for establishing generally safe levels for an individual, but not as the specific levels needed for every individual walking through the door. Keep in mind that the DRIs have not been set to optimize health and do not take into consideration such factors as environmental exposure, medication intake, digestion and absorption efficiency, genetics, food intolerance, and other circumstances that alter nutrient needs.

A FUNCTIONAL APPROACH TO VITAMINS

One only needs to look at the history and identification of most vitamins to understand their profound effects on the physiology of the

TABLE 5.2   *The Four Daily Reference Standards Used to Develop the Dietary Reference Intakes (DRIs)*

- **Estimated Average Requirement (EAR):** the average daily nutrient intake level estimated on deficiency data to meet the needs of 50% of the healthy individuals in a particular life stage and gender group.

- **Recommended Dietary Allowance (RDA):** the average daily nutrient intake level estimated on deficiency data to meet the needs of over 90% of the healthy individuals in a particular life stage and gender group.

- **Adequate Intake (AI):** the recommended average daily intake level based upon observed or experimentally determined approximations for a group of people assumed to be healthy.

- **Tolerable Upper Intake Level (UL):** the highest average daily nutrient intake level under which few or no adverse events (including such events as gastrointestinal disturbance or other more severe effects) have been reported. Intake of a nutrient at or below the UL is considered to pose no risk of adverse health effects to almost all individuals in the general population.

TABLE 5.3 *Summary Table of the DRIs for Vitamins*

Note: RDAs have not been set for all vitamins for the different life stages. When an RDA is not available, the AI is used for that vitamin (denoted by an *). The UL has also not been reported for many vitamins and, in those cases, "nd" (not determined) is shown. For a more complete table see http://www.nap.edu (accessed December 2003).

Vitamin	AGE	RDA/AI*	UL
Vitamin B1 (Thiamin)	Infants (0–12 mo)	0.2–0.3 mg/d*	nd
	Children (1–8 y)	0.5–0.6 mg/d	nd
	Children (9–13 y)	0.9 mg/d	nd
	Males (≥14 y)	1.2 mg/d	nd
	Females (14–18 y)	1.0 mg/d	nd
	Females (<18 y)	1.1 mg/d	nd
	Pregnancy	1.4 mg/d	nd
	Lactation	1.4 mg/d	nd
Vitamin B2 (Riboflavin)	Infants (0–12 mo)	0.3–0.4 mg/d*	nd
	Children (1–8 y)	0.5–0.6 mg/d	nd
	Children (9–13 y)	0.9 mg/d	nd
	Males (≥14 y)	1.3 mg/d	nd
	Females (14 – 18 y)	1.0 mg/d	nd
	Females (<18 y)	1.1 mg/d	nd
	Pregnancy	1.4 mg/d	nd
	Lactation	1.6 mg/d	nd
Vitamin B3 (Niacin)	Infants (0–12 mo)	2–4 mg/d*	nd
	Children (1–8 y)	6–8 mg/d	10–15mg/d
	Children (9–18 y)	12–16 mg/d	20–30 mg/d
	Adults males	16 mg/d	35 mg/d
	Adult females	14 mg/d	35 mg/d
	Pregnancy	18 mg/d	30–35 mg/d
	Lactation	17 mg/d	30–35 mg/day
Vitamin B5 (Pantothenic acid)	Infants (0–12 mo)	1.7–1.8 mg/d*	nd
	Children (1–8 y)	2–3 mg/d*	nd
	Children (9–13 y)	4 mg/d*	nd
	Males (≥14 y)	5 mg/d*	nd
	Females (>14 y)	5 mg/d*	nd
	Pregnancy	6 mg/d*	nd
	Lactation	7 mg/d*	nd

(continues)

Vitamin	AGE	RDA/AI*	UL
Vitamin B6 (Pyridoxine)	Infants (0–12 mo)	0.1 –0.3 mg/d*	nd
	Children (1–8 y)	0.5–0.6 mg/d	30–40 mg/d
	Children (9–13 y)	1.0 mg/d	60 mg/d
	Males (14–50 y)	1.3 mg/d	80–100 mg/d
	Males (>50 y)	1.7 mg/d	100 mg/d
	Females (14 – 18 y)	1.2 mg/d	80 mg/d
	Females (19–50 y)	1.3 mg/d	100 mg/d
	Females (<50 y)	1.5 mg/d	100 mg/d
	Pregnancy	1.9 mg/d	80–100 mg/d
	Lactation	2.0 mg/d	80–100 mg/d
Vitamin B12 (Cobalamin)	Infants (0–12 mo)	0.4–0.5 mcg/d*	nd
	Children (1–8 y)	0.9–1.2 mcg/d	nd
	Children (9–13 y)	1.8 mcg/d	nd
	Males (≥14 y)	2.4 mcg/d	nd
	Females (≥14 y)	2.4 mcg/d	nd
	Pregnancy	2.6 mcg/d	nd
	Lactation	2.8 mcg/d	nd
Folic acid	Infants (0–12 mo)	65–80 mcg/d*	nd
	Children (1–8 y)	150–200 mcg/d	300 mcg/d
	Children (9–18 y)	300–400 mcg/d	600–800 mcg/d
	Adults	400 mcg/d	1,000 mcg/d
	Pregnancy (<18 y)	600 mcg/d	800 mcg/d
	Pregnancy (>18 y)	600 mcg/d	1,000 mcg/d
	Lactation (< 18 y)	500 mcg/d	800 mcg/d
	Lactation (> 18 y)	500 mcg/d	1,000 mcg/d
Biotin	Infants (0–12 mo)	5–6 mcg/d*	nd
	Children (1–8 y)	8–12 mcg/d*	nd
	Children (9–18 y)	20–25 mcg/d*	nd
	Adults	30 mcg/d*	nd
Vitamin C (Ascorbate)	Infants (0–12 mo)	40–50 mg/d*	nd
	Children (1–8 y)	15–25 mg/d	400–650 mg/d
	Children (9–13 y)	45 mg/d	1200 mg/d
	Males (14–18 y)	75 mg/d	1800 mg/d
	Males (>18 y)	90 mg/d	2000 mg/d
	Females (14–18 y)	65 mg/d	1800 mg/d
	Females (>18 y)	75 mg/d	2000 mg/d
	Pregnancy (<18 y)	80 mg/d	1800 mg/d
	Pregnancy (>18 y)	85 mg/d	2000 mg/d
	Lactation (<18 y)	115 mg/d	1800 mg/d
	Lactation (>18 y)	120 mg/d	2000 mg/d

(continues)

Vitamin	AGE	RDA/AI*	UL
Vitamin E	Infants (0–12 mo)	4–5 mg/d*	nd
	Children (1–8 y)	6–7 mg/d	200–300 mg/d
	Children (9–13 y)	11 mg/d	600 mg/d
	Children (14–18 y)	15 mg/d	800 mg/d
	Males (>18 y)	15 mg/d	1000 mg/d
	Females (>18 y)	15 mg/d	1000 mg/d
	Pregnancy (≤18 y)	15 mg/d	800 mg/d
	Pregnancy (>18 y)	15 mg/d	1000 mg/d
	Lactation (≤18 y)	19 mg/d	800 mg/d
	Lactation (>18 y)	19 mg/d	1000 mg/d
Vitamin A (1 mcg=1RE)	Infants (0–12 mo)	400–500 mcg/d*	600 mcg/d
RE= retinal equivalent	Children (1–8 y)	300–400 mcg/d	600–900 mcg/d
	Children (9–13 y)	600 mcg/d	1700 mcg/d
	Males (≥14 y)	900 mcg/d	2800–3000 mcg/d
	Females (≥14 y)	700 mcg/d	2800–3000 mcg/d
	Pregnancy (<18 y)	750 mcg/d	2800 mcg/d
	Pregnancy (>18 y)	770 mcg/d	3000 mcg/d
	Lactation (< 18 y)	1200 mcg/d	2800 mcg/d
	Lactation (> 18 y)	1300 mcg/d	3000 mcg/d
Vitamin D (1 mcg=40 IU)	Infants (0–12 mo)	5 mcg/d*	25 mcg/d
	Children (1–13 y)	5 mcg/d*	50 mcg/d
	Males (14 –50 y)	5 mcg/d*	50 mcg/d
	Males (>50 y)	10–15 mcg/d*	50 mcg/d
	Females (14–50 y)	5 mcg/d*	50 mcg/d
	Females (>50 y)	10–15 mcg/d*	50 mcg/d
	Pregnancy	5 mcg/d*	50 mcg/d
	Lactation	5 mcg/d*	50 mcg/d
Vitamin K	Infants (0–12 mo)	2.0–2.5 mcg/d*	nd
	Children (1–3 y)	30 mcg/d*	nd
	Children (4–8 y)	55 mcg/d*	nd
	Children (9–13 y)	60 mcg/d*	nd
	Males (14–18 y)	75 mcg/d*	nd
	Males (≥18 y)	120 mcg/d	nd
	Females (14–18 y)	75 mcg/d*	nd
	Females (≥18 y)	90 mcg/d*	nd
	Pregnancy (<18 y)	75 mcg/d*	nd
	Pregnancy (>18 y)	90 mcg/d*	nd
	Lactation (< 18 y)	75 mcg/d*	nd
	Lactation (> 18 y)	90 mcg/d*	nd

human body. From reports of beriberi in Asia in 2600 BC to night blindness plaguing 19th century soldiers, the effects of vitamin deficiency and toxicity have led physicians and scientists to search for these vital molecules.[7]

The descriptions that follow include information on each vitamin's role in physiologic functioning. While severe deficiencies may be required to generate frank deficiency diseases, insufficiencies of a vitamin may lead to problems related to less obvious physiologic dysfunction. This decreased functioning may not readily be attributed to a vitamin insufficiency, and the clinician might overlook it as a possible cause of the patient's signs and symptoms. A thorough patient history including diet and lifestyle will help identify this link.

In addition, researchers continue to recognize the importance of vitamin interactions. Consider the recent developments in the homocysteine story, in which researchers have argued the importance of the methylation interactions of vitamins B6, B12, and folic acid in the prevention of heart disease.[8,9,10,11] The homocysteinemia resulting from insufficient supplies of these vitamins in some individuals may lead to coronary artery disease, neurodegenerative disease, or cancer. The role of antioxidant vitamins in keeping other antioxidants from becoming pro-oxidant represents another example of important vitamin interactions.

Individual needs for vitamins vary, based not only on genetic code for physiologic activity, but also on conditional needs for in-creased vitamin availability. The latter situation may arise from increased use of the nutrients in complex physiologic interactions or from loss of vitamin availability due to the presence of substances that antagonize the active vitamin molecule before it can carry on its vital functions. Vitamin availability is also a factor of proper digestion and absorption.

What follows is an outline of each vitamin's structure, absorption in humans, physiologic functioning of the active forms, food sources, therapeutic considerations, safety, and functional medicine considerations. More detailed descriptions are provided in the references cited.

THE WATER-SOLUBLE VITAMINS

Vitamin B1 (Thiamin)

Structure

Thiamin consists of a methylene molecule connecting a pyrimidine and a thiazole ring (Figure 5.1). This vitamin acts as a coenzyme in many important reactions, but it is the thiamin pyrophosphate ester (TPP, thiamin with two phosphate groups) that primarily serves these functions. Adenosine triphosphate (ATP) and magnesium are needed to form this active molecule.[12]

Absorption

The thiamin phosphate esters are hydrolyzed within the proximal small intestine and are absorbed in the jejunum by either an active carrier system or passive diffusion, depending

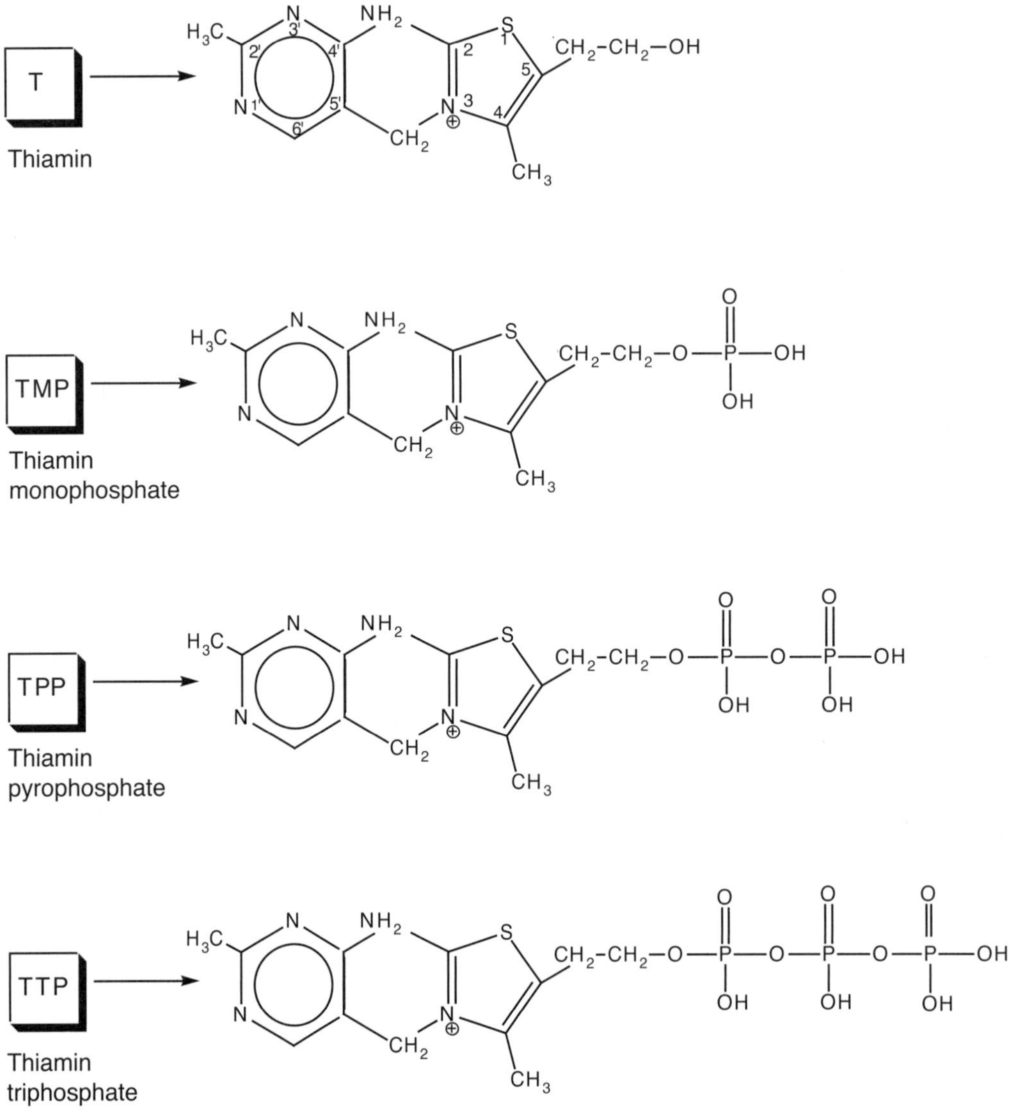

Note: All forms are the same except for the phosphate group.

FIGURE 5.1 *Vitamin B1 (thiamin molecule)*

on the total concentration within the lumen.[13] In adults, the total thiamin content is estimated to be about 30 g; its half-life is 9.5 to 18.5 days.[14] Maintaining this relatively small pool requires regular intake of thiamin. Under conditions of increased energy demand, thiamin requirements may increase accordingly.

Functions

Thiamin is involved in the transfer of aldehyde groups. In serving this purpose, it participates in enzymatic reactions central to energy production, including decarboxylation and transketolation. Thiamin appears to have an important nonenzymatic function as well, as it modulates chloride ion channels in the central nervous system.[15] Thiamin also provides energy for the hexose monophosphate shunt and for the respiratory burst of phagocytes during inflammation.

Vitamin B1 is vitally important in neuronal and neurocognitive functioning.[16] As mentioned above, TPP is important in transketolation, a major source of pentoses for the synthesis of nucleic acids and NADPH. Vitamin B1 is also needed for the synthesis of acetylcholine (ACh) and possibly for the release of ACh at the synaptic junction.

Sources

Thiamin is found in brewer's yeast, wheat germ, peanuts, sunflower seeds, pork, pine nuts, soybeans, and other foods (Table 5.4). Thiamin is destroyed by sulfites, a common food additive, and by moist heat. The use of alkalis such as baking soda with moist heat particularly destroys thiamin.[17] If the diet is high in fats and sugars, thiamin intake will probably be less than adequate.[18]

Therapeutic considerations

Thiamin insufficiency has a marked effect on the central nervous system. Thus, it is used therapeutically in conditions of dementia, neuropathy, fatigue, alcoholism, confusion, depression, pain, memory loss, and ataxia, among others. Because of thiamin's role in energy metabolism, it is used clinically in conditions of impaired detoxification. Severe thiamin deficiency results in the classic symptoms of beriberi (such as fatigue, anorexia, weight loss, gastrointestinal disorders, and weakness). Therapeutic doses are considered to be between 50 and 200 mg/day orally, although up to 8 g daily are often given in conditions of dementia.

Under conditions of increased energy demand and increased caloric intake, thiamin requirements may increase accordingly. Thus, signs and symptoms of insufficiency may be more obvious due to circumstances of increased energy demand. In situations in which vitamin B1 is insufficient (there is a conditional requirement for increased availability), partially metabolized compounds such as pyruvic acid may build up and create the signs and symptoms of thiamin deficiency, such as fatigue.[19] Mental dysfunction may be due to a decrease in the synthesis of ACh due to thiamin insufficiency. As thiamin deficiency increases, marked effects on the central nervous system may develop.

TABLE 5.4   *Thiamin Content of Certain Foods*
Milligrams (mg) per 3 1/2 oz

Yeast, brewer's	15.61	Wild rice	.45
Yeast, torula	14.01	Rye, whole grain	.43
Wheat germ	2.01	Cashews	.43
Sunflower seeds	1.96	Liver, lamb	.40
Rice polishings	1.84	Mung beans	.38
Pine nuts	1.28	Cornmeal, whole ground	.38
Peanuts, with skins	1.14	Lentils	.37
Brazil nuts	.96	Kidneys, beef	.36
Pork, lean	.93	Green peas	.35
Pecans	.86	Macadamia nuts	.34
Soybean flour	.85	Brown rice	.34
Beans, pinto & red	.84	Walnuts	.33
Split peas	.74	Garbanzo beans	.31
Millet	.73	Garlic, cloves	.25
Wheat bran	.72	Liver, beef	.25
Pistachio nuts	.67	Almonds	.24
Navy beans	.65	Lima beans, fresh	.24
Buckwheat	.60	Pumpkin & squash seeds	.24
Oatmeal	.60	Brains, all kinds	.23
Whole wheat flour	.55	Chestnuts, fresh	.23
Whole wheat grain	.55	Soybean sprouts	.23
Lima beans, dry	.48	Peppers, red chili	.22
Hazelnuts	.46	Sesame seeds, hulled	.18
Heart, lamb	.45		

Safety and toxicity

Thiamin toxicity is rare even under conditions of extremely high oral or parenteral intake.[20] However, sensitivity to thiamin may occur depending upon its origin and the susceptibility of the patient. This is true of chemically sensitive patients as well as those with yeast sensitivity. Parenteral forms of thiamin should be preservative-free to minimize the possibility of adverse reactions.

Functional medicine considerations

Keeping in mind the roles of thiamin in physiologic functioning, a patient's diet and lifestyle will often set the stage for the nutrient's role in his or her health. As stated, diets high in fats and sugar should lead clinicians to suspect inadequate thiamin intake. Methods of cooking and intake of prepared foods may also give clues to thiamin insufficiency, as sulfites or excessive cooking of foods may antagonize this vitamin. Other antagonists to thiamin include blueberries, red beet root, Brussels sprouts, and tea. Alcohol consumption may lead to severe vitamin B1 deficiency and Wernecke-Korsakoff syndrome.[21]

A thiamin-deficient patient may experience fatigue, memory loss, depression, headache, confusion, and muscle weakness. More severe deficiencies may result in anorexia, weight loss, gastrointestinal disorders, neurologic problems (including exaggerated deep tendon reflexes and polyneuritis), and cardiovascular problems (including cardiomegaly and tachycardia).

Vitamin B2 (Riboflavin)

Structure

The riboflavin molecule is an isoalloxazine. The coenzyme derivatives include flavin mononucleotide (FMN) and flavin adenine dinucleotide (FAD) (Figure 5.2). Riboflavin can easily be destroyed by strong alkaline substances and by light (both visible and ultraviolet).[22]

Absorption

Hydrolysis of riboflavin's coenzyme derivatives from the diet allows for the absorption

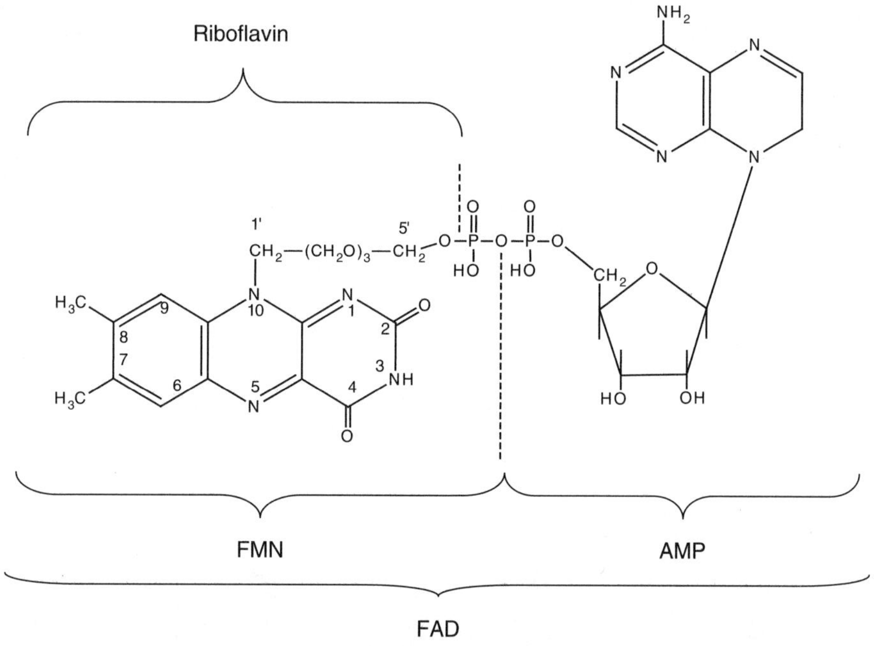

FIGURE 5.2 *Vitamin B2 (riboflavin) and flavin mononucleotide (FMN) as components of flavin-adenine dinucleotide (FAD)*

of this vitamin in the upper intestine by an active phosphorylation transport mechanism. Both ATP and sodium are needed for this absorption. Important dietary considerations in the absorption of vitamin B2 include psyllium gum and alcohol, both of which slow absorption. Antacids may also slow absorption of riboflavin. Riboflavin may be more efficiently absorbed with food and when increased bile salts are present. Some substances may chelate vitamin B2 and reduce its bioavailability. These include copper, zinc, caffeine, theophylline, saccharin, vitamin B3, vitamin C, and tryptophan.[23]

Functions

The major function of riboflavin is to serve as a precursor for the coenzymes FMN and FAD. These enzymes catalyze oxidation reduction and hydrogen ion (or H^+) transfer reactions. Four important roles of riboflavin include the following: 1) energy metabolism as FAD in the respiratory transport chain; 2) drug or xenobiotic metabolism via cyto-

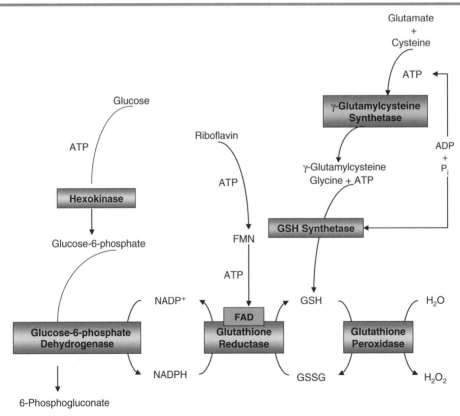

FIGURE 5.3   *Glutathione redox cycle*

chrome P450 enzymes; 3) lipid metabolism; and 4) antioxidant protection by virtue of its role as cofactor in the regeneration of glutathione via glutathione reductase. (Figure 5.3)

Riboflavin inadequacy has been associated with increased lipid peroxidation by virtue of this latter reaction.[24]

Riboflavin is also involved in the metabolism of folic acid, pyridoxine, vitamin K, and niacin.[25] Thus, riboflavin insufficiency can affect a wide array of physiologic functions. Riboflavin deficiency probably occurs only rarely alone.

Sources

Food sources include organ meats, torula yeast, brewer's yeast, almonds, wheat germ, and some mushrooms. See Table 5.5 for additional food sources and amounts.

Therapeutic considerations

Clinical circumstances in which riboflavin may be of value include acne, alcoholism, angular

TABLE 5.5 *Riboflavin Content of Certain Foods*
Milligrams (mg) per 3 1/2 oz

Food	mg	Food	mg
Yeast, torula	5.06	Eggs	.30
Yeast, brewer's	4.28	Split peas	.29
Liver, lamb	3.28	Tongue, beef	.29
Liver, beef	3.26	Brains, all kinds	.26
Liver, pork	3.03	Kale	.26
Liver, calf	2.72	Parsley	.26
Kidneys, beef	2.55	Cashews	.25
Liver, chicken	2.49	Rice bran	.25
Kidneys, lamb	2.42	Veal	.25
Chicken giblets	1.36	Salmon	.23
Heart, veal	1.05	Broccoli	.23
Almonds	.92	Pine nuts	.23
Heart, beef	.88	Sunflower seeds	.23
Heart, lamb	.74	Pork, lean	.22
Wheat germ	.68	Navy beans	.22
Wild rice	.63	Beet and mustard greens	.22
Mushrooms	.46	Lentils	.22
Egg yolks	.44	Prunes	.22
Millet	.38	Rye, whole grain	.22
Peppers, hot red	.36	Pork, lean	.22
Soy flour	.35	Mung beans	.21
Wheat bran	.35	Beans, pinto & red	.21
Mackerel	.33	Black-eyed peas	.21
Collards	.31	Okra	.21
Soybeans, dry	.31		

stomatitis, arthritis, athlete's foot, baldness, cataracts, cheilosis, depression, diabetes, diarrhea, visual disturbances, hysteria, indigestion, light sensitivity, nerve damage, reddening of the eyes (and eyes that tire easily, burn, itch, etc.), scrotal skin changes, seborrheic dermatitis, stress, and failure to detoxify xenobiotics efficiently.[26] Therapeutic range for riboflavin is 50 to 200 mg/day.

Safety and toxicity

When riboflavin intake exceeds 1.3 mg/day, greater quantities of the vitamin are excreted in the urine. However, in cases of increased need, such as in illness or athletic training, less riboflavin is excreted. It is generally agreed that intake of riboflavin many times the RDA does not have adverse consequences.[27]

Functional medicine considerations

A patient's diet and lifestyle may reflect low intake of the listed foods. In addition, food exposed to light may lose riboflavin content; for example, vitamin B2 content may be lower in milk sold in glass bottles or may be reduced in sun-dried fruits and vegetables.[28] A history of chronic alcohol use may be reason to suspect insufficient riboflavin. If the patient also has had chronic drug use or endocrine problems such as decreased thyroid or adrenal activity, the clinician may suspect vitamin B2 insufficiency. Riboflavin insufficiency may also be suspected if the patient presents with cheilosis, oral mucosal inflammation, glossitis, red eyes (that may also be itchy, burning, or photosensitive), dry skin, or depression.[29]

Finally, the range of vitamin B2 functions may indicate an inadequate supply if the patient is fatigued and has increased signs of oxidative stress (including muscle weakness and decreased energy).

Vitamin B3 (Niacin)

Structure

Nicotinic acid and its nicotinamide derivatives are known as niacin or vitamin B3. Niacin is used to form the active cofactors (coenzymes) nicotine adenine dinucleotide (NADH; the ionized form is NAD^+) and nicotine adenine dinucleotide phosphate (NADPH; the ionized form is $NADP^+$).[30] (Figure 5.4) These cofactors are important in many oxidation-reduction reactions in the body, especially those involved in energy.

Absorption

Absorption occurs in the stomach and intestine by both sodium-dependent facilitated diffusion (at lower concentrations) and passive diffusion. The NADH and NADPH forms represent dietary niacin, which is hydrolyzed for absorption. Synthesis of the vitamin occurs from tryptophan, with vitamin B6, riboflavin, and iron as cofactors. Approximately 60 mg of tryptophan are required to form 1 mg of niacin in this way. Thus, the average adult might derive approximately 8 mg of niacin from dietary tryptophan conversion—well below the RDA of 15 to 19 mg per day.

The conversion of extracellular nicotinamide into NADH seems to be under hep-

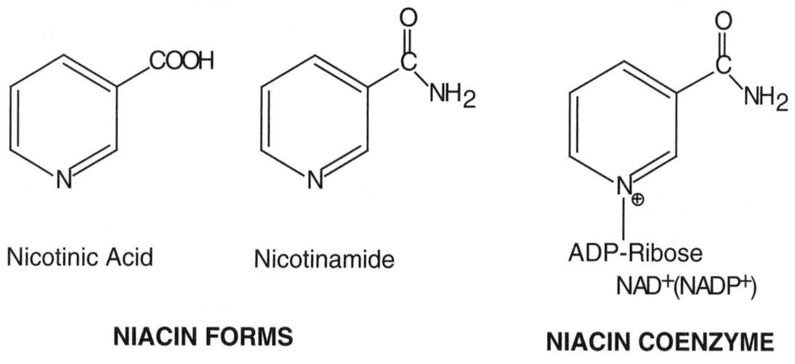

NIACIN FORMS **NIACIN COENZYME**

Nicotinic Acid   Nicotinamide   ADP-Ribose
NAD⁺(NADP⁺)

FIGURE 5.4 *Vitamin B3 (niacin) molecule*

atic control and regulated hormonally. The liver will store excess plasma nicotinamide as unbound NAD. The nicotinamide that forms from this NADH degradation can be reconverted into NADH in most tissues or by microflora in the intestine.[31]

Functions

The body uses NADH as an electron acceptor or as a hydrogen (H^+) donor in many redox reactions. It is a cofactor in the oxidation of some fuel molecules. NADPH donates H^+ in fatty acid or steroid synthesis. Vitamin B3 is also involved in dehydrogenase reactions, such as in the conversion of alpha-ketoglutarate to succinate.

NADH is an important cofactor in nonredox reactions such as the transfer of ADP-ribose catalyzed by poly-ADP-ribose polymerase (PARP) and the formation of cyclic ADP-ribose, which helps move calcium from intracellular storage. The PARP enzyme seems to be important in DNA repair and cell differentiation. Glucose tolerance factor (GTF), which plays an important role in the insulin response, employs niacin (nicotinic acid).[32]

Sources

Food sources of niacin include torula yeast, brewer's yeast, rice bran, wheat bran, and peanuts. Sources of tryptophan include milk, soy, peanuts, eggs, pork, lamb, and beef. For additional sources and amounts, see Table 5.6.

Therapeutic considerations

Niacin deficiency results in pellagra, the signs of which include dermatitis, dementia, diarrhea, and death. Niacin has also been used clinically in a number of circumstances including rheumatoid arthritis and osteoarthritis, diabetes, memory impairment, intermittent claudication, and depression. Niacin has been shown to lower LDL cholesterol, lipoprotein a, triglyceride, and fibrinogen levels, while raising HDL levels.[33] Therapeutic doses of niacin range from 50 to 200 mg per day.

TABLE 5.6 *Niacin Content of Certain Foods*
Milligrams (mg) per 3 1/2 oz

Yeast, torula	44.4	Veal	6.4
Yeast, brewer's	37.9	Kidneys, beef	6.4
Rice bran	29.8	Wild rice	6.2
Rice polishings	28.2	Chicken giblets	6.1
Wheat bran	21.0	Lamb, lean	5.7
Peanuts, with skin	17.2	Chicken, flesh & skin	5.6
Liver, lamb	16.9	Sesame seeds	5.4
Liver, pork	16.4	Sunflower seeds	5.4
Peanuts, without skin	15.8	Beef, lean	5.1
Liver, beef	13.6	Pork, lean	5.0
Liver, calf	11.4	Brown rice	4.7
Turkey, light meat	11.3	Pine nuts	4.5
Liver, chicken	10.8	Buckwheat, whole grain	4.4
Chicken, light meat	10.7	Peppers, red chili	4.4
Trout	8.4	Whole wheat grain	4.4
Halibut	8.3	Whole wheat flour	4.3
Mackerel	8.2	Wheat germ	4.2
Heart, veal	8.1	Barley	3.7
Chicken, flesh only	8.0	Herring	3.6
Swordfish	8.0	Almonds	3.5
Turkey, flesh only	8.0	Shrimp	3.2
Goose, flesh only	7.7	Split peas	3.0
Heart, beef	7.5	Haddock	3.0
Salmon	7.2		

Safety and toxicity

Uncomfortable flushing of skin may occur with as little as 25 mg of niacin, but some individuals may tolerate higher levels. Oral administration of as much as 6 g/day has been taken without side effects.[34] Timed-release niacin has been used to avoid the flushing associated with ingestion of this nutrient. However, hepatic complications have been associated with this form. Liver function should be measured in individuals on high-dose niacin therapy. The use of inositol hexaniacinate rather than niacin may help eliminate some of the side effects experienced with niacin supplementation.[35]

Functional medicine considerations

Clinicians should explore patient use of the drug isoniazid because it competes with the vitamin B6 needed for tryptophan metabolism to niacin. If the patient has been using high levels of niacin, toxicity might be detected by increased liver enzymes. With signs and symptoms of niacin insufficiency, also consider whether vitamin B6, riboflavin, or iron might be less than adequate. These may be the underlying reasons for the niacin insufficiency.

Skin conditions associated with niacin insufficiency include a scaly, dark hyperpigmentation that develops in areas of the body exposed to recurrent trauma, sunlight, or heat. Pale skin will predominate elsewhere. Niacin insufficiency may present with anorexia, nausea, cheilosis, glossitis, stomatitis, confusion, depression, dermatitis, fatigue, headaches, indigestion, insomnia, irritability, muscle weakness, and poor detoxification of xenobiotics.

Vitamin B5 (Pantothenic Acid)

Structure

Pantothenic acid is formed by the combination of beta-alanine and pantoic acid. The Greek *pantos*, meaning "everywhere," reflects the wide distribution of pantothenic acid in nature. A primary biological function of pantothenic acid is to serve as part of the coenzyme A (CoA) molecule. The molecular structure is shown in Figure 5.5.

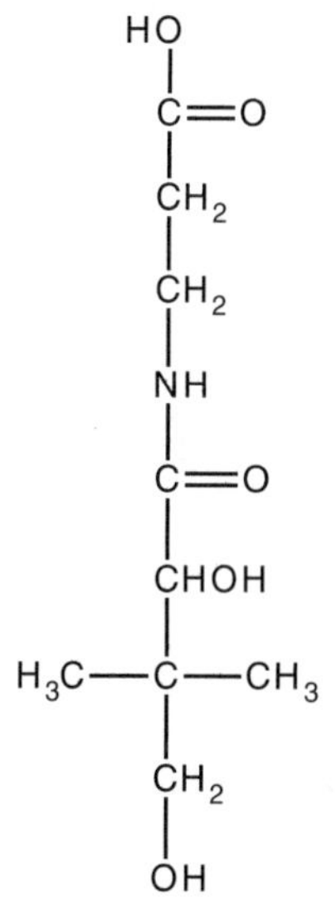

Absorption

Pantothenic acid occurs in food primarily in CoA. During digestion, CoA is hydrolyzed to form pantothenic acid. A sodium-dependent system of transport allows the pantothenic acid to be absorbed. Sodium again plays a role in uptake of vitamin B5 into most cells. Much of the absorption may occur into the mitochondria. Approximately 95 percent of CoA in the body can be found in the mitochondria.[36] Once inside cells, pantothenic

FIGURE 5.5 *Vitamin B5 (pantothenic acid) molecule*

acid is used to synthesize CoA. Cysteine, Magnesium, and ATP are also required for CoA synthesis.

Functions

Pantothenic acid in its biologically active form CoA has numerous functions in the body. These functions include synthesis of several amino acids, steroid hormones, vitamin D, fatty acids, sphingolipids, and the porphyrins. Other functions include oxidation of fatty acids, acetylation of choline, and assisting in pathways involved with metabolism of proteins and carbohydrates. Vitamin B5 works with carnitine and CoQ10 in fatty acid transport and use.

Sources

Food sources include beef, pork, chicken, fish, organ meats, brewer's yeast, torula yeast, oatmeal, and hazelnuts. For additional food sources and amounts, see Table 5.7.

Therapeutic considerations

While frank deficiency of pantothenic acid is uncommon, therapeutic doses appear helpful in a number of conditions requiring enhanced energy production and cell repair.[37] Pantothenic acid supplementation has been used in ulcerative colitis, fatigue, rheumatoid arthritis, infection, adrenal dysfunction, allergies, elevated triglycerides, and problems with impaired detoxification. These uses take into consideration vitamin B5 activity in support of adrenal hormone production, red blood cell production, and energy production. The RDA has not been established for pantothenic acid, but 4 to 7 mg daily is thought to be adequate. Therapeutic doses range from 50 to 1000 mg, although much higher doses have been used without incident. Common therapeutic range is 50 to 250 mg daily.

Safety and toxicity

Pantothenic acid has not been associated with adverse effects. Intake of roughly 10 g of cal-

TABLE 5.7   *Pantothenic Acid Content of Certain Foods*
Milligrams (mg) per 3 1/2 oz

Food	mg	Food	mg
Yeast, brewer's	12.0	Lentils	1.4
Yeast, torula	11.0	Rye flour, whole	1.3
Liver, calf	8.0	Cashews	1.3
Liver, chicken	6.0	Salmon, flesh	1.3
Kidneys, beef	3.9	Camembert cheese	1.2
Peanuts	2.8	Garbanzo beans	1.2
Brains, all kinds	2.6	Wheat germ, toasted	1.2
Heart	2.6	Broccoli	1.2
Mushrooms	2.2	Hazelnuts	1.1
Soybean flour	2.0	Turkey, dark meat	1.1
Split peas	2.0	Brown rice	1.1
Tongue, beef	2.0	Whole wheat flour	1.1
Perch	1.9	Sardines	1.1
Blue cheese	1.8	Peppers, red chili	1.1
Pecans	1.7	Avocados	1.1
Soybeans	1.7	Veal, lean	1.1
Eggs	1.6	Black-eyed peas, dry	1.0
Lobster	1.5	Wild rice	1.0
Oatmeal, dry	1.5	Cauliflower	1.0
Buckwheat flour	1.4	Chicken, dark meat	1.0
Sunflower seeds	1.4	Kale	1.0

cium pantothenate daily for up to six weeks has been utilized without consequence.[38]

Functional medicine considerations

Since it is rare to find vitamin B5 deficiencies, and since B5 is rarely toxic, a functional medicine approach considers possible "sub-clinical" manifestations of B5 insufficiency. Fatigue that may be unexplained by other causes may be addressed with B5 supplementation. Any situation in which low energy production or reduced production of red blood cells or steroid hormones is evident or suspected may warrant B5 supplementation.

Vitamin B6 (Pyridoxine)

Structure

Three primary forms of this nitrogen-containing compound exist: pyridoxine (PN), pyridoxal (PL), and pyridoxamine (PM). The active coenzyme forms of vitamin B6 are pyridoxamine 5' phosphate (PMP) and pyridoxal 5' phosphate (PLP).[39] The structure is shown in Figure 5.6.

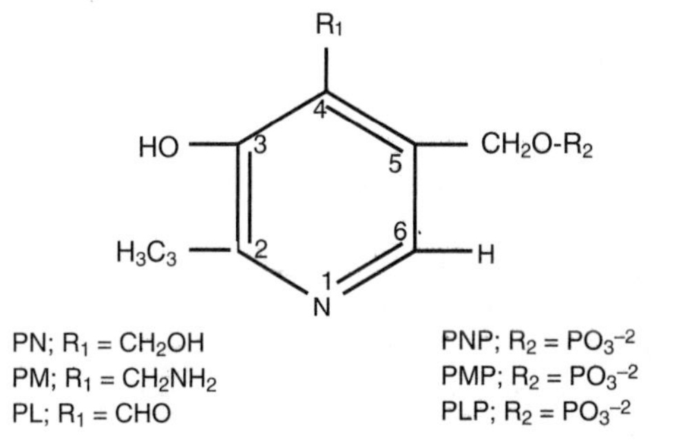

PN; $R_1 = CH_2OH$ PNP; $R_2 = PO_3^{-2}$
PM; $R_1 = CH_2NH_2$ PMP; $R_2 = PO_3^{-2}$
PL; $R_1 = CHO$ PLP; $R_2 = PO_3^{-2}$

FIGURE 5.6 *Vitamin B6 (pyridoxine) molecule*

Absorption

Vitamin B6 is absorbed passively, primarily in the jejunum. Once absorbed, the vitamin is transported in plasma and red blood cells. Much of vitamin B6 from food is converted to PLP the liver, a process that requires zinc, ATP, and FMN. Due to liver regulation of PLP production, possible damage from this highly reactive compound is kept to a minimum.[40]

Functions

This nutrient is involved in roughly 100 enzymatic reactions.[41] Although vitamin B6 is involved in numerous reactions, aminotransfer and decarboxylation are among the most prominent. PLP is considered the active form of vitamin B6. The function of B6 is closely tied to riboflavin status and availability. Approximately 80 to 90 percent of the total body pool of pyridoxine is in muscle.[42]

Vitamin B6 is also involved in the removal of sulfur groups from amino acids, helping to transfer amine groups from one amino acid to another, and participating with folic acid in methylation of choline, serine, and methionine. This latter methylation process is important in ensuring that levels of homocysteine, the precursor to methionine, do not increase beyond normal. Deficiencies in vitamin B6, folic acid, and vitamin B12 will cause homocysteine levels to rise and, in susceptible individuals, increase the risk of atherosclerotic heart disease.

The role of vitamin B6 in decarboxylation reactions makes it important in the conversion of tryptophan to serotonin. Conversion of tryptophan to niacin is also B6-dependent.

PLP plays a role in the production of glucose through gluconeogenesis, and it has been shown to modulate steroid hormone activity by binding to steroid receptors. It may also attach to the DNA receptor for these endocrine messengers and alter the action of the hormone.[43]

Sources

Pyridoxine is the most stable of the vitamers and is almost exclusively found in plant foods, including bananas, walnuts, navy beans, sunflower seeds, and wheat germ. Other vitamers, such as PLP, are found in beef, salmon, and chicken (white meat). For additional sources and amounts, see Table 5.8.

Therapeutic considerations

B6 has been used in the management of asthma, autism, carpal tunnel syndrome, irritability, eczema, EEG abnormalities and con-

TABLE 5.8 *Pyridoxine Content of Certain Foods*
Milligrams (mg) per 3 1/2 oz

Food	mg	Food	mg
Yeast, torula	3.00	Halibut, flesh	.43
Yeast, brewer's	2.50	Kidneys, beef	.43
Sunflower seeds	1.25	Avocados	.42
Wheat germ, toasted	1.15	Kidneys, veal	.41
Tuna, flesh	.90	Whole wheat flour	.34
Liver, beef	.84	Chestnuts, fresh	.33
Soybeans, dry	.81	Egg yolks	.30
Liver, chicken	.75	Kale	.30
Walnuts	.73	Rye flour	.30
Salmon, flesh	.70	Spinach	.28
Trout, flesh	.69	Turnip greens	.26
Liver, calf	.67	Peppers, sweet	.26
Mackerel, flesh	.66	Heart, beef	.25
Liver, pork	.65	Potatoes	.25
Soybean flour	.63	Prunes	.24
Lentils, dry	.60	Raisins	.24
Lima beans, dry	.58	Sardines	.24
Buckwheat flour	.58	Brussels sprouts	.23
Black-eyed peas, dry	.56	Elderberries	.23
Navy beans, dry	.56	Perch, flesh	.23
Brown rice	.55	Cod, flesh	.22
Hazelnuts	.54	Barley	.22
Garbanzos, dry	.54	Cheese, camembert	.22
Pinto beans, dry	.53	Sweet potatoes	.22
Bananas	.51	Cauliflower	.21
Pork, lean	.45	Popcorn, popped	.20
Albacore, flesh	.44	Red cabbage	.20
		Leeks	.20

vulsions, depression, postpartum depression, premenstrual syndrome, atherosclerosis, immunosuppression, diabetes, renal calculi, osteoporosis, and nausea of pregnancy. Therapeutic range for vitamin B6 is considered to be 30 to 500 mg/day. Doses of 250 to 500 mg on a long-term basis may be excessive, and liver enzymes should be monitored.

Safety and toxicity

Levels greater than 2 g/day have been shown to induce neuropathy or sensory neuropathy.[44] Pyridoxal is considered two to five times more toxic than pyridoxamine. Doses of greater than 150 mg may suppress lactation. High doses of PLP have been shown to inhibit sulfotransferases, enzymes that catalyze the transfer of a sulfate group to combine with another molecule.[45] This process is important to detoxification. The same enzymatic step is B6-dependent, so adequacy of B6 must be assured, while avoiding excess. Drugs such as isoniazid and dopamine may interfere with vitamin B6. Food additives such as FD and C yellow #5 may interfere with B6.

Riboflavin and magnesium are required for the conversion of pyridoxine to PLP. Concurrent use of these two nutrients may minimize the likelihood of adverse reactions to pyridoxine.

Functional medicine considerations

Amino acid abnormalities are found in many clinical conditions. Because of the role of pyridoxine in aminotransfer reactions, vitamin B6 status should be considered whenever amino acid abnormalities are encountered. A patient may exhibit signs of frank B6 deficiency including cheilosis, glossitis, fatigue, sleepiness, and stomatitis. In the absence of these symptoms, situations in which vitamin B6 insufficiency should be considered include mood disorders, nervous system dysfunction, pregnancy, the use of oral contraceptives or amphetamines, and cigarette smoking.[46,47]

Vitamin B6 is involved in so many enzymatic reactions in the body and is vital to the production and modulation of so many compounds, that it is necessary to consider a patient's B6 status whenever nutritional imbalances are suspected in the history and physical findings of the patient. This vitamin offers one of the best opportunities to use the detective work necessary to connect seemingly unrelated patterns and findings in the patient's story. It thus lends itself as a model for the weblike approach so critical to the practice of functional medicine.

Vitamin B12 (Cobalamin)

Structure

The terms cobalamin and vitamin B12 are generic references describing the vitamin B12 molecule without the cyanide. The term vitamin B12 is used by chemists to refer to cyanocobalamin. In clinical nutrition and pharmacology the term vitamin B12 usually includes all cobamides active in humans. Coenzyme activity is carried out by methylcobalamin and 5'-deoxyadenoxyl cobalamin (coenzyme B12).[48] The structure is shown in Figure 5.7.

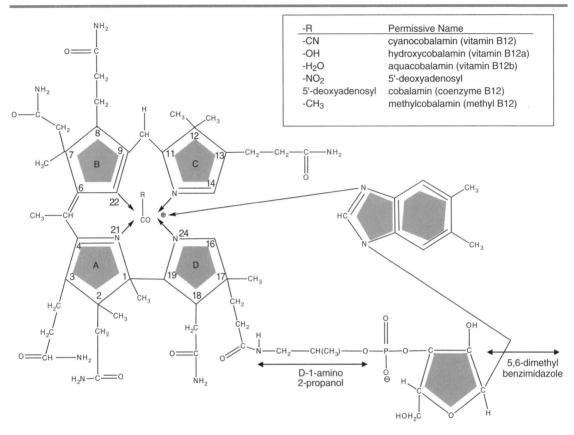

-R	Permissive Name
-CN	cyanocobalamin (vitamin B12)
-OH	hydroxycobalamin (vitamin B12a)
-H2O	aquacobalamin (vitamin B12b)
-NO2	5'-deoxyadenosyl
5'-deoxyadenosyl	cobalamin (coenzyme B12)
-CH3	methylcobalamin (methyl B12)

FIGURE 5.7 *Vitamin B12 (cobalamin) molecule*

Absorption

Vitamin B12 is synthesized by bacteria and exists in all animal foods. It is freed through the process of proteolysis in the stomach. The stomach secretes intrinsic factor (IF), which is necessary for the absorption of B12 in the ileum. Calcium is also needed for this process.[49]

Functions

Vitamin B12 is used by all DNA-synthesizing cells to facilitate the cyclic metabolism of folic acid. Its primary role is as a methyl group donor. For this reason, vitamin B12 is critical to the hemopoietic system. A megaloblastic anemia can occur if vitamin B12 is deficient or IF is deficient. In the latter circumstance, the condition is known as "pernicious anemia."

Vitamin B12 also plays a vital role in nervous system function. For example, glial cells have a relatively small B12 pool. When B12 delivery decreases, they quickly become deficient. This may lead to homocysteine accumulation with neurotoxic consequences.[50] In addition, methionine is needed for the synthesis of choline, a lack of which could lead to impaired fatty acid synthesis and nervous system dysfunction. The role of vitamin B12 in the production of some neurotransmitters may also be evidenced by mood imbalance in susceptible individuals.[51]

Sources

Cyanocobalamin, hydroxocobalamin, adenosylcobalamin, and methylcobalamin are the forms available for supplementation. Methylcobalamin is the form that adds a methyl group to homocysteine, converting it to methionine. Cyanocobalamin is the most common oral

form in use, but it must be converted to an active form. Methylcobalamin is the main active oral form available in the United States.

As stated earlier, vitamin B12 is a product of bacterial metabolism. The best food sources of cobalamins are animal products such as beef liver, beef, poultry, fish, and eggs. These foods contain primarily adenosylcobalamin and hydroxocobalamin. Cow's milk and cow's milk products contain less vitamin B12, and it occurs primarily as hydroxocobalamin and methylcobalamin.[52] For additional sources and amounts, see Table 5.9.

Plants do not contain bioactive forms of B12 unless they are contaminated by microorganisms. Vegetarians commonly attempt to obtain vitamin B12 from sea vegetables such

TABLE 5.9 *Cobalamin Content of Certain Foods*
Micrograms (mcg) per 3 1/2 oz

Liver, lamb	104.0	Eggs	2.0
Clams	98.0	Whey, dried	2.0
Liver, beef	80.0	Beef, lean	1.8
Kidneys, lamb	63.0	Edam cheese	1.8
Liver, calf	60.0	Swiss cheese	1.8
Kidneys, beef	31.0	Brie cheese	1.6
Liver, chicken	25.0	Gruyere cheese	1.6
Oysters	18.0	Blue cheese	1.4
Sardines	17.0	Haddock, flesh	1.3
Heart, beef	11.0	Flounder, flesh	1.2
Egg yolks	6.0	Scallops	1.2
Heart, lamb	5.2	Cheddar cheese	1.0
Trout	5.0	Cottage cheese	1.0
Brains, all kinds	4.0	Mozzarella cheese	1.0
Salmon, flesh	4.0	Halibut	1.0
Tuna, flesh	3.0	Perch, fillets	1.0
Lamb	2.1	Swordfish, flesh	1.0
Sweetbreads (thymus)	2.1		

as wakame or nori. However, these and other related species contain vitamin B12 analogues that do not appear to be metabolically active in humans.

Therapeutic considerations

Vitamin B12 may help manage anemia, asthma, fatigue, hepatitis, dementia, epilepsy, depression, psychosis, irritability, ataxia, numbness, tingling, neuropathy, AIDS, multiple sclerosis, tinnitus, and infertility. Supplemental B12 is commonly given in 1000 to 5000 mcg doses. Injectable forms should be preservative-free if chemical sensitivity is suspected. Oral forms are widely used in Sweden, but less commonly used in the United States. A lack of IF, produced by the parietal cells of the stomach, may be the underlying reason for B12 deficiency in circumstances in which dietary intake appears adequate. If known digestive disturbance exists supplementation with IF or injectable forms should be considered.

Safety and toxicity

Vitamin B12 is extremely safe. No toxicity from high doses of vitamin B12 has ever been reported.[53]

Functional medicine considerations

Patient history should include identifying signs and symptoms of neurological dysfunction, including peripheral neuropathy (numbness, tingling, and neuritis) as well as disorders of mood. If the patient history includes signs and symptoms of anemia, a complete blood count (CBC) should determine whether or not a megaloblastic anemia exists. In cases in which dietary intake appears sufficient, a Schilling test (to test for IF availability) should be considered to determine the exact cause of the B12 deficiency. Individuals who have had vegan dietary habits for a number of years should always be asked about vitamin B12 supplementation. Vitamin B12 stores in the liver may mean that up to five years may pass before problems of B12 shortage are evident.

If the patient is elderly and is exhibiting signs and symptoms of impaired mental function, B12 insufficiency should be considered, as it is a common underlying cause of this problem in the elderly population.

If there is a concern about atherosclerosis, B12 status should be considered since it may help maintain lower plasma levels of homocysteine. In such cases, clinicians should also investigate the status of folic acid and vitamin B6. If the patient has been under a great deal of stress, insufficient vitamin B12 and other B vitamins should be considered if he or she presents with fatigue.

Folic Acid

Structure

Folate is a name given to a family of compounds that share the common molecular architecture called pteroylglutamate. Other names used are folic acid and folacin. The molecule known as 5-methyl-tetrahydropteroylglutamate donates a methyl group to homocysteine to form methionine (Figure 5.8). This methyl-tetrahydrofolate is the most abundant folate in the circulation and it functions with vitamin B12 to transfer a

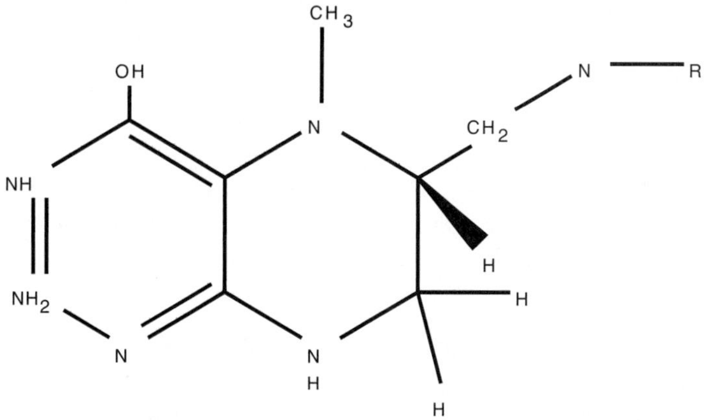

FIGURE 5.8 *Folic acid molecule (5-methyl-tetrahydropteroylglutamate)*

methyl group to homocysteine to produce methionine.[54] The structure is shown in Figure 5.8.

Absorption

Folate is present in the diet primarily as polyglutamate folate. Dietary polyglutamate folate requires enzymatic deconjugation before it can be absorbed. Enzymes responsible for this activity are the pteroylpolyglutamate hydrolases. This enzymatic activity occurs primarily at the brush border of the jejunum. Folate-binding proteins associated with the mucosal membrane sequester the folates, and they are then transported across the membrane by a carrier-mediated process. When the concentration of folate is high in the lumen, a diffusion-mediated transport takes over.[55]

Functions

These molecules primarily serve as one-carbon (or methyl) donors. They may also accept one-carbon groups. Methylation of brain myelin is one crucial reaction in which the folate methyl group transfer is needed. Folate metabolism has been summarized as comprising two crucial groups of reactions that compete in the cell for available folates. These are reactions that lead to the de novo synthesis of methionine and to the synthesis of nucleic acids (purines and thymidylate).

Folic acid is central to all rapidly dividing cells, including blood cells, cells of the gastrointestinal tract, and germinal cells. Synthesis of cysteine from methionine is also folate-dependent. Since formation of the tripeptide glutathione depends upon the presence of adequate cysteine, glutathione formation is indirectly dependent upon adequate folate.

Sources

Folic acid and folicinic acid (5-methyltetrahydrofolate) are supplemental forms. Folic acid derives its name from the Latin folium, which means foliage, an appropriate connection since folic acid is widespread in green leafy plants. It is also high in brewer's yeast, legumes, and rice germ. Diets high in animal protein, except liver, provide little in the way of folate. Folic acid is extremely heat labile and is easily destroyed in cooking. For additional sources and amounts, see Table 5.10.

Therapeutic considerations

Folate has been shown to prevent neural tube defects ranging from spina bifida to anen-cephaly. To achieve this protective effect, folate must be given either preconceptually or within the first weeks of pregnancy.[56] Folic acid abnormalities have also been found in cervical dysplasia, as evidenced by abnormalities in Pap smear results. Supplementation with folate has been shown to normalize abnormal cervical cells.[57]

Folate insufficiency has also been associated with mood disorders such as depression, particularly in the elderly. Folate assessment and therapy should be considered in patients with mood disorders.[58] Frank folic acid defi-

TABLE 5.10   *Folic Acid Content of Certain Foods*
Micrograms (mcg) per 3 1/2 oz

Brewer's yeast	2022	Peanuts, roasted	56
Black-eyed peas	440	Peanut butter	56
Rice germ	430	Broccoli	53
Soy flour	425	Barley	50
Wheat germ	305	Split peas	50
Liver, beef	295	Whole wheat cereal	49
Liver, lamb	275	Brussels sprouts	49
Soy beans	225	Almonds	45
Liver, pork	220	Whole wheat flour	38
Bran	195	Oatmeal	33
Kidney beans	180	Cabbage	32
Mung beans	145	Dried figs	32
Lima beans	130	Avocado	30
Navy beans	125	Green beans	28
Garbanzo beans	125	Corn	28
Asparagus	110	Coconut, fresh	28
Lentils	105	Pecans	27
Walnuts	77	Mushrooms	25
Spinach, fresh	75	Dates	25
Kale	70	Blackberries	14
Filbert nuts	65	Ground beef	7
Beet & mustard greens	60	Orange	5
Textured vegetable protein	57		

ciency presents as macrocytic anemia. In the absence of an assessment of the patient's vitamin B12 status, folic acid supplementation for macrocytic anemia should always be accompanied by B12.

Folic acid is clinically useful in managing homocysteinemia. Accumulation of homocysteine (HCys metabolism shown in Figure 5.9) may contribute to vascular damage. Homocysteinemia may exist in individuals who are homozygous or heterozygous for this trait. Supplementation may help reduce homocysteine levels.

Doses of folate ranging from 400 mcg to 10 mg have been used clinically. A more common therapeutic range is 400 to 1000 mcg per day.

Safety and toxicity

Supplemental doses have been recommended not to exceed 400 mcg/day, because folic acid

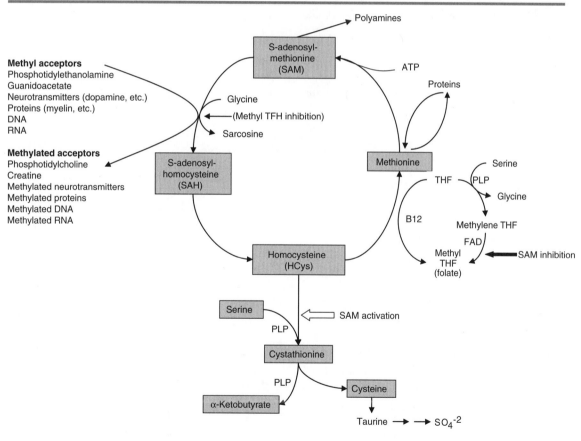

FIGURE 5.9 *Homocysteine metabolism in animals*

supplementation may mask the symptoms of B12 deficiency. Thus, if folate is provided and B12 deficiency is undetected, neurological damage (e.g., to myelin) may continue to progress. When this relationship is taken into consideration, levels of folate beyond 400 mcg daily (e.g., 400 to 1000 mcg) may be used. As stated, folate supplementation should probably be accompanied by simultaneous B12 supplementation to avoid this adverse consequence.

Groff et al. have reviewed the question of folate toxicity at high doses and note that doses of 400 mg/day for five months, 10 mg/day for four months, and 10 mg/day for five years have been used in adults with no adverse effects. However, high doses (up to 15 mg/day) may incite hypersensitivity responses in some individuals. Symptoms include insomnia, irritability, and gastrointestinal problems.[59] Care should also be taken not to have folate intake greater than 12 mg/day if certain anticonvulsants (such as phenytoin) are being taken.

Functional medicine considerations

Dietary history should explore intake of folic acid-rich foods. If intake is low, the patient's complaints should be considered in light of potential folic acid deficiency or insufficiency. Signs and symptoms of anemia may be present (fatigue, shortness of breath, pale skin and mucosa). Gastrointestinal difficulties such as diarrhea or decreased appetite may suggest folic acid insufficiency if other causes are ruled out. Difficulties in the genital tract (especially cervical cellular changes) should also heighten suspicion of folate insufficiency.[60]

Patient intake of anticonvulsants should also direct the investigation into a possible folate insufficiency, as these drugs interfere with folate metabolism.[61] The intimate relationship between folic acid and vitamin B12 should remain in the clinician's mind as patient assessment progresses. If heart disease is suspected, an assessment of homocysteine levels may justify folate supplementation.

Biotin

Structure

Biotin has a cyclic structure. While eight isomers exist, only one is enzymatically active. This structure is known as biotin or D-biotin.[62] The biotin molecule is shown in Figure 5.10.

Absorption

Biotin is absorbed in the intestines by way of a specific transporter molecule. The process is not completely understood, but it is known that another mediator carries biotin from enterocytes. This mechanism is impaired by

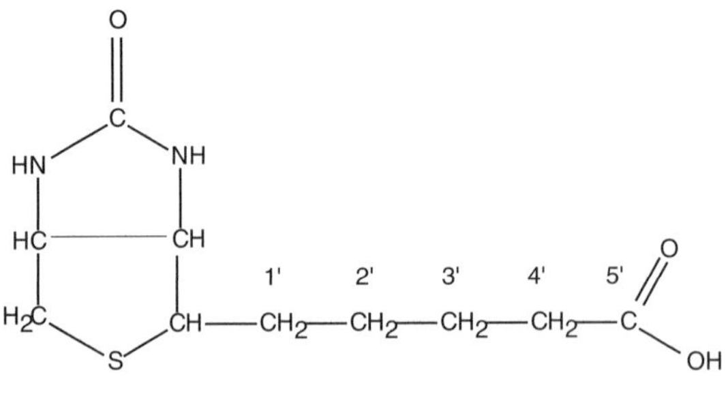

FIGURE 5.10 *Biotin molecule*

chronic alcohol intake.[63] Raw egg whites contain avidin (a glycoprotein that may irreversibly bind biotin), which may prevent its absorption. However, absorption may be enhanced by the effects of a vegetarian diet on gut flora.[64]

Functions

Biotin is a B vitamin that receives little attention in nutrition texts. It is widely available in foods, but its bioavailability is highly variable (100 percent from corn, 0 percent from wheat).[65] Biotin is crucial to several enzyme systems involved in carboxylation. Examples include pyruvate carboxylase, involved in energy metabolism, and acetyl CoA carboxylase, which commits acetate units in fatty acid synthesis.

Biotin deficiency has been observed to lead to accumulation of odd-numbered fatty acids (15:0, 17:0, etc.) in liver, red cells, and plasma.[66] Biotin deficiency may also lead to accumulation of lactic acid in the central nervous system due to inefficient pyruvate carboxylase activity.[67] Symptoms include hypotonia, seizures, and ataxia. Biotin is also involved in the promotion of healthy hair and nails, a benefit that may come from its ability to positively affect the metabolism of oils in the integumentary system.[68] Biotin is also involved in creating the active form of folacin.[69]

Sources

Biotin is widely distributed in foods like brewer's yeast, liver, soybean, egg yolk, rice polish, peanuts, and walnuts (Table 5.11).

Therapeutic considerations

Classic biotin deficiency is characterized by alopecia, scaly dermatitis, nausea, depression,

TABLE 5.11 *Biotin Content of Certain Foods*
Micrograms (mcg) per 3 1/2 oz

Food	mcg	Food	mcg
Brewer's yeast	200	Oatmeal	24
Liver, lamb	127	Sardines, canned	24
Liver, pork	100	Whole egg	22
Liver, beef	96	Black-eyed peas	18
Soy flour	70	Split peas	18
Soybeans	61	Almonds	18
Rice bran	60	Cauliflower	17
Rice germ	58	Mushrooms	16
Rice polishings	57	Whole wheat cereal	16
Egg yolk	52	Salmon, canned	15
Peanut butter	39	Textured vegetable protein	15
Walnuts	37	Bran	14
Peanuts, roasted	34	Lentils	13
Barley	31	Brown rice	12
Pecans	27		

hallucinations, muscle pain, and localized paresthesia.[70] In infants, cradle cap appears to be a common manifestation of biotin insufficiency. This may be due, in part, to the influence of biotin on fatty acid biosynthesis. Seborrheic dermatitis (the adult version of cradle cap) usually requires the supplementation of a B-vitamin complex to improve fatty acid metabolism. Biotin alone may not be sufficient.[71] Normal intestinal bacteria are largely responsible for biotin. Supplemental range for biotin is from 300 to 600 mcg, though doses up to 3000 mcg are commonly used.

Safety and toxicity

Biotin has been used at doses of 10 mg daily for over six months with no toxicity. Excess biotin is readily excreted in urine.

Functional medicine considerations

In addition to ascertaining whether the patient's diet has enough biotin (deficiencies are actually rare), the clinician should ask the patient about intake of raw egg white. As noted above, interference with the absorption of biotin can occur under the influence of raw egg whites. Excessive animal products in the diet and exclusion of vegetables and fruit may interfere with gut flora and its role in biotin synthesis.

Dandruff or scaly, yellow skin lesions should raise suspicion of a biotin insufficiency. The patient may also have brittle nails. There may also be significant hair loss with a biotin insufficiency. Complaints of nausea, reduced appetite, or depression should also prompt consideration of biotin status.

The role of biotin in energy metabolism should also be considered when the patient presents with fatigue or muscle weakness. In addition, glucose metabolism problems for which insulin resistance is suspected may warrant biotin supplementation because of its ability to increase both insulin sensitivity and glucokinase activity.[72]

Vitamin C (Ascorbate)

Structure

Ascorbate exists in three primary forms: ascorbic acid, semidehydroascorbate, and dehydroascorbate. Ascorbic acid is the reduced form; it progresses to dehydroascorbate as it gives up its electrons. Molecular structure of ascorbic acid is shown in Figure 5.11.

Absorption

Unlike most other mammals, humans are unable to synthesize vitamin C from glucose because of their lack of one vital enzyme. Thus, humans must ingest vitamin C, which can be absorbed by an active transporter in the intestines.

Functions

Since vitamin C loses an electron easily, it serves as a good electron donor. Therefore, it reduces several oxidizing agents in the body. Of particular importance is its antioxidant function with lipids. Low density lipoproteins (LDLs) are also protected from free radical damage by this vitamin.[73] Vitamin C acts as a substrate or cosubstrate for eight different enzymes that affect collagen synthesis,

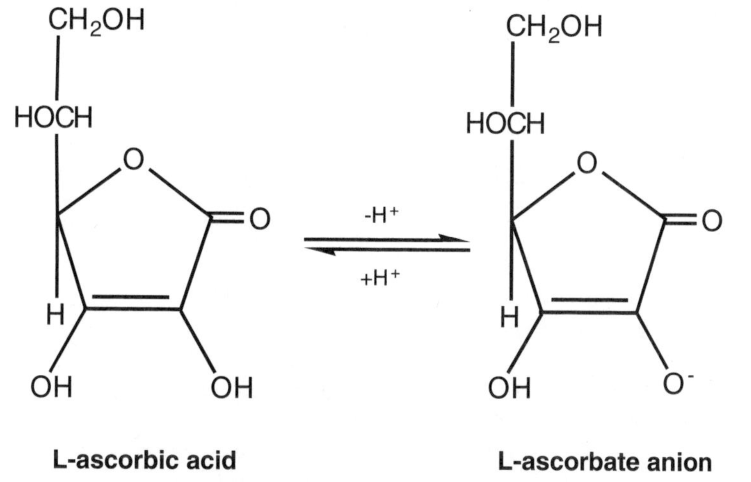

FIGURE 5.11 *Ascorbic acid molecule*

carnitine synthesis, catecholamine synthesis, peptide amidation, and tyrosine metabolism.

In collagen synthesis, vitamin C helps form hydroxyproline from proline. Thus, vitamin C helps to form strong connective tissue, repair wounds, improve gum health, and reduce bruising.[74]

As an antioxidant, ascorbate reduces hydroxyl radical, superoxide, hypochlorite, and other radical species.[75] Ascorbic acid is able to regenerate vitamin E by donating a hydrogen ion to the oxidized tocopheroxyl radical.

Sources

Vitamin C is often derived from corn-based material, which may present problems for sensitive patients. Additional sources include potato, citrus, Acerola cherry, and sago palm. Salts of ascorbic acid (sodium, magnesium, potassium, and calcium) are commonly used in supplementation.

Food sources of vitamin C include Acerola cherries, red chili peppers, green peppers, guavas, papaya, oranges, cantaloupe, broccoli, cauliflower, Brussels sprouts, grapefruit, and strawberries. Vitamin C content declines rapidly in foods once they've been picked or sliced. Thus, fresh foods eaten immediately after harvest are the richest sources. For additional sources and amounts, see Table 5.12.

Therapeutic considerations

Scurvy is the classic deficiency disease associated with vitamin C. This disease occurs when the total body pool of vitamin C falls to about 300 mg. Scurvy is rare in the United States. Fatigue is one of the first deficiency signs of vitamin C deficiency. Other signs

TABLE 5.12   *Ascorbic Acid Content of Certain Foods*
Milligrams (mg) per 3 1/2 oz

Acerola	1300	Liver, calf	36
Peppers, red chili	369	Turnips	36
Guavas	242	Mangoes	35
Peppers, red sweet	204	Asparagus	33
Kale leaves	186	Cantaloupes	33
Parsley	172	Swiss chard	32
Collard leaves	152	Green onions	32
Turnip greens	139	Liver, beef	31
Peppers, green sweet	128	Okra	31
Broccoli	113	Tangerines	31
Brussels sprouts	102	New Zealand spinach	30
Mustard greens	97	Oysters	30
Watercress	79	Lima beans, young	29
Cauliflower	78	Black-eyed peas	29
Persimmons	66	Soybeans	29
Cabbage, red	61	Green peas	27
Strawberries	59	Radishes	26
Papayas	56	Raspberries	25
Spinach	51	Chinese cabbage	25
Oranges & juice	50	Yellow summer squash	25
Cabbage	47	Loganberries	24
Lemon juice	46	Honeydew melon	23
Grapefruit & juice	38	Tomatoes	23
Elderberries	36		

associated with vitamin C insufficiency include bleeding gums, sublingual hemorrhages, impaired wound healing, joint pain, loose teeth, easy bruising, frequent infections, and cardiovascular disease.

Vitamin C is helpful in supporting certain activities of the immune system including enhancement of white blood cell activity and the production of immune-mediating chemicals. When the body is under a great deal of stress, both emotional and environmental, vitamin C may be excessively excreted, and greater intake may be necessary to maintain immune function and the other vitamin C functions.[76]

Because vitamin C can regenerate vitamin E, it is important to consider its inclusion in any therapeutic antioxidant combination.

Levin et al. have suggested that adults receive at least 200 mg/day of vitamin C and that an "upper safe" recommendation be set at 1000 mg/day.[77] However, many clinicians have observed benefits using doses ranging from 1000 to 20,000 mg daily. Rea reports on the use of large doses of vitamin C for several months with notable clinical benefit.[78]

Safety and toxicity

Vitamin C is considered extremely safe. Suggested problems of rebound scurvy, destruction of vitamin B12, and other complications have not been supported by data. However, individuals with glucose-6-phosphate dehydrogenase deficiency have been shown to experience red cell hemolysis upon intravenous administration of large doses of vitamin C.[79] Individuals who are homozygous for hemochromatosis may experience increased iron uptake with vitamin C ingestion. It is not known whether those who are heterozygous experience problematic increased iron uptake. While concerns have been raised over the a bility of vitamin C to cause renal stones, a review by The New York Academy of Sciences showed this was not a problem.[80] A more recent review of 20,000 patients found no cases of stones associated with vitamin C use.[81]

Functional medicine considerations

Vitamin C insufficiency should be suspected when the patient is fatigued, especially if ecchymoses or petechiae accompany the fatigue. After ruling out other possible causes of these symptoms, including blood pathologies, vitamin C support should be considered.

Other possible symptoms of vitamin C insufficiency include gingivitis, poor wound healing, a history of recurrent infections and colds, amino acid imbalances, and follicular hyperkeratosis, especially on the buttocks and lower extremities.[82]

THE FAT-SOLUBLE VITAMINS

Vitamin E

Structure

Vitamin E is a general designation given to a family of compounds consisting of eight different vitamers. Four of these compounds, known as tocopherols, consist of a chromane ring and a saturated side chain. The natural tocopherols are designated *alpha, beta, gamma,* and *delta.* Four other vitamers are known as tocotrienols. These are structurally similar, with the exception being unsaturated side chains. They too are labeled *alpha, beta, gamma,* and *delta* (Figure 5.12).

Alpha tocopherol is considered the most bioactive. *Beta* tocopherol possesses 25 to 50 percent bioactivity, *gamma* tocopherol has 10 to 35 percent bioactivity, and *alpha* tocotrienol has roughly 30 percent.[83] The antioxidant activity of the vitamers is in the following order of greatest to least: [84]

> *alpha* tocopherol
> *beta* tocopherol
> *alpha* tocotrienol
> *gamma* tocopherol
> *delta* tocopherol

Absorption

Vitamin E found in the diet is primarily *alpha* and *gamma* tocopherols. These compounds must be acted on by bile acids from the liver. Absorption then occurs in cells of the intestinal mucosa by passive diffusion or in micelles. Like dietary fats, vitamin E is incorporated into chylomicrons (primarily hepatocytes) for

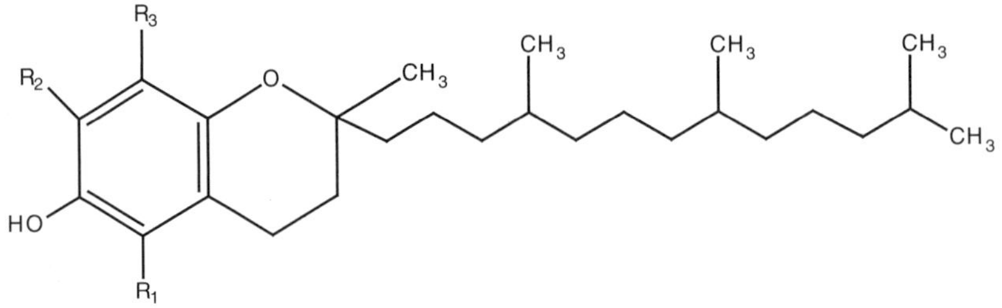

Compound	R_1	R_2	R_3
α-tocopherol	CH_3	CH	CH_3
β-tocopherol	CH_3	H	CH_3
γ-tocopherol	H	CH_3	CH_3
δ-tocopherol	H	H	CH_3

FIGURE 5.12   *Vitamin E molecules (tocopherols)*

transport. The hepatocytes are responsible for vitamin E incorporation into very-low-density lipoproteins, which transport it to other tissue.[85] Vitamin E is stored in adipose tissue, but its primary site is the lipid membrane of cells.

Functions

The primary function of vitamin E is to prevent peroxidation of unsaturated fatty acids that form the structural component of phospholipid membranes. Cells with a high content of polyunsaturated fatty acids have a high vitamin E requirement and are particularly susceptible to oxidative damage. Those with high polyunsaturate content include erythrocytes, neurons, and lung epithelium. These are all tissues with high oxygen expo-

sure. Phagocytic cells must also possess rich stores of vitamin E to protect against auto-oxidation by the oxidants produced in the respiratory burst.

Vitamin E also plays a role in protecting vitamin A and increasing its storage.[86] It should be noted that vitamin C can regenerate the tocopheroxyl radical, restoring vitamin E to its normal antioxidant state. The ability of one antioxidant to regenerate another reflects the interdependence among antioxidant nutrients. Antioxidants, therefore, are best given in conjunction with others rather than individually.

Sources

Vitamin E is generally available as the d-isomers—d-*alpha* tocopherol, d-*alpha* tocopheryl acetate, or d-*alpha* tocopheryl succi-nate—which are considered natural forms of *alpha* tocopherol. Synthetic forms are desig-nated dl-. Thus, dl-*alpha* tocopherol contains a racemic mixture of the natural d-form and the synthetic l-form. D-forms are generally preferred in clinical practice, while natural vitamin E supplements ideally contain the other vitamers, including *gamma*, *beta*, and *delta* tocopherol. A mixture of the tocotri-enols is also desirable.

Vitamin E is contained in highest amounts in plant foods, especially the oils of seeds and nuts (Table 5.13). Wheat germ is an excellent source of vitamin E. Green leafy vegetables also contain vitamin E. Animal flesh is not a good source of vitamin E, as it is concentrated in the fatty portion of the ani-mal. Cooking or processing foods can sub-stantially lower vitamin E amounts. Vitamin E supplements are sometimes made from the byproducts of vegetable oil refining.[87]

Therapeutic considerations

Vitamin E has been employed in a variety of conditions in which antioxidant activity or lipid membrane repair is needed. Conditions include neuropathy, multiple sclerosis, Parkinson's dis-ease, tardive dyskinesia, immunosuppression, intermittent claudication, mitochondrial oxida-tive phosphorylation disorders, macular degen-eration, infertility, myopathy, epilepsy, diabetes, autoimmune disorders, liver disease, periodon-tal disease, Alzheimer's disease, and others.

Deficiencies in vitamin E are difficult to di-agnose, as the range of actions of this vitamin

TABLE 5.13 *Vitamin E Content of Certain Foods*
Milligrams (mg) per 100 grams (g)

Wheat germ oil	216.0	Bran	3.0
Sunflower seeds	90.0	Asparagus	2.9
Sunflower seed oil	88.0	Salmon	2.5
Safflower oil	72.0	Brown rice	2.5
Almonds	48.0	Rye, whole	2.3
Sesame oil	45.0	Rye bread, dark	2.2
Peanut oil	34.0	Pecans	1.9
Corn oil	29.0	Wheat germ	1.9
Wheat germ	22.0	Rye & wheat crackers	1.9
Peanuts	18.0	Whole wheat bread	1.4
Olive oil	18.0	Carrots	1.0
Soybean oil	14.0	Peas	.99
Peanuts, roasted	13.0	Walnuts	.92
Peanut butter	11.0	Bananas	.88
Butter	3.6	Eggs	.83
Spinach	3.2	Tomatoes	.72
Oatmeal	3.0	Lamb	.29

is quite diverse. For example, a patient may have a hemorrhage resulting from the loss of integrity of red blood cell membrane and depend upon vitamin E for protection from lipid peroxidation. Any physiologic processes that depend on the integrity of the cellular membrane may also be disrupted with an insufficient supply of vitamin E. Insufficient vitamin E may also result in DNA damage and decreased energy production from the mitochondria, a process that is particularly susceptible to oxidant damage. In a developing baby, the effects of a vitamin E deficiency on the nervous system may include reduced or absent deep tendon reflexes, impaired vibratory sensation, and other posterior column abnormalities.[88]

Vitamin E's role as an antioxidant has raised speculation about whether a higher risk for age-related disorders might be considered a vitamin E deficiency disease.[89]

Therapeutic range for vitamin E is 100 to 1,200 IU per day. Increased intake of polyunsaturated fatty acids necessitates an increase in vitamin E intake.

Safety and toxicity

Vitamin E is considered one of the safest vitamins. Some hypertensives may experience increased blood pressure with increasing vitamin E intake. Gradual increase in dose is recommended. Patients on anticoagulants should use vitamin E with caution as vitamin E may augment anticoagulant activity. The effect of long-term ingestion of synthetic (l-form) vitamin E is unknown.

Functional medicine considerations

If vitamin E availability is insufficient, the patient may present with a history of exposure to free-radical promoting agents. The history may also indicate difficulty digesting and absorbing fatty foods. If other symptoms of malabsorption are present (such as gluten-sensitive enteropathy), vitamin E insufficiency should be suspected as well. The patient may also complain of weakness or poor coordination.

In situations in which oxidative stress is suspected, antioxidant combinations, including vitamin E, should be considered in nutritional support. Oxidative stress can cause destruction of membrane lipids through formation of radicals (Figure 5.13). Susceptibility to infections, poor wound healing, and fatigue may all be signs of vitamin E insufficiency.

Vitamin A

Structure

Vitamin A is a fat-soluble nutrient generally identified as all-*trans* retinol (Figure 5.14). The vitamin A family includes the aldehydes retinal and retinoic acid. The carotenoids are another group of nutrients in the vitamin A family. Although carotenoids are widespread in nature, less than 10 percent have vitamin A activity. Of these, *beta*-carotene, *alpha*-carotene, and *gamma*-carotene have the highest activity.

Absorption

Preformed vitamin A exists in the retinyl form. Once proteolysis releases preformed

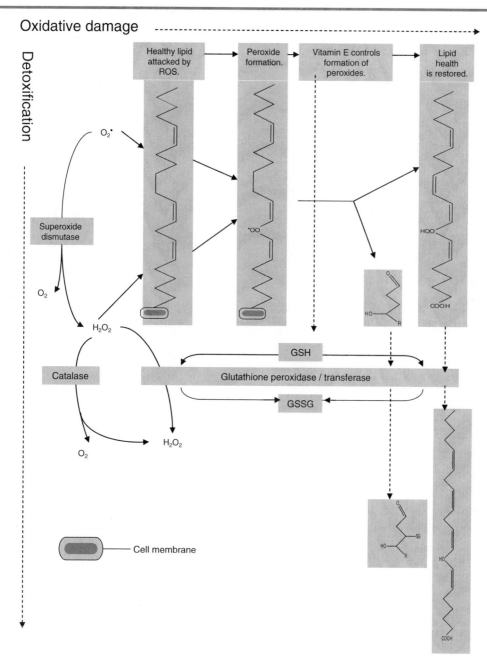

Oxidative damage

Detoxification

Healthy lipid attacked by ROS.

Peroxide formation.

Vitamin E controls formation of peroxides.

Lipid health is restored.

$O_2^{\bullet}$

Superoxide dismutase

O_2

H_2O_2

Catalase

O_2

H_2O_2

GSH

Glutathione peroxidase / transferase

GSSG

Cell membrane

FIGURE 5.13   *Role of Vitamin E in oxidative stress reactions*

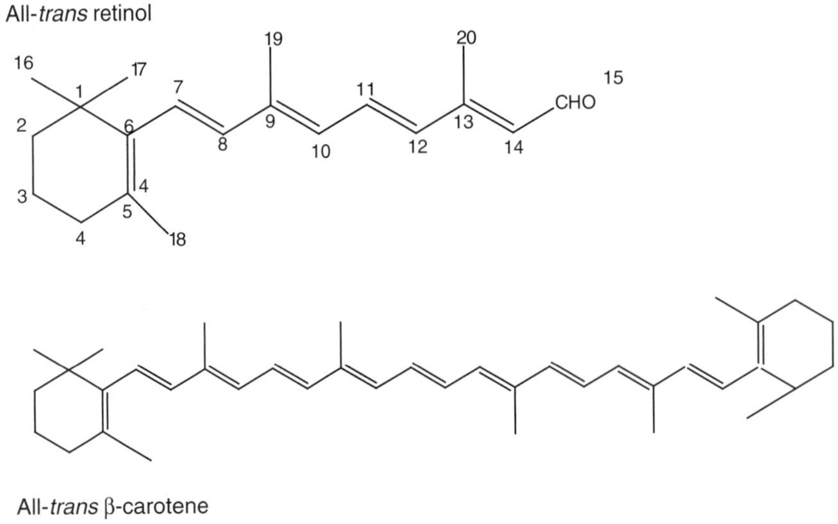

All-*trans* retinol

All-*trans* β-carotene

FIGURE 5.14   *Vitamin A (all-trans retinol) molecule*

vitamin A and carotenoids from food, they are micellized and absorbed in the intestines.[90] The carotenoids in the diet are much more dependent on the presence of fat in the meal than is preformed vitamin A (primarily from animal tissue).[91]

Provitamin carotenoids, including *beta*-carotene, undergo oxidative cleavage to produce, ultimately, all-*trans* retinal. Reduction and acylation of this molecule produces the retinyl ester. The retinyl ester is incorporated into chylomicrons for transport. Vitamin A is stored primarily in the liver. About 80 to 90 percent of vitamin A is absorbed from an oral dose, while 5 to 50 percent of *beta*-carotene is absorbed.[92,93]

Functions

The primary functions of vitamin A are related to vision, immune function, bone development, cellular differentiation, growth, and reproduction. Vitamin A is also required for detoxification of xenobiotics such as PCBs and dioxin. Epithelial tissue cannot be properly maintained without sufficient vitamin A. Thus all mucous membranes, the cornea of the eye, the skin, and all organs in which tissue turnover is great rely on vitamin A. If vitamin A status is not adequate, keratin may be secreted in these tissues, rendering them hard, dry, and unable to carry out normal functions. The result is a greater susceptibility to infection.[94]

Sources

The richest food sources of vitamin A are liver, egg yolks, whole milk, butter, and fish liver. Carotenes are found in dark-green leafy vegetables and yellow and orange vegetables, such as squash, yams, sweet potatoes, and carrots. For additional sources and amounts, see Table 5.14.

Therapeutic considerations

The therapeutic range is 4000 IU for adult females, 5000 IU for adult males. The designation IU (international unit) has been replaced with retinol equivalent. One microgram of retinol equals one retinol equivalent.

Signs and symptoms of vitamin A deficiency include night blindness, poor dark

TABLE 5.14 *Vitamin A Content of Certain Foods*
IU per 3 1/2 oz

Food	IU	Food	IU
Liver, lamb	50,500	Whitefish	2,260
Liver, beef	43,900	Green onions	2,000
Liver, calf	22,500	Romaine lettuce	1,900
Peppers, red chili	21,600	Papayas	1,750
Dandelion greens	14,000	Nectarines	1,650
Liver, chicken	12,100	Prunes	1,600
Carrots	11,000	Pumpkin	1,600
Apricots, dried	10,900	Swordfish	1,580
Collard greens	9,300	Cream, whipping	1,540
Kale	8,900	Peaches	1,330
Sweet potatoes	8,800	Acorn squash	1,200
Parsley	8,500	Eggs	1,180
Spinach	8,100	Chicken	1,080
Turnip greens	7,600	Cherries, sour red	1,000
Mustard greens	7,000	Butterhead lettuce	970
Swiss chard	6,500	Asparagus	900
Beet greens	6,500	Tomatoes, ripe	900
Chives	5,800	Peppers, green chili	770
Butternut squash	5,700	Kidneys	690
Watercress	4,900	Green peas	640
Mangoes	4,800	Elderberries	600
Peppers, sweet red	4,450	Watermelon	590
Hubbard squash	4,300	Rutabagas	580
Cantaloupe	3,400	Brussels sprouts	550
Butter	3,300	Okra	520
Endive	3,300	Yellow cornmeal	510
Apricots	2,700	Yellow squash	460
Broccoli spears	2,500		

adaptation, follicular hyperkeratosis, poor wound healing, dry eyes, and infection susceptibility. Vitamin A has been used successfully in the treatment of infections, such as measles in childhood. High doses (50,000 to 100,000 IU per day for one to two days) are used for a short period in instances such as these.[95,96]

Diabetics have a decreased ability to change carotene into retinol. Thus, low-grade deficiencies may develop within individuals with diabetes mellitus.[97] Other problems that may occur in vitamin A-deficient individuals include weight loss and anorexia, decreased steroid synthesis, and poor tooth and bone function. During an infection, vitamin A stores are soon depleted. If not replaced, the infection can worsen. Exposure to toxic chemicals requires increased vitamin A intake because of increased use in the function of xenobiotic detoxification.[98]

Vitamin A may also be useful in skin disorders related to hyperkeratosis, such as acne and psoriasis. The carotenes have shown some promise in the prevention of both cancer and cardiovascular disease, as well as in enhancement of immune function. An insufficient level of beta-carotene has also been linked with increased vaginal candidiasis.[99] Most carotenoids can serve as singlet oxygen quenchers and as antioxidants.[100]

Safety and toxicity
Vitamin A is well known for its potential for toxicity; however, only an estimated 200 cases of vitamin A toxicity are reported worldwide each year.[101] Because of teratogenic effects, vitamin A should not be used in doses above the RDA during pregnancy.

Patients with liver disease are susceptible to vitamin A toxicity and should be monitored when they are taking the vitamin. Oral contraceptives significantly elevate plasma vitamin A levels. In an individual with a healthy liver, doses should be considered potentially toxic if they exceed 50,000 IU a day for several years.

Emerging evidence from epidemiological studies suggests a diet high in vitamin A [greater than 3000 IU vitamin A (retinol/retinal) per day] over a sustained period of time may increase bone fracture rate.[102] In this analysis, however, beta-carotene intake was not associated with increased fracture risk.

Symptoms of vitamin A toxicity include weight loss, appetite loss, dry shedding skin, hair loss, fatigue, bone pain, headache, irritability, increased intracranial pressure (bulging fontanels in infants), and joint pain. Most signs of toxicity subside once vitamin A intake is discontinued.

Functional medicine considerations
In situations in which vitamin A is insufficient, the patient's history may indicate fatigue, poor fat absorption and metabolism, symptoms of steroid hormone dysfunction, or poor night vision. There may be a history of recurrent infections or the inability to fight off colds.

In the presence of possible vitamin A toxicity (headache, fatigue, emotional lability, and dry skin), a patient should be asked about all supplements that may contain vitamin A, and his or her history of taking the supplement. Patient history should be explored carefully for exposure to environmental toxins in the home, workplace, or elsewhere. A history or current evidence of liver pathology may warrant investigation into vitamin A intolerance or insufficiency. A woman who presents with a history of recurrent yeast vaginitis should be questioned about dietary sources of vitamin A and about her fat digestion. On examination, the teeth may be crooked, and the mouth may be dry. There may be dry patches on the conjunctivae. The skin may show hyperkeratosis.

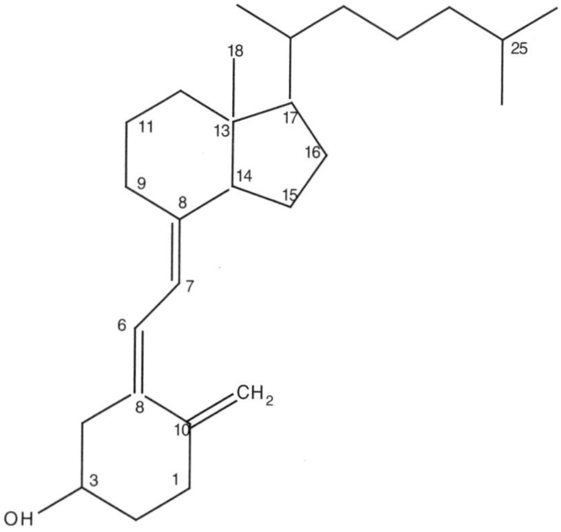

FIGURE 5.15 *Vitamin D3 molecule*

Vitamin D

Structure

Vitamin D, also known as calciferol, is a secosteroid. Its designation as vitamin D was based on its role as a dietary factor that aided in the cure of rickets. Currently, it is thought that vitamin D is more hormone-like in its action and not a true vitamin. The active form is known as calcitriol or 1,25 dihydroxycholecalciferol. Vitamin D remains stable with heat and oxidation.[103] The structure is shown in Figure 5.15.

Absorption

Vitamin D is not required in the diet if there is sufficient sunlight to allow the production of vitamin D from provitamin D molecules in the skin. This process may be hampered by skin pigments and keratin or other substances that block UV light.[104] The molecule produced by this photochemical reaction is converted in the liver to 25, hydroxycholecalciferol (25-(OH)D$_3$). The kidney then converts 25-(OH)D$_3$ to 1,25 dihydroxycholecalciferol (1,25-(OH)$_2$D$_3$), the active form of vitamin D. Boron may be important in converting 25-(OH)D$_3$ to 1,25-(OH)$_2$D$_3$. Parathyroid hormone will stimulate synthesis of 1,25-(OH)$_2$D3 in kidneys when blood calcium levels are low.[105] Vitamin D metabolism is depicted in Figure 5.16.

Functions

Many tissues possess receptors for this hormone-like vitamin. The primary roles of calcitriol are regulation of calcium and phosphorus absorption in the intestine, parathyroid-directed regulation of calcium balance,

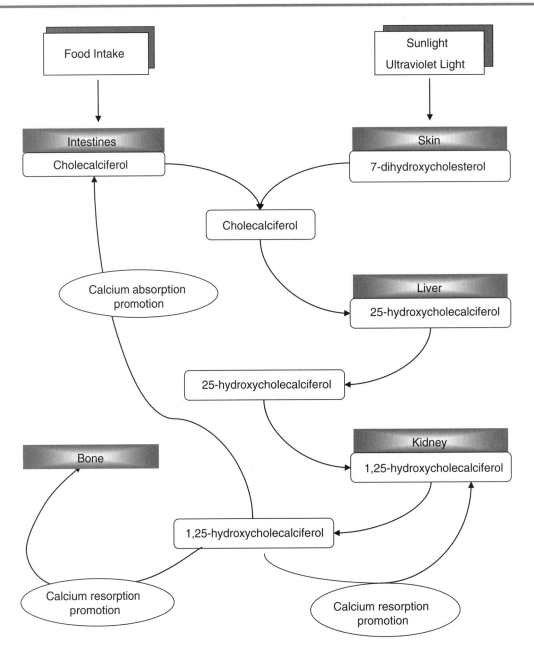

FIGURE 5.16 *Vitamin D metabolism*

and stimulation of bone cell mineralization. This last function may be due to vitamin D's ability to promote calcium uptake by osteoclasts and osteoblasts.

Sources

The most common supplemental form is vitamin D2 (ergocalciferol). Calcitriol (1,25-(OH)2D3) is prescribed for those with renal disease, since such patients are unable to convert vitamin D2 to this active form. Vitamin D from animal foods occurs in liver, eggs, fatty fish, butter, and fortified foods like milk. Vegetables are low in vitamin D. However, the common plant sterol ergosterol can be activated by irradiation to vitamin D2. Ten minutes of summer sun exposure to the face and hands results in the endogenous production of roughly 400 IU of cholecalciferol.[106] For additional sources and amounts, see Table 5.15.

TABLE 5.15 *Vitamin D Content of Certain Foods IU* per 100 grams*

Sardine, canned	500
Salmon	350
Tuna	250
Shrimp	150
Butter	90
Sunflower seeds	90
Liver	50
Eggs	50
Milk, fortified	40
Mushrooms	40
Natural cheese	30

*40 IU = 1 microgram

Therapeutic considerations

The primary signs associated with vitamin D deficiency are rickets in children and osteomalacia in adults. Prior to the advent of vitamin D fortification, these disorders were somewhat common. Today they are rare. Presently, vitamin D deficiency is most notable in the elderly and in individuals who may receive inadequate sunlight stimulation. In fact, vitamin D levels in blood decline measurably as the season progresses from fall to winter.

It should be noted that in individuals with poor fat absorption, vitamin D may be deficient (e.g., with gluten-sensitive enteropathy), as the vitamin will be found in the steatorrheic stool of these individuals.[107]

Safety and toxicity

A high level of vitamin D from endogenous synthesis due to sunlight exposure is closely regulated and does not produce toxicity.[108] Early uses of vitamin D (2,000 to 3,000 IU/day) for the purpose of infant feeding resulted in soft-tissue calcification and other severe complications. Large single doses of vitamin D or prolonged modest doses (>1200 IU/day) should be avoided.

Functional medicine considerations

Patients who live in areas with minimum sunlight or who are seldom exposed to the sun (such as those in nursing homes) should be evaluated for vitamin D deficiency. Any history of liver or kidney disorder should also be taken into consideration when assessing the effects of vitamin D status on the individual's health.

Patients should be questioned about all sources of vitamin D, including all supplements that contain the vitamin. Many individuals take a multitude of supplements, and they may be unaware of the amount of vitamin D they are actually taking in.

Individuals with problems related to parathyroid function should also be assessed, as there may be a breakdown of the feedback mechanism for decreased blood calcium levels, prompting a failure of the kidneys to respond to the additional need. The complex endocrine interactions of this vitamin make it important to consider its role in the health of several organ systems (GI, liver, kidney, and integumentary). Recently published research has expanded the important functional interactions of Vitamin D in the prevention of cancers, type 1 diabetes, heart disease, osteoporosis and persistent, nonspecific musculoskeletal pain.[109,110]

Vitamin K

Structure

The term vitamin K describes compounds possessing a 1,4-napthaquinone ring. Phylloquinone (K1) is a naturally occurring form of vitamin K found in plants. Menaquinone (K2) is a variant form synthesized by bacteria and found in animal foods. Menadione (K3) is a synthetic form of vitamin K that must be alkylated for use by the body. Structures are shown in Figure 5.17.

Absorption

Absorption of vitamin K, like that of other fat-soluble vitamins, depends on normal fat absorption. Vitamin K is absorbed in the upper two-thirds of the small intestine and is transported in chylomicrons. Integrity of colonic microflora is important for maintenance of vitamin K status. It has been estimated that bacterial manufacture of vitamin K may account for up to 50 percent of vitamin K needs.[111] Thus, both exogenous and endogenous sources are necessary to preserve vitamin K levels. Menaquinones produced in the gut are absorbed via a mechanism that is not yet clearly understood.[112]

Functions

The primary function of vitamin K is to aid in the formation of clotting factors and bone proteins. The clotting factors include: factor II (prothrombin), factor VII, factor IX, and factor X. The carboxylation of these factors enables the formation of calcium-binding sites in necessary blood clotting. Vitamin K's carboxylation function also helps form osteocalcin, a calcium-binding protein necessary for the mineralization of bone. Antagonists to biological activity of vitamin K include Coumadin (from sweet clover) and heparin.[113]

Sources

The most common supplemental form is vitamin K1, often derived from chlorophyll. Water-soluble and fat-soluble forms of chlorophyll-derived vitamin K are available (Table 5.16). Fat-soluble chlorophyll appears to provide the broadest benefit.

Therapeutic considerations

The primary uses of vitamin K are hemorrhagic disease prevention in newborns and

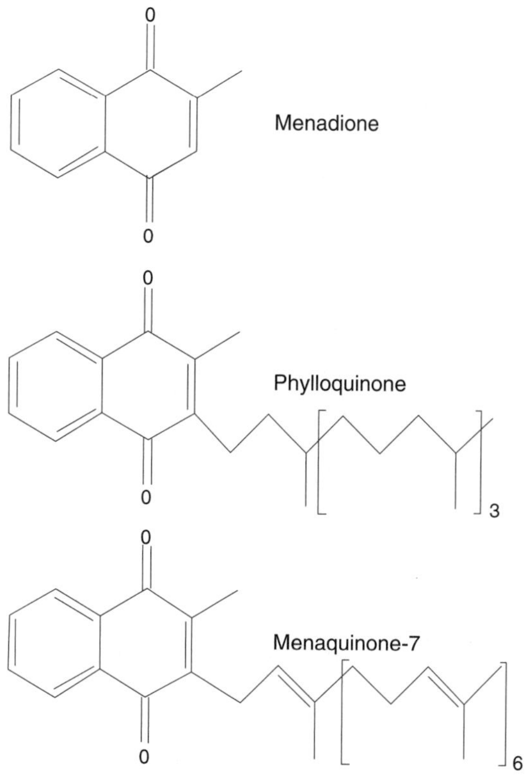

FIGURE 5.17 *Vitamin K molecule*

correction of vitamin K deficiency induced by antibiotic drugs or disruption of intestinal bacteria. A 1994 report suggests the use of vitamin K in the clinical management of menorrhagia.[142] As a result of the role vitamin K plays in osteocalcin synthesis and bone formation, long-term vitamin K insufficiency may impair bone integrity and growth. Patients with secondary fractures due to osteoporosis demonstrated low levels of vitamin K.[115]

A subclinical deficiency of vitamin K may be difficult to detect since the clotting mechanism would not be affected. Diets low in dark green, leafy vegetables quite likely result in subclinical deficiencies.[116] It is uncommon to find frank deficiencies of this vitamin because of its synthesis by intestinal bacterial. Long-term salicylate use may increase the need for vitamin K. The vitamin may be used in osteoporosis and menorrhagia, given its activities in bone mineralization and in clotting.[117]

Therapeutic doses of vitamin K commonly range from 100 to 500 mcg/day. Infants

TABLE 5.16 *Vitamin K Content of Certain Foods*
IU per 3 1/2 oz

Turnip greens	650	Whole wheat	17
Broccoli	200	Green beans	14
Lettuce	129	Pork	11
Cabbage	125	Eggs	11
Liver, beef	92	Corn oil	10
Spinach	89	Peaches	8
Watercress	57	Beef	7
Asparagus	57	Liver, chicken	7
Cheese	35	Raisins	6
Butter	30	Tomato	5
Liver, pork	25	Milk	3
Oats	20	Potato	3
Green peas	19		

typically receive a one-time IM dose of 1 mg to prevent hemorrhagic disease.

Safety and toxicity

Phylloquinone produces no signs of toxicity even when given in large amounts. However, the synthetic vitamin K3 (menadione) binds with sulfhydryl groups such as those found in the tripeptide glutathione. Glutathione may become oxidized and result in oxidation of membrane phospholipids.[118] Excess of vitamins A and E antagonize vitamin K. Administration of vitamin K may antagonize the action of anticoagulant drugs such as Coumadin.

Functional medicine considerations

Although diet does not play a major role in vitamin K status with regard to frank deficiencies, a patient's gastrointestinal health should be explored. Problems with fat absorption, general malabsorption, or bacterial

imbalances may lead the clinician to suspect decreased vitamin K levels in light of any signs or symptoms of vitamin K deficiency.

If a patient is on any medications that antagonize vitamin K activity or are antagonized by vitamin K, this should be noted for both assessment and treatment. A history of easy bruising or recurrent menorrhagia should warrant consideration of vitamin K status. If problems with bone mineralization exist, vitamin K as well as the minerals needed for this process should be assessed. Knowledge of the patient's GI history, medication, and supplementation intake are vital to understanding the interactions of various substances on vitamin K status.

SUMMARY

Vitamins play an essential role in most metabolic processes governing human physiology. It is not as simple as stating that a particular vitamin is needed for a single function. The complex interactions of vitamins in digestion, absorption, synthesis, and the activities of other vitamins make it imperative that the status of all vitamins be kept at levels necessary for proper physiologic functioning.

The intake of foods or substances that antagonize the absorption or activity of one vitamin may ultimately show itself as a deficiency symptom of another vitamin. Gastrointestinal

dysfunction or imbalances in normal bacterial colonies may disrupt this weblike interplay of active molecules and contribute to symptoms not readily attributed to vitamin insufficiency.

It should not be assumed that consistent intake of the DRIs of vitamins through food or supplementation would alone rule out the possibility that a patient's signs and symptoms are related to vitamin insufficiency. The patient's history must be explored carefully, keeping the relationships of the vitamins in mind.

CHAPTER 5 REFERENCES

1. Garrison R, Somer E. Nutrition Desk Reference. New Canaan, Conn.: Keats Publishing; 1995:65.
2. Groff JL, Gropper SS, Hunt SM. Advanced Nutrition and Human Metabolism. Minneapolis, Minn: West Publishing Company; 1995:222.
3. Groff JL, Gropper SS, Hunt SM. Advanced Nutrition and Human Metabolism. Minneapolis, Minn: West Publishing Company; 1995:222.
4. Williams RJ, Deason G. Individuality in vitamin C needs. Proc Natl Acad Sci. 1967;57:1638–1641.
5. Williams RJ, Pelton RB. Individuality in nutrition: effects of vitamin A-deficient and other deficient diets on experimental animals. Proc Natl Acad Sci. 1966;55:126–134.
6. Williams RJ. Nutrition Against Disease. New York, NY: Pitman Publishing Corporation; 1971:24.
7. Ziegler EE, Filer LJ, eds. Present Knowledge in Nutrition. Washington, DC: ILSI Press; 1996:109,160.
8. Alfthan G, Aro A, Gey K. Plasma homocysteine and cardiovascular disease mortality. Lancet. 1997; 349:397.
9. Stacey M. The fall and rise of Kilmer McCully. New York Times Magazine. Aug 10, 1997:25–29.
10. Verhoef P, Kok FJ, Kruyssen DA, et al. Plasma total homocysteine, B vitamins, and risk of coronary atherosclerosis. Arterioscler Thromb Vasc Biol. 1997;17(5):989–995.
11. Rimm EB, Willett WC, Hu FB, et al. Folate and vitamin B6 from diet and supplements in relation to risk of coronary heart disease among women. JAMA. 1998;279(5):359–364.
12. Rimm EB, Willett WC, Hu FB, et al. Folate and vitamin B6 from diet and supplements in relation to risk of coronary heart disease among women. JAMA. 1998;279(5):359–364.
13. Rimm EB, Willett WC, Hu FB, et al. Folate and vitamin B6 from diet and supplements in relation to risk of coronary heart disease among women. JAMA. 1998;279(5):359–364.
14. Ariaey-Nejad MR, Balaghi M, Baker EM, Sauberlich E. Thiamin metabolism in man. Am J Clin Nutr. 1970;23:764–778.
15. Ziegler EE, Filer LJ, eds. Present Knowledge in Nutrition. Washington, DC: ILSI Press; 1996:161.
16. Garrison R., Somer E. Nutrition Desk Reference. New Canaan, Conn: Keats Publishing; 1995:103.

17. Garrison R., Somer E. Nutrition Desk Reference. New Canaan, Conn: Keats Publishing; 1995:103.

18. Garrison R., Somer E. Nutrition Desk Reference. New Canaan, Conn: Keats Publishing; 1995:103.

19. Garrison R., Somer E. Nutrition Desk Reference. New Canaan, Conn: Keats Publishing; 1995:103.

20. Claus D, Eggers R, Warecka K, Neundorfer B. Thiamin deficiency and nervous system function disturbances. Eur Arch Psychiatry Neurol Sci. 1985;234:390–394.

21. Ziegler EE, Filer LJ, eds. Present Knowledge in Nutrition. Washington, DC: ILSI Press; 1996:163.

22. Ziegler EE, Filer LJ, eds. Present Knowledge in Nutrition. Washington, DC: ILSI Press; 1996:167.

23. Ziegler EE, Filer LJ, eds. Present Knowledge in Nutrition. Washington, DC: ILSI Press; 1996:168.

24. Dutta P, Serafi J, Haplin D, Pinto J, Rivlin R. Acute ethanol exposure alters hepatic glutathione metabolism in riboflavin deficiency. Alcohol. 1995;12:43-47.

25. Rivlin RS. Disorders of vitamin metabolism: deficiencies, metabolic abnormalities and excesses. In: Wyngaarden JH, Smith LH, Jr, Bennett JC, Plum F, eds. Cecil Textbook of Medicine, 19th ed. Philadelphia, Pa: WB Saunders; 1991:1170–1183.

26. Rea WJ. Chemical Sensitivity, vol 4. Boca Raton, FL: CRC Press, Inc.; 1997:2590.

27. Food and Nutrition Board, National Research Council. Recommended Dietary Allowances, 10th ed. Washington, DC: National Academy Press; 1989:132–137.

28. Ziegler EE, Filer LJ, eds. Present Knowledge in Nutrition. Washington, DC: ILSI Press; 1996:171.

29. Garrison R. Somer E. Nutrition Desk Reference. New Canaan, Conn: Keats Publishing; 1995:108.

30. Ziegler EE, Filer LJ, eds. Present Knowledge in Nutrition. Washington, DC: ILSI Press; 1996:184.

31. Ziegler EE, Filer LJ, eds. Present Knowledge in Nutrition. Washington, DC: ILSI Press; 1996:185.

32. Ziegler EE, Filer LJ, eds. Present Knowledge in Nutrition. Washington, DC: ILSI Press; 1996:187.

33. DiPalma JR, Thayer WS. Use of niacin as a drug. Annu Rev Nutr. 1991;11:169–87.

34. Physician's Desk Reference. 47th ed. Montvale, NJ: Medical Economics Data Production Co.; 1993: 2491.

35. Murray M. Encyclopedia of Nutritional Supplements. Rocklin, Ca: Prima Publishing; 1996:97.

36. Ziegler EE, Filer LJ, eds. Present Knowledge in Nutrition. Washington, DC: ILSI Press; 1996: 236.

37. Fidanza A. Therapeutic action of pantothenic acid. Int J Vit Nutr Res. 1983;24(suppl):53–67.

38. Bender DA. Nutritional Biochemistry of the Vitamins. New York, NY: Cambridge University Press; 1992:341–59.

39. Ziegler EE, Filer LJ, eds. Present Knowledge in Nutrition. Washington, DC: ILSI Press; 1996:174.

40. Ziegler EE, Filer LJ, eds. Present Knowledge in Nutrition. Washington, DC: ILSI Press; 1996:176.

41. Korpela TK, Christen P, eds. Biochemistry of vitamin B6. Proceedings of the 7th International Congress on Chemical and Biological Aspects of Vitamin B6 Catalysis. Birkhauser Congress Reports, Life Sciences, vol. 2. Birkhauser Verlag, Basel. 1987.

42. Coburn SP. Location and turnover of vitamin B6 pools and vitamin B-6 requirements of humans. Ann NY Acad Sci. 1990;585:76–85.

43. Ziegler EE, Filer LJ, eds. Present Knowledge in Nutrition. Washington, DC: ILSI Press; 1996:178.

44. Schaumberg H, Kaplan J, Windebank A, et al. Sensory neuropathy from pyridoxine abuse. A new megavitamin syndrome. N Engl J Med. 1983;309:445–448.

45. Bartzatt R, Beckmann JD. Inhibition of phenol sulfotransferase by pyridoxal phosphate. Biochem Pharmacol. 1994;47(11):2087–2095.

46. Ziegler EE, Filer LJ, eds. Present Knowledge in Nutrition. Washington, DC: ILSI Press; 1996:179.

47. Garrison R. Somer E. Nutrition Desk Reference. New Canaan, Conn: Keats Publishing; 1995:116.

48. Herbert V. Vitamin B12. In: Ziegler EE, Filer LJ Jr., eds. Present Knowledge in Nutrition. Washington, DC: International Life Sciences Institute Press; 1996:191-205.

49. Herbert V. Vitamin B12. In: Ziegler EE, Filer LJ Jr., eds. Present Knowledge in Nutrition. Washington, DC: International Life Sciences Institute Press; 1996:191–205.

50. Herbert V. Vitamin B12. In: Ziegler EE, Filer LJ Jr., eds. Present Knowledge in Nutrition. Washington, DC: International Life Sciences Institute Press; 1996:191–205.

51. Garrison R. Somer E. Nutrition Desk Reference. New Canaan, Conn: Keats Publishing; 1995:125.

52. National Research Council. Recommended Dietary Allowances, 10th ed. Washington, DC: National Academy Press; 1989:158–165.

53. National Research Council. Recommended Dietary Allowances, 10th ed. Washington, DC: National Academy Press; 1989:158–165.

54. Ziegler EE, Filer LJ, eds. Present Knowledge in Nutrition. Washington, DC: ILSI Press; 1996:207.

55. Gregory JF. Bioavailability of folate. Eur J Clin Nutr. 1997;51:S54–S59.

56. Werler MM, Shapiro S, Mitchell AA. Periconceptional folic acid exposure and risk of occurrent neural tube defects. JAMA. 1993; 269: 1257–1261.

57. Butterworth C, Hatch K, Gore H, Mueller H, Krumdieck CL. Improvement in cervical dysplasia associated with folic acid therapy in users of oral contraceptives. Am J Clin Nutr. 1982; 35:73–82.

58. Crellin R, Bottiglieri T, Reynolds EH. Folates and psychiatric disorders: clinical potential. Drugs. 1993; 45:623–636.

59. Groff JL, Gropper SS, Hunt SM. Advanced Nutrition and Human Metabolism. Minneapolis, Minn: West Publishing Co.; 1995:268–269.

60. Murray M. Encyclopedia of Nutritional Supplements. Rocklin, Ca: Prima Publishing; 1996:20.

61. Garrison R. Somer E. Nutrition Desk Reference. New Canaan, Conn: Keats Publishing; 1995:120.

62. Ziegler EE, Filer LJ, eds. Present Knowledge in Nutrition. Washington, DC: ILSI Press; 1996:220.

63. Ziegler EE, Filer LJ, eds. Present Knowledge in Nutrition. Washington, DC: ILSI Press; 1996: 225–226.

64. Murray M. Encyclopedia of Nutritional Supplements. Rocklin, Ca: Prima Publishing; 1996:111.

65. Groff JL, Gropper SS, Hunt SM. Advanced Nutrition and Human Metabolism. Minneapolis, Minn: West Publishing Co.; 1995:257.

66. Kramer TR, Briske-Anderson M, Johnson B, Holman RT. Effects of biotin deficiency on polyunsaturated fatty acid metabolism in rats. J Nutr. 1984;114:2047–2052.

67. Mock DM. Biotin. In Brown M, ed. Present Knowledge in Nutrition. 6th ed. Washington, DC: International Life Sciences Institute. 1989: 189–207.

68. Murray M. Encyclopedia of Nutritional Supplements. Rocklin, Ca: Prima Publishing; 1996:113.

69. Garrison R. Somer E. Nutrition Desk Reference. New Canaan, Conn: Keats Publishing; 1995:129.

70. Groff JL, Gropper SS, Hunt SM. Advanced Nutrition and Human Metabolism. Minneapolis, Minn: West Publishing Company; 1995:261.

71. Murray M. Encyclopedia of Nutritional Supplements. Rocklin, Ca: Prima Publishing; 1996:113.

72. Murray M. Encyclopedia of Nutritional Supplements. Rocklin, Ca: Prima Publishing; 1996:113.

73. Garrison R, Somer E. Nutrition Desk Reference. New Canaan, Conn: Keats Publishing; 1995:133.

74. Murray M. Encyclopedia of Nutritional Supplements. Rocklin, Ca: Prima Publishing; 1996:61.

75. Levin M, Rumsey S, Wang Y, et al. Vitamin C. In: Ziegler EE, File, LJ, Jr. eds. Present Knowledge in Nutrition. Washington, DC: International Life Sciences Institute Press. 1996:146–159.

76. Murray M. Encyclopedia of Nutritional Supplements. Rocklin, Ca: Prima Publishing; 1996:62.

77. Murray M. Encyclopedia of Nutritional Supplements. Rocklin, Ca: Prima Publishing; 1996:62.

78. Rea WJ. Chemical Sensitivity. Volume 4. Boca Raton, Fla: CRC Press, Inc. 1997; 2598.

79. Mehta, JB, Singhal SB, Mehta BC. Ascorbic acid-induced haemolysis in G-6-PD deficiency. Lancet. 1990;336:944.

80. Burns JJ, Rivers JM, Machlin LJ, eds. Third Conference on Vitamin C. New York: The New York Academy of Sciences; 1987.

81. Rea WJ. Chemical Sensitivity, vol 4. Boca Raton, Fla: CRC Press, Inc.; 1997:2600.

82. Ziegler EE, Filer LJ, eds. Present Knowledge in Nutrition. Washington, DC: ILSI Press; 1996:152.

83. Dillard CJ, Gavino VC, Tappel AL. Relative antioxidant effectiveness of alpha-tocopherol and gamma-tocopherol in iron-loaded rats. J Nutr. 1983;131:2266–2273.

84. Farrell PM, Roberts RJ. Vitamin E. In: Shils ME, Olson JA, Shike M, eds. Modern Nutrition in Health and Disease. 8th ed., Philadelphia, Pa: Lea and Febiger, 1994:326–341.

85. Ziegler EE, Filer LJ, eds. Present Knowledge in Nutrition. Washington, DC: ILSI Press; 1996:130-131.

86. Garrison R, Somer E. Nutrition Desk Reference. New Canaan, Conn: Keats Publishing; 1995:84.

87. Garrison R, Somer E. Nutrition Desk Reference. New Canaan, Conn: Keats Publishing; 1995:88.

88. Ziegler EE, Filer LJ, eds. Present Knowledge in Nutrition. Washington, DC: ILSI Press; 1996:133.

89. Garrison R, Somer E. Nutrition Desk Reference. New Canaan, Conn: Keats Publishing; 1995:86.

90. Ziegler EE, Filer LJ, eds. Present Knowledge in Nutrition. Washington, DC: ILSI Press; 1996:109.

91. Garrison R. Somer E. Nutrition Desk Reference. New Canaan, Conn: Keats Publishing; 1995:66.

92. Blomhoff R, Green MH, Norum KR. Vitamin A: physiological and biochemical processing. Annu Rev Nutr. 1992;12:37–57.

93. National Research Council. Recommended Dietary Allowances, 10th ed. Washington, DC: National Academy Press; 1989:78–92.

94. Garrison R, Somer E. Nutrition Desk Reference. New Canaan, Conn: Keats Publishing; 1995:67.

95. Fawzi WW, Chalmer TC, Herrera MG, Mosteller F. Vitamin A supplementation and child mortality. JAMA. 1993;269:898–903.

96. Arieta AC, Zaleska M, Stutman HR, Marks MI. Vitamin A levels in children with measles in Long Beach, California. J Pediatr. 1992; 121:75–78.

97. Garrison R. Somer E. Nutrition Desk Reference. New Canaan, Conn: Keats Publishing; 1995:67.

98. Murray M. Encyclopedia of Nutritional Supplements. Rocklin, Ca: Prima Publishing; 1996:24.

99. Murray M. Encyclopedia of Nutritional Supplements. Rocklin, Ca: Prima Publishing; 1996:32–35.

100. Ziegler EE, Filer LJ, eds. Present Knowledge in Nutrition. Washington, DC: ILSI Press; 1996:109.

101. Werbach MR. Nutritional Influences on Mental Illness: A Sourcebook of Clinical Research. Tarzana, Ca: Third Line Press, Inc.; 1991:20.

102. Feskanich D, Singh V, Willett WC, Colditz GA. Vitamin A intake and hip fractures among postmenopausal women. JAMA 2002;287: 47–54.

103. Garrison R, Somer E. Nutrition Desk Reference. New Canaan, Conn: Keats Publishing; 1995:79.

104. Garrison R, Somer E. Nutrition Desk Reference. New Canaan, Conn: Keats Publishing; 1995:79.

105. Garrison R, Somer E. Nutrition Desk Reference. New Canaan, Conn: Keats Publishing; 1995:80.

106. DeLuca HD. Vitamin D. NutrToday. 1993; 28:6–11.

107. Garrison R. Somer E. Nutrition Desk Reference. New Canaan, Conn: Keats Publishing; 1995:81.

108. Webb AR. Hoick MF. The role of sunlight in cutaneous production of vitamin D3. Annu Rev Nutr. 1988; 8:375–399.

109. Holick MF. Vitamin D: importance in the prevention of cancers, type 1 diabetes, heart disease, and osteoporosis. Am J Clin Nutr 2004; 79:362–71

110. Plotnikoff GA, et al. Prevalence of severe hypovitaminosis D in patients with persistent, nonspecific musculoskeletal pain. Mayo Clin Proc. 2003;78:1463–70

111. National Research Council. Recommended Dietary Allowances, 9th ed. Washington, DC: National Academy Press; 1980:69–71.

112. Ziegler EE, Filer LJ, ed. Present Knowledge in Nutrition. Washington, DC: ILSI Press; 1996:138.

113. Garrison R. Somer E. Nutrition Desk Reference. New Canaan, Conn: Keats Publishing; 1995:91.

114. Gubner R, Ungerleider HE. Vitamin K therapy in menorrhagia. South Med J. 1944;37: 556–558.

115. Bitensky L, Hart JP, Catterall A, et al. Circulating vitamin K levels in patients with fractures. J Bone Joint Surg. 1988;70B:663–664.

116. Garrison R, Somer E. Nutrition Desk Reference. New Canaan, Conn: Keats Publishing; 1995:93.

117. Murray M. Encyclopedia of Nutritional Supplements. Rocklin, Ca: Prima Publishing; 1996:57.

118. Esmon CT. Cell mediated events that control blood coagulation and vascular injury. Annu Rev Cell Biol. 1993;9:1–26.

6

Minerals

HUMAN PHYSIOLOGIC FUNCTION involves approximately 18 different minerals. These inorganic substances often play critical roles, such as acting as coenzymes in a number of reactions. In addition to initiating or facilitating biochemical reactions, minerals can alter electrical currents to generate nerve impulses, open channels for transport across otherwise selectively permeable cellular membranes, and initiate muscle contraction. Minerals can hold molecules together to form carrier structures, vitamin structures, or compounds that are part of hormones, and mineral content affects excretory and immune function. In fact, nearly every system in the body relies on these 18 inorganic substances to carry out normal physiologic functions.

While many more than 18 minerals play physiologic roles in the body, only those that are considered "essential" are generally discussed. As essential minerals, they are important constituents of other essential nutrients and are needed for an important structural or regulatory function. Essential minerals cannot be missing from the diet without deficiency symptoms appearing.[1]

Many minerals now considered essential have only been known to be critical to the diet since the early 20th century. Researchers are still testing other minerals that may be essential, exploring safe and toxic mineral doses, and investigating how the elements interact in the body. This chapter explores the roles of established essential minerals by outlining each mineral's absorption and regulation processes, functions, food sources, therapeutic considerations, and safety. Each discussion concludes with a functional medicine approach to correcting mineral insufficiency.

MINERAL CLASSIFICATION

Because minerals are required in relatively small amounts, they are classified as micronutrients. They may be further categorized as those the body needs in quantities of 100 mg or more per day (*major* minerals) and those requiring less intake (*minor* or *trace* minerals), which the body needs in microgram (mcg) amounts. Major minerals are present in the body in amounts greater than 5 grams; trace minerals exist in amounts less than 5 grams. Table 6.1 lists minerals generally classified as major or minor. Recommended Dietary Intakes (RDIs) for the most commonly supplemented minerals are provided in Table 6.2. (See Chapter 5 for a discussion of RDIs.)

Mineral intake varies based on an individual's dietary habits, gastrointestinal absorption, mineral content of the soil, and influence of other substances or other minerals. Although a diet may seem complete with regard to a particular mineral, poor absorption or other factors may result in low-level deficiency symptoms. In other cases, an excess may occur from imbalanced intake of an antagonist mineral, or other underlying cause, and create symptoms of overdose. However, the body attempts to maintain a balanced concentration of minerals in the absence of interfering conditions or substances.[2]

Calcium

The body contains more calcium than any other mineral. Ninety-five to 99 percent of the body's total calcium forms the mineral matrix of bone tissue. The other 1 to 5 percent plays a critical role in nervous system function, blood clotting, and muscle contractions.[3]

TABLE 6.1   *Major and Minor Minerals*

Major	Minor
Calcium	Arsenic
Phosphorus	Boron
Magnesium	Chromium
Potassium	Cobalt
Sodium	Copper
Chloride	Fluoride
	Iodine
	Iron
	Manganese
	Molybdenum
	Nickel
	Selenium
	Silicon
	Tin
	Vanadium
	Zinc

Absorption and Regulation

Two processes are involved in the absorption of calcium through the intestines. In the duodenum and jejunum, an active transcellular process allows calcium to be absorbed. In the ileum, it is absorbed by a positive paracellular transport mechanism. The active process is mediated by calcitriol (1, 25-dihydroxycholecalciferol). Endogenous calcium is excreted into the intestines. Its resorption depends on the same factors responsible for absorption. Urinary resorption of calcium depends on parathyroid hormone and calcitriol.[4] These processes are all part of a complex system of calcium regulation involving release,

TABLE 6.2   *Summary Table of the Dietary Recommended Intakes (DRIs) for Minerals*

Note 1: Recommended Dietary Allowances (RDAs) have not been set for all minerals for different life stages. When an RDA is not available, the Adequate Intake (AI) is used for that vitamin (denoted by an *). The Upper Limit (UL) indicates the level at which adverse events have been noted. The UL has not been reported for many minerals and, in those cases, nd (not determined) is shown. For a more complete table see http://www.nap.edu (accessed December 2003).

Note 2: The UL for magnesium is only representative of intake from supplemental sources above the dietary intakes; the RDA and AI for magnesium represent recommended dietary intakes.

Mineral	AGE	RDA/AI*	UL
Calcium	Infants (0–12 mo)	210–270 mg/d*	nd
	Children (1–8 y)	500–800 mg/d*	2500 mg/d
	Children (9–18 y)	1300 mg/d*	2500 mg/d
	Adults (19–50 y)	1000 mg/d*	2500 mg/d
	Adults (> 50 y)	1200 mg/d*	2500 mg/d
	Pregnancy (≤18 y)	1300 mg/d*	2500 mg/d
	Pregnancy (>18 y)	1000 mg/d*	2500 mg/d
	Lactation (≤18 y)	1300 mg/d*	2500 mg/d
	Lactation (>18 y)	1000 mg/d*	2500 mg/d
Phosphorus	Infants (0–12 mo)	100–275 mg/d*	nd
	Children (1–8 y)	460–500 mg/d	3000 mg/d
	Children (9–18 y)	1250 mg/d	4000 mg/d
	Adults (>19 y)	700 mg/d	4000 mg/d
	Pregnancy (≤18 y)	1250 mg/d	3500 mg/d
	Pregnancy (>18 y)	700 mg/d	3500 mg/d
	Lactation (≤18 y)	1250 mg/d	4000 mg/d
	Lactation (>18 y)	700 mg/d	4000 mg/d
Magnesium	Infants (0–6 mo)	30 mg/d*	nd
	Infants (7–12 mo)	75 mg/d*	nd
	Children (1–3 y)	80 mg/d	65 mg/d
	Children (4–8 y)	130 mg/d	110 mg/d
	Children (9–13 y)	240 mg/d	350 mg/d
	Males (14–18 y)	410 mg/d	350 mg/d
	Males (>19 y)	400–420 mg/d	350 mg/d
	Females (14–18 y)	360 mg/d	350 mg/d
	Females (>19 y)	310–320 mg/d	350 mg/d
	Pregnancy (<18 y)	400 mg/d	350 mg/d
	Pregnancy (>18 y)	350 mg/d	350 mg/d
	Lactation (<18 y)	360 mg/d	350 mg/d
	Lactation (>18 y)	310 mg/d	350 mg/d

(continues)

Mineral	AGE	RDA/AI*	UL
Chromium	Infants (0–6 mo)	0.2 mcg/d*	nd
	Infants (7–12 mo)	5.5 mcg/d*	nd
	Children (1–3 y)	11 mcg/d*	nd
	Children (4–8 y)	15 mcg/d*	nd
	Males (9–18 y)	25 mcg/d*	nd
	Males (19–50 y)	35 mcg/d*	nd
	Males (>50 y)	30 mcg/d*	nd
	Females (9–18 y)	21 mcg/d*	nd
	Females (19–50 y)	25 mcg/d*	nd
	Females (>50 y)	20 mcg/d*	nd
	Pregnancy (≤18 y)	29 mcg/d*	nd
	Pregnancy (>18 y)	30 mcg/d*	nd
	Lactation (≤18 y)	44 mcg/d*	nd
	Lactation (>18 y)	45 mcg/d*	nd
Zinc	Infants (0–6 mo)	2 mg/d*	4 mg/d
	Infants (7–12 mo)	3 mg/d	5 mg/d
	Children (1–3 y)	3 mg/d	7 mg/d
	Children (4–8 y)	5 mg/d	12 mg/d
	Children (9–13 y)	8 mg/d	23 mg/d
	Males (14–18 y)	11 mg/d	34 mg/d
	Males (>19 y)	11 mg/d	40 mg/d
	Females (14–18 y)	9 mg/d	34 mg/d
	Females (>19 y)	8 mg/d	40 mg/d
	Pregnancy (≤18 y)	12 mg/d	34 mg/d
	Pregnancy (>18 y)	11 mg/d	40 mg/d
	Lactation (≤18 y)	13 mg/d	34 mg/d
	Lactation (>18 y)	12 mg/d	40 mg/d
Copper	Infants (0–12 mo)	200–220 mcg/d*	nd
	Children (1–3 y)	340 mcg/d	1000 mcg/d
	Children (4–8 y)	440 mcg/d	3000 mcg/d
	Children (9–13 y)	700 mcg/d	5000 mcg/d
	Adolescents (14–18 y)	890 mcg/d	8000 mcg/d
	Adults(>19 y)	900 mcg/d	10 000 mcg/d
	Pregnancy (≤18 y)	1000 mcg/d	8000 mcg/d
	Pregnancy (>18 y)	1000 mcg/d	10 000 mcg/d
	Lactation (≤18 y)	1300 mcg/d	8000 mcg/d
	Lactation (>18 y)	1300 mcg/d	10 000 mcg/d
Iodine	Infants (0–12 mo)	110–130 mcg/d*	nd
	Children (1–8 y)	90 mcg/d	200–300 mcg/d
	Children (9–13 y)	120 mcg/d	600 mcg/d

(continues)

Mineral	AGE	RDA/AI*	UL
	Adolescents (14–18 y)	150 mcg/d	900 mcg/d
	Adults(>19 y)	150 mcg/d	1100 mcg/d
	Pregnancy (≤18 y)	220 mcg/d	900 mcg/d
	Pregnancy (>18 y)	220 mcg/d	1100 mcg/d
	Lactation (≤18 y)	290 mcg/d	900 mcg/d
	Lactation (>18 y)	290 mcg/d	1100 mcg/d
Iron	Infants (0–6 mo)	0.27 mg/d*	40 mg/d
	Infants (7–12 mo)	11 mg/d	40 mg/d
	Children (1–3 y)	7 mg/d	40 mg/d
	Children (4–8 y)	10 mg/d	40 mg/d
	Children (9–13 y)	8 mg/d	40 mg/d
	Males (14–18 y)	11 mg/d	45 mg/d
	Males (>19 y)	8 mg/d	45 mg/d
	Females (14–18 y)	15 mg/d	45 mg/d
	Females (19–50 y)	18 mg/d	45 mg/d
	Females (> 50 y)	8 mg/d*	45 mg/d
	Pregnancy	27 mg/d	45 mg/d
	Lactation (≤18 y)	10 mg/d	45 mg/d
	Lactation (>18 y)	9 mg/d	45 mg/d
Manganese	Infants (0–6 mo)	0.003 mg/d*	nd
	Infants (7–12 mo)	0.6 mg/d*	nd
	Children (1–8 y)	1.2–1.5 mg/d*	2–3 mg/d
	Children (9–13 y)	1.6–1.9 mg/d*	6 mg/d
	Males (14–18 y)	2.2 mg/d*	9 mg/d
	Males (>19 y)	2.2–2.3 mg/d*	11 mg/d
	Females (14–18 y)	1.6 mg/d*	9 mg/d
	Females (>19 y)	1.8 mg/d*	11 mg/d
	Pregnancy (<18 y)	2.0 mg/d*	9 mg/d
	Pregnancy (>18 y)	2.0 mg/d*	11 mg/d
	Lactation (<18 y)	2.6 mg/d*	9 mg/d
	Lactation (>18 y)	2.6 mg/d*	11 mg/d
Molybdenum	Infants (0–12 mo)	2–3 mcg/d*	nd
	Children (1–3 y)	17mcg/d	300 mcg/d
	Children (4–8 y)	22 mcg/d	600 mcg/d
	Children (9–13 y)	34 mcg/d	1100 mcg/d
	Adolescents (14–18 y)	43 mcg/d	1700 mcg/d
	Adults(>19 y)	45 mcg/d	2000 mcg/d
	Pregnancy (≤18 y)	50 mcg/d	1700 mcg/d
	Pregnancy (>18 y)	50 mcg/d	2000 mcg/d
	Lactation (≤18 y)	50 mcg/d	1700 mcg/d
	Lactation (>18 y)	50 mcg/d	2000 mcg/d

(continues)

Mineral	AGE	RDA/AI*	UL
Selenium	Infants (0–6 mo)	15 mcg/d*	45 mcg/d
	Infants (7–12 mo)	20 mcg/d*	60 mcg/d
	Children (1–3 y)	20 mcg/d	90 mcg/d
	Children (4–8 y)	30 mcg/d	150 mcg/d
	Children (9–13 y)	40 mcg/d	280 mcg/d
	Adolescents (14–18 y)	55 mcg/d	400 mcg/d
	Adults (>19 y)	55 mcg/d	400 mcg/d
	Pregnancy	60 mcg/d	400 mcg/d
	Lactation	70 mcg/d	400 mcg/d
Vanadium	Infants (0–12 mo)	nd	nd
	Children (1–18 y)	nd	nd
	Adults (>19 y)	nd	1.8 mg/d
	Pregnancy	nd	nd
	Lactation	nd	nd
Boron	Infants (0 –12 mo)	nd	nd
	Children (1–3 y)	nd	3 mg/d
	Children (4–8 y)	nd	6 mg/d
	Children (9–13 y)	nd	11 mg/d
	Adolescents (14–18 y)	nd	17 mg/d
	Adults (>18 y)	nd	20 mg/d
	Pregnancy ($\leq$ 18 y)	nd	17 mg/d
	Pregnancy (> 18 y)	nd	20 mg/d
	Lactation ($\leq$ 18 y)	nd	17 mg/d
	Lactation (> 18 y)	nd	20 mg/d

resorption, and excretion. This system keeps available calcium (outside the bone matrix) within optimal range. Calcium's many important regulatory functions require these mechanisms for homeostasis.

Calcium homeostasis is maintained with help from parathyroid hormones (PTH), calcitonin (CT), and calcitriol. A negative feedback mechanism regulates the production and secretion of these substances.[5] PTH stimulates an increase in circulating calcium (with an increase in bone resorption of calcium). When enough calcium is in the blood, PTH stops stimulating bone resorption.

Calcium absorption may be impaired by excess dietary fat. Excess dietary fiber, caffeine, and ethanol may increase fecal excretion of calcium. Excess dietary protein may increase renal loss of calcium. Glucose and aspartame may also increase urinary loss.[6] Note that surprising results show some types of fiber may actually enhance absorption of calcium and other minerals.[7] High-protein foods may cause calcium imbalance and increase bone demineralization.

Absorption of calcium is enhanced by substances that increase its solubility, including hydrochloric acid, ascorbic acid, citric acid, glycine, and lysine. Substances that interfere with calcium absorption include phytic acid, oxalic acid, and cocoa.[8]

Functions

The development of bone tissue and teeth requires sufficient calcium intake, absorption, and homeostatic mechanisms. The body goes to great lengths to maintain adequate plasma levels of calcium, which may lead to the resorption of mineral from the bone matrix.

Both striated (skeletal and cardiac) and smooth muscles require calcium to trigger ATP for energy needed in the contraction process. A number of neurotransmitters require calcium for release at the synaptic cleft, which enables nerve impulse transmission.

Calcium helps regulate ion transport in cell membranes. Within the cell itself, calcium levels are tightly regulated by calmodulin, which ensures the appropriate composition of fluids.

Lesser known functions of calcium are its participation in blood-clotting, including activation of prothrombin, conversion of fibrinogen to fibrin,[9] and activation of multiple enzymes.

The role of calcium in maintaining normal blood pressure is controversial. Supplementation with calcium has been effective in reducing high blood pressure in some studies, but not in others.[10] However, hypertensive patients with insulin resistance have shown an increase in insulin sensitivity with oral calcium supplementation.[11] A positive correlation also exists between higher calcium levels and some increased risks for myocardial infarction (serum cholesterol, serum glucose, and hypertension).[12]

Sources

Dairy is a major food source of calcium. However, a number of plants also contain high levels of calcium, which is important to note because many individuals are sensitive to dairy. Cabbage family plants (e.g., kale and collards) have very absorbable calcium. Spinach, although it has a rich supply of calcium, has oxalic acid, which reduces calcium absorption. Table 6.3 lists food sources of calcium, and Table 6.4 lists sources of nondairy calcium.

Therapeutic considerations

Pregnant or lactating women require 1200 mg of calcium per day. Calcium deficiencies may seriously affect bone tissue because the body uses calcium from bone to maintain adequate blood levels. For children, deficiency may result in rickets; for adults, osteomalacia. Teeth are not nearly as affected unless the calcium deficiency occurs during their development.[13] In addition to the effects on bone, a deficiency will result in a loss of other calcium-dependent functions as well (e.g., control of muscle contractions). Thus, muscle spasms, twitches, and hypertension may result from low calcium availability.[14]

TABLE 6.3   *Food Sources of Calcium*

Milligrams (mg) per 100 grams edible portion (100 grams = 3 1/2 oz)

1093	Kelp	51	Dried prunes
925	Swiss cheese	51	Pumpkin & squash seeds
750	Cheddar cheese	50	Cooked dry beans
352	Carob flour	49	Common cabbage
296	Dulse	48	Soybean sprouts
250	Collard leaves	46	Hard winter wheat
246	Turnip greens	41	Orange
245	Barbados molasses	39	Celery
234	Almonds	38	Cashews
210	Brewer's yeast	38	Rye grain
203	Parsley	37	Carrot
200	Corn tortillas (lime added)	35	Quinoa
187	Dandelion greens	34	Barley
186	Brazil nuts	32	Sweet potato
151	Watercress	32	Brown rice
129	Goat's milk	29	Garlic
128	Tofu	28	Summer squash
126	Dried figs	27	Onion
121	Buttermilk	26	Lemon
120	Sunflower seeds	26	Fresh green peas
120	Yogurt	25	Cauliflower
119	Beet greens	25	Lentils, cooked
119	Wheat bran	22	Corn meal, whole grain
118	Whole milk	22	Sweet cherry
114	Buckwheat, raw	22	Asparagus
110	Sesame seeds, hulled	22	Winter squash
106	Ripe olives	21	Strawberry
103	Broccoli	20	Millet
99	English walnut	19	Mung bean sprouts
94	Cottage cheese	18	Rye flour, dark
93	Spinach	18	Peanut butter
85	Filbert butter	17	Pineapple
73	Soybeans, cooked	16	Grapes
73	Pecans	16	Beets
72	Wheat germ	14	Cantaloupe
69	Peanuts	14	Jerusalem artichoke
68	Miso	13	Tomato
68	Romaine lettuce	12	Eggplant
67	Dried apricots	12	Chicken
66	Rutabaga	11	Orange juice
62	Raisins	10	Avocado
60	Black currant	10	Beef
59	Dates	9	Rye flour, light
57	Shrimp	9	Brown rice, cooked
56	Green snap beans	8	Banana
53	Sunflower seed butter	7	Apple
51	Globe artichoke	3	Sweet corn

TABLE 6.4 *Nondairy High-Calcium Foods*
Approximate milligrams (mg) calcium content per 8 oz (1 cup)

Vegetables		Fish	
1093	Kelp	1000	Sardines, canned with bones
450	Mustard greens, cooked	680	Mackerel, canned with bones
450	Turnip greens, cooked	490	Salmon with bones
330	Bok choy, cooked	300	Raw oysters
320	Bean sprouts		
260	Collard greens, cooked		
250	Spinach, cooked		

Nuts		Grains	
900	Sesame seeds	300	Tapioca, dried
660	Almonds	**Beans**	
600	Chestnuts		
450	Filberts	450	Soybeans, cooked
280	Walnuts	400	Tofu
260	Sunflower seeds	340	Garbanzo beans, cooked

Nut Butters		Nut Milks	
426	Sesame	400	Sesame butter (100 gm) + 2 Tbsp molasses + water
270	Almond	300	Almond (100 gm) + honey + water
		200	Filbert + maple syrup + water

Safety and toxicity

Calcium toxicity is not generally a problem since its levels in the body are so well regulated and maintained within normal range.

Functional medicine considerations

A patient diet history that includes excess caffeine, alcohol, or both may suggest the possibility of insufficient calcium stores. Clinicians should consider patient complaints of muscle cramps, twitches, or symptoms of hypertension (e.g., headache, dizziness) as possible signs of this insufficiency.

A diet high in protein or fiber or both may contribute to excessive calcium excretion. Elderly individuals, especially those females at high risk for osteoporosis, should have their calcium status assessed. Risks for osteoporosis include family history of osteoporosis, white or Asian heritage, small bone structure, short stature, lack of physical exercise, nulliparity, smoking, and excess alcohol intake. Low estrogen levels (typically present in individuals with signs of early or normal menopause, excess exercise, or exceptional leanness) may interfere with bone metabolism and increase calcium excretion.[15]

A history of fractures, gastrointestinal dysfunction, or even blood clotting problems may also indicate that calcium has not been absorbed adequately and that blood levels may be low. Since blood levels are readily maintained, a serum screening test indicating abnormally high levels of calcium may indicate problems in parathyroid hormone metabolism or a neoplasm. However, chronically high or low serum calcium levels should not be ignored when considering a possible calcium imbalance. They should be examined in light of other blood parameters and signs and symptoms. Therapeutic intervention with calcium and vitamin D may benefit patients with bone density loss.[16]

Phosphorus

Another key inorganic component of bone and teeth is phosphorus. In addition to its role in forming the mineral matrix of bone, phosphorus contributes to other critical life-maintaining compounds. Examples of such molecules include phospholipids, nucleic acids, cyclic adenosine monophosphate, cyclic quinine monophosphate, and 2,3-disphosphoglycerate (regulates oxygen release from hemoglobin). Energy is stored within the molecule adenosine triphosphate (ATP). Serum phosphate levels help regulate calcitriol production.[17]

Calcium absorption may be affected by phosphorus intake, as noted previously. However, unless the kidneys are not able to produce calcitriol sufficiently, calcium levels remain normal because of the increased activity of homeostatic mechanisms. Phosphorus concentration in plasma is about half that of calcium.

Absorption and regulation
Regulation of phosphorus occurs through renal absorption, interaction with calcium, PTH, and vitamin D. While about 70 percent of dietary intake is absorbed, it may be inhibited by excessive iron intake. Aluminum will bind phosphorus in the intestine and prevent its absorption. Calcitonin lowers plasma levels of calcium and phosphorus. Urinary excretion is the primary regulatory mechanism of phosphorus.[18]

Functions
Phosphorus is the source of metabolic energy, which is stored in phosphate bonds. Phosphorus also helps regulate a number of enzymes and participates in buffer systems within the body. Its role in the structure of every cell in the body makes phosphorus not only an important molecule but also the second most abundant mineral found in the human body. The genetic code depends on the structure of nucleic acids of which phosphorus is an important component. Development and repair of body tissue also depend on phosphorus.

Numerous phosphorylation processes help carry out cellular functions and enzymatic reactions. Lipid metabolism relies on phosphorus as well, and lipid-phosphorus structures are important components of cell membranes and nervous system structures.[19]

Sources

Animal tissues have an abundance of phosphorus. Individuals also get phosphorus from soft drinks and fast foods (often excessively). The result may be reduced calcium absorption, as noted above. Table 6.5 lists foods that contain phosphorus.

Therapeutic considerations

Deficiencies in phosphorus may result from excess calcium intake or vitamin D deficiency. Rickets can result from low serum phosphorus as well as low serum calcium. Symptoms of deficiency may include anorexia, weakness, fragile bones, and joint stiffness. Over consumption of antacids has been known to cause phosphorus deficiency because antacids often inhibit absorption.[20]

Safety and toxicity

No toxic levels have been reported. Nonetheless, imbalanced calcium levels may occur with excessive intake of phosphorus. The typical American diet, with high amounts of soda drinks and fast food, can lead to excess phosphorus-to-calcium ratios.

Functional medicine considerations

A patient's dietary history should be obtained to determine whether or not he or she is consuming high amounts of animal products, fast foods, or sodas. If so, consideration should be given to the signs and symptoms of calcium insufficiency as outlined earlier. If the patient consumes large amounts of antacids, signs and symptoms of phosphorus deficiency should be carefully considered.

Magnesium

As with many vitamins and minerals, magnesium deficiency symptoms were first identified in patients having either underlying diseases or in those whose alcohol intake had caused serious depletion of the nutrient. However, dysfunctions related to inadequate magnesium levels continue to be identified. Little doubt exists about magnesium's participation in at least 300 intermediary enzymatic reactions. For example, for glucose to be converted to phosphorus, magnesium is needed in seven important enzymatic reactions. Magnesium is also required in fatty acid synthesis and oxidation and in protein synthesis.

Formation of cAMP requires magnesium as do over 100 protein kinase reactions. These functions of magnesium also make it an important modulator of cardiac physiology.[21] Muscles contain 27 percent of all magnesium in the body, with bones containing 60 percent (some of it bound to phosphorus).

Absorption and regulation

Magnesium is best absorbed in the lower small intestine and the colon by passive transport, facilitated diffusion, and active cellular transport. How much magnesium is absorbed may therefore depend on how much

TABLE 6.5   *Food Sources of Phosphorus*

Milligrams (mg) per 100 grams edible portion (100 grams = 3 1/2 oz)

1753	Brewer's yeast	78	Broccoli
1276	Wheat bran	77	Figs, dried
1144	Pumpkin & squash seeds	69	Yams
1118	Wheat germ	67	Soybean sprouts
837	Sunflower seeds	64	Mung bean sprouts
693	Brazil nuts	63	Dates
592	Sesame seeds, hulled	63	Parsley
554	Soybeans, dried	62	Asparagus
504	Almonds	59	Bamboo shoots
478	Cheddar cheese	56	Cauliflower
457	Pinto beans, dried	53	Potato with skin
409	Peanuts	51	Okra
400	Wheat	51	Spinach
380	English walnut	44	Green beans
376	Rye grain	44	Pumpkin
373	Cashews	42	Avocado
353	Beef liver	40	Beet greens
338	Scallops	39	Swiss chard
311	Millet	38	Winter squash
290	Barley, pearled	36	Carrot
289	Pecans	36	Onions
267	Dulse	35	Red cabbage
240	Kelp	33	Beets
239	Chicken	31	Radish
221	Brown rice	29	Summer squash
205	Eggs	28	Celery
202	Garlic	27	Cucumber
175	Crab	27	Tomato
152	Cottage cheese	26	Banana
150	Beef or lamb	26	Persimmon
119	Lentils, cooked	26	Eggplant
116	Mushrooms	26	Lettuce
116	Fresh peas	24	Nectarine
111	Sweet corn	22	Raspberries
101	Raisins	20	Grapes
93	Whole cow's milk	20	Orange
88	Globe artichoke	17	Olives
87	Yogurt	16	Cantaloupe
80	Brussels sprouts	10	Apple
79	Prunes, dried	8	Pineapple

was consumed, the needs of the body, intestinal transit time, and H_2O absorption in the colon.[22] Calcitriol does not seem to affect magnesium absorption and regulation.[23] The kidneys help regulate magnesium concentrations by excreting it in response to changing plasma levels. Lactose as well as other carbohydrates may increase magnesium absorption. Alcohol and caffeine cause an increase in urinary excretion but evidently do not affect the status unless they are excessive.[24]

Functions

Magnesium is necessary for muscle relaxation, neuromuscular junction activity, protein synthesis, fat synthesis, and energy production (often complexed with ATP, ADP, or AMP). Magnesium is also important in removing excess ammonia through its role in forming urea.[25]

The functions of magnesium in the body relate primarily to its role as an enzymatic cofactor or in energy molecule complexes. The Δ6 desaturase enzyme required in the metabolism of fatty acids depends on magnesium.

It may be that magnesium plays some role in platelet aggregation, as evidenced by the increase in this activity in subjects with whom magnesium infusion was used. While homeostatic changes occurred as a result, normal physiologic ranges remained.[26]

One of the enzymes in which magnesium plays an important role is sodium/potassium ATPase, which activates and regulates cellular energy metabolism, transport across membranes, and vascular tone. Blood vessels may contract excessively if magnesium is not available. Magnesium supplementation has been shown to decrease vasoconstriction in cerebral vascular accidents (CVAs).[27]

Therapeutic considerations

Deficient or insufficient magnesium may create a number of clinical signs and symptoms. Table 6.7 indicates a number of conditions that may improve with magnesium supplementation.

Deficiencies are more likely to occur in elderly and pregnant populations and are often the result of decreased absorption or increased excretion. Signs and symptoms include weakness, heart irregularities, muscle cramps or twitches, insomnia, mental confusion, fatigue, irritability, and decreased appetite.[28]

Studies have illustrated that low levels of magnesium exist in diabetics[29] and in patients with systemic lupus erythematosus.[30] In patients with non-insulin-dependent diabetes (NIDDM), supplemental magnesium has been shown to improve cellular uptake of glucose by insulin.[31]

Magnesium supplementation may prevent vasoconstriction of intracranial vessels after CVA (specifically subarachnoid hemorrhage).[32] Magnesium was also found to lower blood pressure in healthy subjects; this study speculated that the lowered blood pressure was due to the suppression of adrenergic activity and to natriuresis. This same study observed an

improvement in serum lipid concentrations because of an increase in lecithin-cholesterol
acyltransferase (LCAT).[33]

Sources

Magnesium exists in whole grains, nuts and
legumes, and seafood. It is an important com-

TABLE 6.6   *Food Sources of Magnesium*

Milligrams (mg) per 100 grams edible portion (100 grams = 3 1/2 oz)

760	Kelp	37	Common beans, cooked
490	Wheat bran	37	Barley
336	Wheat germ	36	Dandelion greens
270	Almonds	36	Garlic
267	Cashews	35	Raisins
258	Blackstrap molasses	35	Fresh green peas
231	Brewer's yeast	34	Potato with skin
229	Buckwheat	34	Crab
225	Brazil nut	33	Banana
220	Dulse	31	Sweet potato
184	Filberts	30	Blackberry
175	Peanuts	25	Beets
162	Millet	24	Broccoli
160	Wheat germ	24	Cauliflower
142	Pecan	23	Carrot
131	English walnut	22	Celery
115	Rye	21	Beef
111	Tofu	20	Asparagus
106	Beet greens	19	Chicken
90	Coconut meat, dry	18	Green pepper
88	Soybeans, cooked	17	Winter squash
88	Spinach	16	Cantaloupe
88	Brown rice	16	Eggplant
71	Dried figs	14	Tomato
65	Swiss chard	13	Cabbage
62	Apricots, dried	13	Grapes
58	Dates	13	Milk
57	Collard leaves	13	Pineapple
51	Shrimp	13	Mushroom
48	Sweet corn	12	Onion
45	Avocado	11	Orange
45	Cheddar cheese	11	Iceberg lettuce
41	Parsley	9	Plum
40	Prunes, dried	8	Apple
38	Sunflower seeds		

ponent of chlorophyll and is found in large amounts in green vegetables. Magnesium supplementation is best absorbed in small amounts throughout the day.[34] Magnesium citrate and magnesium glycinate are the most absorbable forms of supplemental magnesium. Food sources of magnesium are listed in Table 6.6.

Safety and toxicity

Diarrhea can result if more than 600 mg of supplemental magnesium are taken per day. Toxicity can result in more severe symptoms including drowsiness, lethargy, and weakness. The elderly, whose renal function may be generally reduced, may be more likely to have symptoms, especially because they often consume large amounts of magnesium-containing antacids and laxatives. The central nervous system can also be affected by hypermagnesemia.[35]

Functional medicine considerations

Several situations may indicate magnesium insufficiency or excess. If patients are elderly, their history of taking antacids and laxatives containing magnesium should be explored. Also, digestive problems resulting from myriad causes, including poor dentition and factors interfering with magnesium absorption, should be considered.

While these same concerns may arise in non-elderly individuals, any potential source of supplemental magnesium should also be explored if magnesium excess is suspected (often indicated by diarrhea, somnolence, and lethargy). A history of allergies or other im-

TABLE 6.7 *Conditions that May Involve Magnesium Deficiency*

Angina	Glaucoma
Asthma	High blood pressure
Cardiomyopathy	Hypoglycemia
Cardiovascular disease	Insulin resistance
Cardiac arrhythmia	Intermittent
Congestive heart	claudication
failure	Kidney stones
Diabetes	Migraines
Dysmenorrhea	Osteoporosis
Fatigue	Premenstrual
Fibromyalgia	syndrome
	Stroke

mune system disorders or inflammatory responses should lead the clinician to consider a magnesium insufficiency in part because of poor Δ6 desaturase activity.

If a patient's history or lab results suggest insulin insensitivity, exploring magnesium levels in cells may help remedy the situation. In addition, considering magnesium's important role, disorders of energy production indicated by fatigue, muscle weakness, depression, or sleep disruptions should prompt clinicians to investigate magnesium status.

Sodium, Chloride, and Potassium

To better understand the role of these three minerals (electrolytes), it is useful to describe the fluid compartments in the body. The extracellular compartment in which cells are bathed makes up approximately one-third of the body's extracellular fluid (ECF). The other two-thirds resides inside cells (intracellular fluids or ICF). The major solutes in the ECF are sodium and chloride, while potassium is the major component of the ICF. The percentage of fluid constituents may change somewhat in various tissue types because of the varying H_2O concentrations.[36] The differences represent important factors in regulatory and homeostatic mechanisms, including nerve transmission and muscle contractions.

Absorption and regulation

The upper small intestine is the site of greatest absorption for these electrolytes. The kidneys eliminate them, and balance is maintained by regulatory mechanisms. Renal disease may interfere with renal elimination of the electrolytes, whereas diarrhea, excessive vomiting, or Addison's disease (lack of mineral corticoids from the adrenal glands) may result in excess loss of electrolytes and subsequent hypotension. If it is severe enough, shock or even death may result.[37]

The absorption and renal excretion of sodium and chloride are controlled by active and passive transport mechanisms. In addition, salt appetite and thirst are behavioral mechanisms that help in this regulation. Hormones that influence the balance of sodium, chloride, and water include the renin-angiotensin-aldosterone axis, vasopressin, and others. The autonomic nervous system (sympathetic branch) also helps regulate sodium and chloride by altering blood flow through the kidneys, releasing renin from juxtaglomerular apparatus, or directly stimulating receptors in the renal tubules. Finally, renal mechanisms also help control sodium and chloride.[38]

Potassium exists primarily in the ICF. An increase or decrease in ECF potassium concentration may result from increases or decreases in potassium intake, increases or decreases in potassium excretion from the kidneys, or a shift in potassium concentration on the outside or inside of the cellular membrane. Regulation of potassium occurs by mechanisms similar to those for sodium and chloride.

Functions

As an important electrolyte, potassium passes across the cellular membrane fairly easily, more easily than sodium. Potassium, as has been noted, participates in nerve transmission, muscle contractions, glycogen and glucose metabolism, and maintenance of cellular integrity. Sodium also plays important roles in transport of carbon dioxide, muscle contraction, nerve transmission, and amino acid transport.[39]

Sources

Potassium is found in many foods. Some of the better sources are potatoes, bananas, and other fruits (Table 6.8).

Table salt is the major source of sodium, but other good sources of sodium exist as well (Table 6.9). American diets are often higher in foods containing sodium than those containing potassium. Over time this can result in potassium insufficiencies and imbalances in fluid concentrations (Table 6.10).

Therapeutic considerations

A potassium deficiency can result in changes in the central nervous system, muscle weakness, bradycardia, bone fragility, and even death. Situations that might result in potassium deficiencies include diarrhea, vomiting, renal disease, aging, starvation, burns, and some diuretics. If an individual is dehydrated, there is the risk of increased loss of potassium in the urine. A magnesium deficiency will contribute to potassium loss; this same deficiency also makes it difficult for the cells to regain potassium stores.[40] Diabetes may result in loss of both potassium and sodium through increased urinary flow.[41]

A deficiency of sodium rarely occurs. Starvation, vomiting, or diarrhea may cause

TABLE 6.8   *Food Sources of Potassium*
Milligrams (mg) per 100 grams edible portion (100 grams = 3 1/2 oz)

8060	Dulse	295	Cauliflower
5273	Kelp	282	Watercress
920	Sunflower seeds	278	Asparagus
827	Wheat germ	268	Red Cabbage
773	Almonds	264	Lettuce
763	Raisins	251	Cantaloupe
727	Parsley	249	Lentils, cooked
715	Brazil nuts	244	Tomato
674	Peanuts	243	Sweet potato
648	Dates	234	Papaya
640	Figs, dried	214	Eggplant
604	Avocado	213	Green pepper
603	Pecans	208	Beets
600	Yams	202	Peach
550	Swiss chard	202	Summer squash
540	Soybeans, cooked	200	Orange
529	Garlic	199	Raspberries
470	Spinach	191	Cherries
450	English walnuts	164	Strawberry
430	Millet	162	Grapefruit juice
416	Beans, cooked	158	Grapes
414	Mushrooms	157	Onions
407	Potato with skin	146	Pineapple
382	Broccoli	144	Milk, whole
370	Banana	141	Lemon juice
370	Meats	130	Pear
369	Winter squash	129	Eggs
366	Chicken	110	Apple
341	Carrots	100	Watermelon
341	Celery	70	Brown rice, cooked
322	Radishes		

TABLE 6.9   *Food Sources of Sodium*

Milligrams (mg) per 100 grams edible portion (100 grams = 3 1/2 oz)

3007	Kelp	49	Turnip
2400	Green olives	47	Carrot
1428	Dill pickles	47	Yogurt
828	Ripe olives	45	Parsley
747	Sauerkraut	43	Artichoke
700	Cheddar cheese	34	Dried figs
265	Scallops	30	Lentils, dried
229	Cottage cheese	30	Sunflower seeds
210	Lobster	27	Raisins
147	Swiss chard	26	Red cabbage
130	Beet greens	19	Garlic
130	Buttermilk	19	While beans
126	Celery	15	Broccoli
122	Eggs	15	Mushrooms
110	Cod	13	Cauliflower
71	Spinach	10	Onion
70	Lamb	10	Sweet potato
65	Pork	9	Brown rice
64	Chicken	9	Lettuce
60	Beef	6	Cucumber
60	Beets	5	Peanuts
60	Sesame seeds	4	Avocado
52	Water cress	3	Tomato
50	Whole cow's milk	2	Eggplant
2132	Salt, 1 tsp.		
1319	Soy sauce, 1 tbsp.		

decreased sodium in the ECF, which causes H_2O to pass into the cell. Symptoms of this H_2O toxicity include loss of appetite, muscle twitching, and apathy. If both sodium and H_2O are lost in these situations, ECF fluids diminish and low blood volume results. Muscles may cramp, and veins may collapse under such circumstances.[42] Potassium supplementation has been shown to have a low-

ering effect on blood pressure.[43] A deficiency of chloride can also result from vomiting or diarrhea. Acid/base disturbances can be a consequence of this situation.

Safety and toxicity

Potassium is safe in excess except for individuals with kidney disease. These patients may experience disturbances of heart function

TABLE 6.10 *Foods with High Amounts of Added Sodium Chloride*

Bouillon cubes	Luncheon meats
Canned fish	Meat tenderizers
Canned or frozen vegetables	Packaged spice mixes
Canned or packaged soups	Potato chips, corn chips, pretzels, etc.
Catsup, barbecue sauce	Processed cheeses
Commercial peanut butter	Salted crackers
Commercial salad dressings	Salted nuts
Cured, smoked, or canned meats	

from even normal potassium intake and may need to restrict intake. Potassium intake may also need to be restricted when the individual takes potassium-sparing diuretics or ACE inhibitors (angiotensin-converting enzyme inhibitors). High levels of potassium might also result from adrenal dysfunction or rapid protein catabolism.

Functional medicine considerations

The standard American diet ingested over a long period of time may account for some signs and symptoms of potassium excess or potassium deficiency. A history of renal problems or a recent history of excessive diarrhea or vomiting should prompt clinicians to investigate electrolyte status, especially if hypotension, muscle weakness, or heart disturbances are identified.

Sodium/potassium ratios should also be considered when the patient has hypertension. If a magnesium deficiency has been determined, especially in diabetes cases (due to increased urine flow), potassium status should be determined, as it may also be deficient as a result.

Chromium

Absorption and regulation

Very little chromium is absorbed. Chromium in the diet as well as prior chromium status will affect the absorption. Other substances that affect its absorption include amino acids, ascorbic acid, and starch—all of which increase its absorption; zinc may decrease its absorption. Some medications can also affect chromium absorption (e.g., antacids may reduce absorption, while aspirin may increase it).[44]

Functions

Chromium is the major component in glucose tolerance factor (GTF), along with niacin (vitamin B3) and the amino acids glycine, glutamic acid, and cysteine. Chromium, via GTF, has a strong insulin-enhancing activity. The mineral might help bind insulin to its receptors in the cellular membrane. Chromium may have an effect on lipid metabolism as well. Some studies show increases in high-density lipoprotein cholesterol with chromium supplementation.[45] The immune response may also benefit from chromium, as it may decrease serum cortisol and increase immunoglobulins.

Sources

Chromium is found more in meats and whole grains than in fruits or vegetables. Table 6.11 lists some sources of chromium.

Therapeutic considerations

A chromium deficiency may result in elevated blood sugar and insulin levels. Cells may become less sensitive to insulin as a result. A highly refined diet is lower in chromium due to its removal in the refining process.[46] Chromium supplementation may help reduce body fat.[47]

Safety and toxicity

Chromium is very safe and can be tolerated at amounts higher than the estimated safe amounts.

Functional medicine considerations

When taking a patient history and determining the cause of symptoms typical of decreased insulin sensitivity, clinicians should

TABLE 6.11   *Food Sources of Chromium*

Micrograms (mcg) per 100 grams edible portion (100 grams = 3 1/2 oz)

112	Brewer's yeast*	11	Scallops
57	Beef, round	11	Swiss cheese
55	Calf's liver*	10	Banana
42	Whole wheat bread*	10	Spinach
38	Wheat bran	10	Pork chop
30	Rye bread	9	Carrots
30	Fresh chili	8	Navy beans, dry
26	Oysters	7	Shrimp
24	Potatoes	7	Lettuce
23	Wheat germ	5	Orange
19	Green pepper	5	Lobster tail
16	Hen's eggs	5	Blueberries
15	Chicken	4	Green beans
14	Apple	4	Cabbage
13	Butter	4	Mushrooms
13	Parsnips	3	Beer
12	Cornmeal	3	Strawberries
12	Lamb chop	1	Milk

Note: The above values show total chromium content of these foods and do not indicate the amount that may be biologically active as the Glucose Tolerance Factor (GTF). Those foods marked with an * are high in GTF.

examine the possibility of a chromium insufficiency. Other components of GTF may also be insufficient. Therapeutic intervention would then include all components.

Zinc

Zinc is important to the functioning of many enzymes. Zinc also assists in many hormone activities (thymic hormones, growth hormones, and insulin).[48] As a result, zinc is critical to immune function.

Absorption and regulation

Zinc is primarily absorbed in the upper small intestine. The intestine also plays a key role in controlling how much zinc is absorbed based on previous absorption. Some endogenous zinc may be released if there is an inadequate amount of zinc in the intestines. Inorganic iron in the diet may decrease zinc absorption, as may calcium supplements. Alcohol, infection, surgery, and other physiologic factors may alter the absorption of zinc. Cytokines, especially interleukins 1 and 6, may affect zinc metabolism by increasing its uptake by the liver. Fecal zinc excretion helps maintain homeostatic levels.[49]

Functions

As stated, zinc is a cofactor in a number of enzymatic reactions. In addition, zinc is important for protein and DNA synthesis, wound healing, bone structure, immune function, and skin oil gland function.[50] Zinc is also important for healthy prostate tissue.

Sources

Oysters are a well-known source of zinc. Zinc is also found in red meat and other shellfish. While zinc is high in whole grains, legumes, and nuts, it is not as absorbable from these sources, due to its binding with phytic acid.[51] Table 6.12 lists good food sources of zinc.

Therapeutic considerations

Symptoms of zinc deficiency typically include skin changes, hair loss, recurrent infections, and diarrhea. While it is not common to find severe zinc deficiencies, simple zinc insufficiencies are common. These may be associated with sleep disturbances, slow wound healing, dandruff, rheumatoid arthritis, reduced appetite, and inflammatory bowel disease, among others. Minor skin disorders may also occur, such as acne or psoriasis.

Rheumatoid arthritis patients have been shown to have insufficient intake of zinc, copper, B6, and magnesium.[52] Zinc has also been found deficient in non-insulin-dependent diabetics.[53] Zinc may also help relieve the common cold; zinc lozenges have been used with positive results in individuals with colds.[54]

Safety and toxicity

Zinc supplementation should be kept at 15 mg a day or below for general, chronic consumption. Short-term supplementation at higher levels may be beneficial in certain patients, but should be kept below 80 mg per day. If safe levels are not adhered to, a copper deficiency anemia may result, because zinc

TABLE 6.12   *Food Sources of Zinc*

Milligrams (mg) per 100 grams edible portion (100 grams = 3 1/2 oz)

148.7	Fresh oysters	1.7	Haddock
6.8	Ginger root	1.6	Green peas
5.6	Ground round steak	1.5	Shrimp
5.3	Lamb chops	1.2	Turnips
4.5	Pecans	0.9	Parsley
4.2	Split peas, dry	0.9	Potatoes
4.2	Brazil nuts	0.6	Garlic
3.9	Beef liver	0.5	Whole wheat bread
3.5	Nonfat dry milk	0.4	Black beans
3.5	Egg yolk	0.4	Raw milk
3.2	Whole wheat	0.4	Pork chop
3.2	Rye	0.4	Corn
3.2	Oats	0.3	Grape juice
3.2	Peanuts	0.3	Olive oil
3.1	Lima beans	0.3	Cauliflower
3.1	Soy lecithin	0.2	Spinach
3.1	Almonds	0.2	Cabbage
3.0	Walnuts	0.2	Lentils
2.9	Sardines	0.2	Butter
2.6	Chicken	0.2	Lettuce
2.5	Buckwheat	0.1	Cucumber
2.4	Hazelnuts	0.1	Yams
1.9	Clams	0.1	Tangerine
1.7	Anchovies	0.1	String beans
1.7	Tuna		

Black pepper, paprika, mustard, chili powder, thyme, and cinnamon are also high in zinc.

and copper compete for absorption. In addition, too much zinc can result in a depressed immune function.[55] Toxic effects may include dizziness, vomiting, lethargy, and anemia.

Functional medicine considerations

If a patient is HIV positive, a clinician should consider that zinc has been shown to be deficient in individuals with AIDS. Smokers also have lower zinc levels, and zinc may help protect against damage to blood vessel walls.[56] A patient's supplementation history should explore zinc intake and copper intake. If the patient has a history of recurrent infections, skin conditions, slow wound healing, or disrupted inflammatory response, zinc status should be assessed.

Copper

Copper is found in concentrations of 1–2 mcg per gram in living organisms. The highest concentrations in humans can be found in the kidneys, liver, brain, and bone. The copper in humans is almost exclusively in a +2 or +1 valence state.[57]

Absorption

The duodenum and jejunum are responsible for the absorption of copper, and this occurs with relatively high efficiency (35 to 70 percent). Mucosal cells take up copper most often by facilitated diffusion. Albumin carries the plasma copper to the liver to be incorporated into ceruloplasmin.[58]

Copper shares an absorption carrier with zinc and calcium. Thus, excess amounts of either of these two minerals may antagonize the absorption of copper. Iron may also interfere with copper absorption, but only in extreme situations. Amino acids and citrate in the diet can act as chelating agents to enhance copper absorption, while fiber and bile may act as inhibiting agents. Little copper is excreted in the urine; most of it is removed through the digestive tract.[59]

Erythrocuprein binds copper in red blood cells. This protein is involved in some antioxidant activity. Estrogens will increase serum copper concentrations.[60] Molybdenum, in combination with sulfate, may block copper usage or encourage its excretion.

Functions

Copper is important in a number of enzyme systems, including 11 oxidase systems, such as cytochrome oxidase, superoxide dismutase, and lysyl oxidase. Hemoglobin synthesis also relies on copper. In the aerobic production of energy, copper contributes in two ways: 1) by facilitating an electron shift of iron and 2) by oxidizing cytochrome C.[61]

Sources

Many foods contain copper, but the richest sources include shellfish and legumes. Table 6.13 gives a list of copper-containing foods.

Therapeutic considerations

Because of copper's importance to iron utilization in red blood cells, a copper deficiency may result in iron deficiency anemia.

Another important function of copper is its role in the activity of lysyl oxidase, an enzyme needed for the cross-linking of collagen and elastin. A deficiency in copper may result in poor collagen integrity, evidenced by the breaking of blood vessels and bone and joint problems. Lipid problems may also arise with a copper deficiency.[62]

Low copper status is also associated with reduced skin pigmentation, central nervous system impairment, and osteoporosis. Inadequate copper limits its role in energy production and enzymatic reactions.[63] Copper has been used supplementally in disease prevention and in bracelets worn by individuals with rheumatoid arthritis, the latter possibly due to its activity in antiinflammatory and antioxidant compounds.[64]

Safety and toxicity

In high doses (60 mg) copper may act as an emetic. In doses of approximately 3.5 grams,

TABLE 6.13 *Food Sources of Copper*

Milligrams (mg) per 100 grams edible portion (100 grams = 3 1/2 oz)

13.7	Oysters	0.4	Gelatin
2.3	Brazil nuts	0.3	Shrimp
2.1	Soy lecithin	0.3	Olive oil
1.4	Almonds	0.3	Clams
1.3	Hazelnuts	0.3	Carrots
1.3	Walnuts	0.3	Coconut
1.3	Pecans	0.3	Garlic
1.2	Split peas, dry	0.2	Millet
1.1	Beef liver	0.2	Whole wheat
0.8	Buckwheat	0.2	Chicken
0.8	Peanuts	0.2	Eggs
0.7	Cod liver oil	0.2	Corn oil
0.7	Lamb chops	0.2	Ginger root
0.5	Sunflower oil	0.2	Molasses
0.4	Butter	0.2	Turnips
0.4	Rye grain	0.1	Green peas
0.4	Pork loin	0.1	Papaya
0.4	Barley	0.1	Apple

Black pepper, thyme, paprika, bay leaves, and active dry yeast are also high in copper.

copper may be lethal.[65] Copper levels are excessive in Wilson's disease, a genetic disorder, and in hemochromatosis. Severe liver, kidney, and brain damage can occur if excess copper is not chelated and removed from the body. Excess copper in the bloodstream may result in epigastric pain, headache, and diarrhea, as well as hemolytic anemia.[66]

Functional medicine considerations

While copper deficiencies and toxicities are not common, a patient's history may lead the clinician to suspect them if symptoms are otherwise not explained. Copper pipes in the home, supplementation, high copper food in-take, and a family history of Wilson's disease or hemochromatosis may indicate copper toxicity (if the patient complains of the symptoms listed above).

High intake of zinc, antacids, vegetarian diet (high in legumes and vegetables), poor digestion, or molybdenum supplementation may warrant investigation into copper levels, as the patient may not be absorbing the copper, or its actions may be antagonized. Symptoms of copper deficiency (as listed above) in conjunction with these historical details may increase the suspicion of low copper levels. Decreased immune function, as evidenced by recurrent bacterial infection, may also suggest low copper levels and may contribute to low antibody response to infection.[67]

Iodine

The body uses iodine primarily as a component of thyroid hormones.

Absorption

Organic iodine substances are degraded in the gut to inorganic iodide, which is quickly and efficiently absorbed. The blood contains the absorbed free iodide, and the kidneys and thyroid rapidly pick up this free form. The kidney clears some of this iodide, depending on plasma supply. Uptake by the thyroid depends on previous iodine intake. If iodine has been deficient, as much as 80 percent of the available amount will be taken up by the thyroid.

Use of available iodine in synthesis of thyroid hormones is governed by a negative feedback loop involving the pituitary gland and its product, thyroid-stimulating hormone (TSH), and the hypothalamus and its product, thyroid-releasing hormone (TRH). These factors and not absorption or excretion generally govern iodine uptake and use by the thyroid. Iodine is stored primarily in the thyroid gland as mono- and diiodotyrosine and thyroxine with some triiodothyronine.

Functions

As stated above, iodine is used for the production of thyroid hormones such as thyroxine 3,5,3',5' tetraiodothyronine (T4) and 3,5,3' triiodothyronine (T3). Since thyroid hormones are needed to increase cellular reactions, including oxygen consumption and basal metabolic rate, and to influence growth and differentiation, iodine obviously plays a major role in these activities.[68]

Selenium is needed in the deiodinase enzyme to convert T4 to T3 in the liver. A selenium deficiency can cause thyroid enlargement. Also, thyroperoxidase needs iron for its activity. Without enough iron, thyroid metabolism is impaired.

Sources

Iodine is abundant in sea vegetables and seafood. It is also added to most salt, so most Americans get more than adequate amounts. Sea salt does not have much iodine. Food sources of iodine are listed in Table 6.14.

Therapeutic considerations

Iodine deficiency may result in goiters (due to enlargement of the thyroid via hypertrophy and/or hyperplasia) and hypothyroidism. Goiters may also be caused by excessive consumption of cabbage, rutabagas, cauliflower, and soybeans, all of which contain substances that may interfere with iodine used by the thyroid.

Severe iodine deficiency in an infant can result in cretinism, growth retardation, and even mortality.[69] Since iodine works with neutrophil peroxidases in bactericidal activity, iodine deficiency may result in decreased immune function of neutrophils.[70]

TABLE 6.14   *Food Sources of Iodine*

Micrograms (mcg) per 100 grams edible portion (100 grams = 3¹/2 oz)

90	Clams	11	Cheddar cheese
65	Shrimp	10	Pork
62	Haddock	10	Lettuce
46	Halibut	9	Spinach
50	Oysters	9	Green peppers
50	Salmon	9	Butter
37	Sardines, canned	7	Milk
19	Beef liver	6	Cream
16	Pineapple	6	Cottage cheese
16	Tune, canned	6	Beef
14	Eggs	3	Lamb
11	Peanuts	3	Raisins
11	Whole wheat bread		

Safety and toxicity

Thyroid hormone secretion may be inhibited by excess iodine intake in hyperthyroid individuals.[71] Also, there are reports of acne-like skin lesions erupting from high levels of dietary iodine intake.[72]

Functional medicine considerations

Symptoms of low thyroid function include fatigue, constipation, depression, dry skin, weight gain, and cold intolerance. While iodine deficiency may not necessarily be the cause of hypothyroidism, it should be explored especially in light of dietary considerations. A history of recurrent bacterial infections may be the presenting symptom, and poor iodine status should be ruled out, if other symptoms lead to suspicion of deficiency.

Iron

Since iron status is relatively easy to assess through blood tests, iron has been well studied.

Iron-containing compounds may be either directly functional or useful in transport and storage. The functional compounds have metabolic or enzymatic function in the body; and two-thirds of total body iron is used in this latter category of compound. A high percentage of that amount is in the form of hemoglobin, as iron is necessary for the structure of the heme portion of hemoglobin (Figure 6.1).

Absorption

Iron absorption occurs primarily in the duodenum by an active process that moves it into the blood. Transferrin, one of the transport/storage compounds, carries iron to cells and bone marrow. Absorption is increased when needed and decreased when erythropoiesis is reduced. Excess iron is then stored rather than excreted; ferritin and hemosiderin are the main storage compounds.

Iron absorption may be inhibited by phytic acid, polyphenolic compounds, calcium, and partially digested proteins. Ascor-

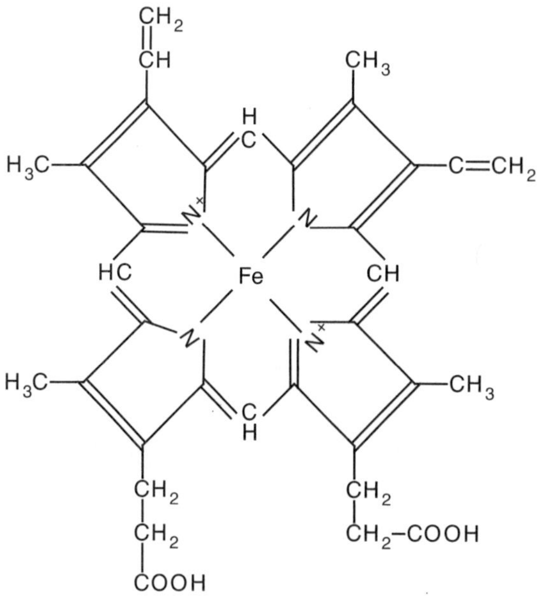

FIGURE 6.1 showing chemical structure of heme:

CH_2
‖
CH CH_3

H_3C—

            $\overset{H}{C}$

H_3C— $C{=}CH_2$

        N^+ N

HC   Fe   CH

        N N^+

H_3C— CH_3

            $\overset{C}{H}$

    CH_2 CH_2

    CH_2 CH_2–COOH

    COOH

FIGURE 6.1 *Chemical structure of heme*

bic acid (as well as meat eaten during the meal) will enhance iron absorption. Cysteine also helps iron absorption.[73]

Functions

As stated, iron is primarily used as part of the hemoglobin and myoglobin, which carry and release O_2 in tissue. Other cellular activities also need iron, as do enzymes in the Krebs cycle. Other functions of iron include helping to maintain normal immune function and collagen synthesis.

While bacteria are able to sequester iron from the human iron stores, oral iron supplementation does not increase the risk of infection. On the contrary, iron supplementation may enhance enzymes needed for optimal lymphocyte and neutrophil functioning.[74] In addition, iron deficiency results in decreased anatomical development of immune tissue, reduction in antibody and interleukin synthesis, and decreased protein synthesis. Granulocyte phagocytosis is also reduced in iron deficiency.[75]

Sources

Heme iron is found in animal tissue and is absorbed better than other iron forms. Non-heme iron is found in plant tissue and is not well absorbed. Table 6.15 lists food sources of iron.

Therapeutic considerations

Iron deficiency can result in severe anemia, decreased energy levels, decreased immune function, and learning disabilities. By the time iron deficiency anemia is observed, iron-dependent enzymatic activity has already been reduced. Serum ferritin and total-iron-binding capacity tests help find the earlier deficits.

Decreased iron is most common in low-income elderly individuals. Absorption may be inhibited in elderly individuals in general because of hypochlorhydria or other interfering factors (see above).[76] Blood loss that is constant and low grade may be a cause of iron deficiency. Symptoms of low iron status (before anemia) may include increased blood glucose, impaired growth, and recurrent infections.[77]

Safety and toxicity

Since iron is not easily excreted, excess iron can build up. Excess intake (diet or

TABLE 6.15   *Food Sources of Iron*

Milligrams (mg) per 100 grams edible portion (100 grams = 3 1/2 oz)

100.0	Kelp	1.3	Artichoke
17.3	Brewer's yeast	1.3	Mung bean sprouts
16.1	Blackstrap molasses	1.2	Salmon
14.9	Wheat bran	1.1	Broccoli
11.2	Pumpkin & squash seeds	1.1	Currants
9.4	Wheat germ	1.1	Whole wheat bread
8.8	Beef liver	1.1	Cauliflower
7.1	Sunflower seeds	1.0	Cheddar cheese
6.8	Millet	1.0	Strawberries
6.2	Parsley	1.0	Asparagus
6.1	Clams	0.9	Blackberries
4.7	Almonds	0.8	Red cabbage
3.9	Dried prunes	0.8	Pumpkin
3.8	Cashews	0.8	Mushrooms
3.7	Lean beef	0.7	Banana
3.5	Raisins	0.7	Beets
3.4	Jerusalem artichoke	0.7	Carrot
3.4	Brazil nuts	0.7	Eggplant
3.3	Beet greens	0.7	Sweet potato
3.2	Swiss chard	0.6	Avocado
3.1	Dandelion greens	0.6	Figs
3.1	English walnut	0.6	Potato
3.0	Dates	0.6	Corn
2.9	Pork	0.5	Pineapple
2.7	Cooked dry beans	0.5	Nectarine
2.4	Sesame seeds, hulled	0.5	Watermelon
2.4	Pecans	0.5	Winter squash
2.3	Eggs	0.5	Brown rice, cooked
2.1	Lentils	0.5	Tomato
2.1	Peanuts	0.4	Orange
1.9	Lamb	0.4	Cherries
1.9	Tofu	0.4	Summer squash
1.8	Green peas	0.3	Papaya
1.6	Brown rice	0.3	Celery
1.6	Ripe olives	0.3	Cottage cheese
1.5	Chicken	0.3	Apple

supplementation) may lead to hemosiderosis, a condition in which transferrin is saturated and iron is deposited in soft tissue. A more severe condition of iron deposition in soft tissue is hemochromatosis. Alcoholism may put one at risk for this condition. Excess iron may be associated with increased free radical production and an increased risk of cancer and heart disease.[78] This increase in free radicals may also exacerbate joint inflammation and degradation in rheumatoid arthritis.

Functional medicine considerations

In assessing whether iron deficiency may be the cause of symptoms such as fatigue, lack of energy, shortness of breath, or chronic infection, patient history should be explored for frank or occult bleeding, vegetarian diet, malabsorption, or hypochlorhydria.

Signs and symptoms of possible iron overload (as discussed earlier) should also warrant iron status assessment. Dietary supplementation, factors that enhance absorption, family history of hemochromatosis, and/or alcoholism should be explored if toxicity is suspected. Use of iron pans and food storage bins should also raise suspicion if symptoms of overload are present.[79]

Manganese

Manganese is important in a wide range of metabolic functions. Small amounts of manganese can be found in bones, pituitary gland, liver, and elsewhere.

Absorption

While the details of manganese absorption are not entirely understood, studies demonstrate efficiency of absorption to be between 1 and 25 percent.[80] It is believed that the entire small intestine absorbs manganese. It is also believed that homeostasis occurs primarily through excretion, because absorption is not altered by the amount of manganese ingested.

Absorption is inhibited by phytate. Other minerals such as iron, calcium, and phosphorus create a greater need for manganese, but only iron alters absorption significantly. Aluminum reduces tissue stores of manganese. Although uptake mechanisms are not clear, manganese is similar to iron in physiochemistry. It appears that they compete for absorption, as manganese absorption is decreased when iron content of the meal is high.[81]

Most of the manganese is then taken to the liver and goes into several metabolic pools (lysosomes, mitochondria, nucleus, new proteins, and free manganese). Transferrin transports manganese to other tissues. Manganese is not stored well, and much is excreted in feces via bile.[82]

Functions

Manganese helps with carbohydrate metabolism, bone development, prothrombin synthesis, protein digestion, collagen formation, fatty acid synthesis, and protein synthesis. In addition, manganese is a cofactor in a number of enzymes important in energy production and antioxidant defense (e.g., superoxide dismutase).[83]

Sources

Table 6.16 lists food sources of manganese.

Therapeutic considerations

Deficiency symptoms include impaired growth, poor carbohydrate and fat metabolism, and skeletal problems. Manganese is important in utero for the development of the otoliths needed in the inner ear for equilibrium.

Studies have found that adults who are deficient in manganese report loss of hair color, skin rash, decreased hair and nail growth, and decreased HDL cholesterol.[84]

Safety and toxicity

Manganese ingestion through diet and supplemental intake is generally very safe. However, if iron intake is low, the possibility of iron deficiency may result from manganese supplementation, as manganese competes for absorption with iron. Some individuals with amyotrophic lateral sclerosis have been found to have increased levels of manganese in the brain. However, the relationship is not conclusive.[85] Manganese toxicity may result in extrapyramidal effects similar to those of Parkinson's disease.

TABLE 6.16 *Food Sources of Manganese*
Milligrams (mg) per 100 grams edible portion (100 grams = 3 1/2 oz)

3.5	Pecans	0.13	Swiss cheese
2.8	Brazil nuts	0.13	Corn
2.5	Almonds	0.11	Cabbage
1.8	Barley	0.10	Peach
1.3	Rye	0.09	Butter
1.3	Buckwheat	0.06	Tangerine
1.3	Split peas, dry	0.06	Peas
1.1	Whole wheat	0.05	Eggs
0.8	Walnuts	0.04	Beets
0.8	Fresh spinach	0.04	Coconut
0.7	Peanuts	0.03	Apple
0.6	Oats	0.03	Orange
0.5	Raisins	0.03	Pear
0.5	Turnip greens	0.03	Lamb chops
0.5	Rhubarb	0.03	Pork chops
0.4	Beet greens	0.03	Cantaloupe
0.3	Brussels sprouts	0.03	Tomato
0.3	Oatmeal	0.02	Whole milk
0.2	Cornmeal	0.02	Chicken breasts
0.2	Millet	0.02	Green beans
0.19	Gorgonzola cheese	0.02	Apricot
0.16	Carrots	0.01	Beef liver
0.15	Broccoli	0.01	Scallops
0.14	Brown rice	0.01	Halibut
0.14	Whole wheat bread	0.01	Cucumber

Cloves, ginger, thyme, bay leaves, and tea are also high in manganese.

Functional medicine considerations

If an individual has iron deficiency anemia and the reasons are not clear, it may be prudent to explore manganese status and/or manganese intake to determine whether competition resulting in iron deficiency exists. Manganese status should also be explored in individuals who complain of a lack of energy. If free radical toxicity is suspected, manganese status relative to the activity of superoxide dismutase should be explored.

Molybdenum

Since molybdenum changes its oxidative state readily, it can act as an electron transfer agent in oxidation/reduction reactions. Much molybdenum in the body is in a bound cofactor form attached to the mitochondrial membrane. It is then transformed to an active enzyme molecule.[86] More research about molybdenum still needs to be conducted.

Absorption

Molybdenum from food is easily absorbed in the stomach and proximal small intestine. Molybdenum may be transported by both diffusion and active transport. Excretion through the kidneys is the major regulatory mechanism for molybdenum.

Functions

The primary role of molybdenum is acting as a coenzyme for a number of enzymes, including xanthine oxidase (uric acid formation), aldehyde oxidase (alcohol detoxification), and sulfite oxidase (detoxification of sulfite).

Sources

Table 6.17 indicates food sources of molybdenum, although the soil content of molybdenum may vary, as with other minerals.

Therapeutic considerations

Because of the need for molybdenum in the detoxification of sulfite (by sulfite oxidase), a molybdenum deficiency may result in sulfite toxicity, which may manifest as tachycardia, headache, and disorientation.[87] Molybdenum supplementation may be useful in patients with sulfite sensitivity. Molybdenum's role as a cofactor in detoxification enzymes may help prevent some cancers, such as esophageal cancer. Combining molybdenum with fluoride may help reduce dental caries more than fluoride alone.[88]

Safety and toxicity

Molybdenum is a very safe mineral with rare toxicity, probably owing to excretory regulation. Large, regular doses of 10–15 mg per day may cause some individuals to experience symptoms similar to gout because of increases in uric acid production.[89]

Functional medicine considerations

If the patient is aware or suspicious of sulfite sensitivity, molybdenum status should be assessed. In these cases, there is the possibility that molybdenum may be insufficient to

TABLE 6.17   *Food Sources of Molybdenum*
Micrograms (mcg) per 100 grams edible portion (100 grams = 3 1/2 oz)

155	Lentils	31	Cottage cheese
135	Beef liver	30	Beef
130	Split peas	30	Potatoes
120	Cauliflower	25	Onions
110	Green peas	25	Coconut
109	Brewer's yeast	25	Pork
100	Wheat germ	24	Lamb
100	Spinach	21	Green beans
77	Beef kidney	19	Crab
75	Brown rice	19	Molasses
70	Garlic	16	Cantaloupe
60	Oats	14	Apricots
53	Eggs	10	Raisins
50	Rye bread	10	Butter
45	Corn	7	Strawberries
42	Barley	5	Carrots
40	Fish	5	Cabbage
36	Whole wheat	3	Whole milk
32	Whole wheat bread	1	Goat milk
32	Chicken		

detoxify the sulfites. In cases in which alcohol consumption is excessive, molybdenum may support detoxification mechanisms.

Selenium

Selenium is considered an essential mineral. It is important for the role it plays in antioxidant activities, working as a component of glutathione peroxidase with vitamin E.

Absorption and regulation

Food sources of selenium are in the form of seleno amino acids such as selenomethionine and selenocysteine. Supplemental selenium is often an inorganic form. Absorption of selenium is usually relatively efficient.

Selenium regulation keeps levels of the reactive molecule selenocysteine low and selenium in homeostasis by excretion of metabolites. Selenocysteine may be the primary compound in which selenium has biological activity.[90]

Functions

Selenium is important as a cofactor of glutathione peroxidase. It works with vitamin E in the vital antioxidant systems of the body.

Selenium also helps prevent cancer and heart disease and reduces heavy metal toxicity. This trace mineral is also important in sulfur amino acid metabolism.[91]

Sources

Selenium is found in meats and seafood. While it is also found in vegetables and grains, the soil content will determine the content of these food sources. Table 6.18 lists food sources of selenium.

Therapeutic considerations

Selenium supplementation may help decrease the risk of cancer because of its role in supporting DNA repair. The antioxidant action of selenium may also help prevent heart disease and decrease asthma symptoms.

The deficiency symptoms of selenium are similar to vitamin E symptoms—conditions related to poor antioxidant activity. If the soil is deficient in selenium, there is risk for cardiac conditions such as cardiomyopathy, and

TABLE 6.18   *Food Sources of Selenium*
Microgram (mcg) per 100 grams edible portion (100 grams = 3 1/2 oz)

146	Butter	25	Garlic
141	Smoked herring	24	Barley
123	Smelt	19	Orange juice
111	Wheat germ	19	Gelatin
103	Brazil nuts	19	Beer
89	Apple cider vinegar	18	Beef liver
77	Scallops	18	Lamb chop
66	Barley	18	Egg yolk
66	Whole wheat bread	12	Mushrooms
65	Lobster	12	Chicken
63	Bran	10	Swiss cheese
59	Shrimp	5	Cottage cheese
57	Red swiss chard	5	Wine
56	Oats	4	Radishes
55	Clams	4	Grape juice
51	King crab	3	Pecans
49	Oysters	2	Hazelnuts
48	Milk	2	Almonds
43	Cod	2	Green beans
39	Brown rice	2	Kidney beans
34	Top round steak	2	Onion
30	Lamb	2	Carrots
27	Turnips	2	Cabbage
26	Molasses	1	Orange

there is increased risk of cancer. In addition, immune function will be reduced.

Studies also indicate that selenium is helpful in decreasing symptoms associated with rheumatoid arthritis, including reducing inflammatory markers and decreasing tenderness and swelling in joints.[92]

Recent arguments in favor of selenium and vitamin E supplementation for pregnant women suggest that cerebral palsy might be prevented with these antioxidants.[93]

Selenium enhances immune function by helping phagocytes in microbicidal activity through improved glutathione peroxidase activity. Selenium helps with metabolism of hydroperoxides produced as part of inflammation, and helps modulate the phagocytic respiratory burst.[94]

Safety and toxicity

Selenium can be toxic in amounts greater than 900 mcg per day. It is recommended, however, that in the absence of further studies, individuals should not take supplemental selenium greater than 200 mcg per day unless a physician advises doing so. Excess selenium might interfere with enzyme systems related to sulfur metabolism. Liver disease and impaired bone and tooth growth may result as well.[95]

Functional medicine considerations

Individuals whose histories indicate recurrent infections, difficulties controlling inflammatory disorders, fatigue, or other indicators of oxidative stress should have selenium status assessed. Where family history of cancer is evident, selenium supplementation may be warranted, especially if the patient's diet is low in selenium or poor soil content is suspected.

Vanadium

Vanadium has only recently begun to be viewed as an essential nutrient. Most of the current research on vanadium has examined its role in glucose metabolism.

Absorption

Very little ingested vanadium actually is absorbed. The absorption probably takes place in the upper GI tract. It is rapidly removed and kept in the kidneys, liver, testes, bone, and spleen. Vanadium may bind with iron-containing proteins as part of its metabolism and retention in organs. Most vanadium is excreted in the urine.[96]

Functions

It is possible that vanadium is involved in the metabolism of lipids and catecholamines, and it may help form red blood cells and affect the function of the thyroid gland. Some recent studies indicate vanadium may help protect against cancer, in the management of diabetes, and in cell division.[97] One of the most promising effects studied recently is the improvement of insulin sensitivity with vanadium supplementation.[98]

Sources

Table 6.19 lists sources of vanadium in foods.

Therapeutic considerations

Deficiency symptoms have not actually been noted for vanadium in humans. However, animal studies have demonstrated some deficiency symptoms including increased abortion, decreased milk production, hepatic lipid changes, growth impairment, and thyroid metabolic changes.[99]

The principal therapeutic use for vanadium at this time is as a glucose metabolism regulator. However, vanadium may also help to inhibit cholesterol synthesis.

Safety and toxicity

Symptoms of excess vanadium may include increased blood pressure, decreased coenzymes A and Q1O, and interference with cellular energy production. Bipolar disorder may be a toxic side effect, as increased vanadium in the hair samples of such individuals has been found.[100] Toxicity may begin at 10-20 mg per day.

Functional medicine considerations

A history of or current diagnosis of NIDDM should prompt clinicians to consider vanadium assessment and supplementation. If cholesterol levels are also high, vanadium status should be explored. Low levels of vanadium may indicate that a nutritional therapeutic approach to lowering the cholesterol levels would be helpful. The patient who presents with symptoms of Syndrome X, the constellation of symptoms associated with insulin insensitivity and increased fasting/postprandial serum insulin, may also benefit from vanadium supplementation.

TABLE 6.19 *Food Sources of Vanadium*
Microgram (mcg) per 100 grams edible portion (100 grams = 3 1/2 oz)

100	Buckwheat	10	Cabbage
80	Parsley	10	Garlic
70	Soybeans	6	Tomatoes
64	Safflower oil	5	Radishes
42	Eggs	5	Onions
41	Sunflower seed oil	5	Whole wheat
35	Oats	4	Lobster
30	Olive oil	4	Beets
15	Sunflower seeds	3	Apples
15	Corn	2	Plums
14	Green beans	2	Lettuce
11	Peanut oil	2	Millet
10	Carrots		

Boron

Boron is a trace mineral that is important for maintaining healthy bone.

Absorption

Boron is rapidly absorbed, and its homeostasis is maintained by urinary excretion. Since boron is primarily bound to oxygen in organic tissue, it is probably converted to $B(OH)_3$ in the gastrointestinal tract.

Function

It is quite possible that boron modulates cell signaling by assisting in transmembrane ion movement, thus exerting an influence on cellular response to hormones. Evidence points to the need for boron in the body's absorption of calcium and for protection against calcium loss, possibly by enhancing estrogen activity in bone.[101,102]

Sources

If the soil contains adequate levels of boron, fruits and vegetables will be the primary sources of this mineral.

Therapeutic considerations

Boron is considered important for bone and joint health. Safe and adequate dose is 1.5–3.0 mg per day.

Calcium metabolism may be impaired if boron is deficient. The result would be bone mineral loss and central nervous system dysfunction as calcium levels in the brain are reduced.[103]

Safety and toxicity

Boron is relatively safe. However, nausea, vomiting, diarrhea, dermatitis, and lethargy may occur if doses of boron exceed 300 mg per day.[104]

Functional medicine considerations

Boron should be considered in situations where fruit and vegetable intake is low and in women who are menopausal.

SUMMARY

Perhaps nowhere in human nutrition is understanding nutrient interactions more important than in the area of minerals. The observation that "mineral A" may interfere or enhance the absorption of "mineral B," together with a clear understanding of the physiologic roles played by "mineral B" may present clinicians with an entirely new way of viewing their patients' symptoms.

The knowledge that mineral cofactors play a key role in many biochemical processes, understanding the specific roles for these nutrients, and recognizing possible symptoms experienced by the patient as a shortage or excess of the nutrients, will help clinicians develop a more in-depth view of the dysfunctions that might lead to symptoms and to disease processes. With appropriate assessment of mineral status, adequate and individually designed nutritional therapies can be applied with the goal of improving underlying function for optimal biochemical activities.

CHAPTER 6 REFERENCES

1. Garrison R, Somer E. Nutrition Desk Reference. 3rd ed. New Canaan, Conn; Keats Publishing; 1995:147.
2. Garrison R, Somer E. Nutrition Desk Reference. 3rd ed. New Canaan, Conn; Keats Publishing; 1995:147.
3. Garrison R, Somer E. Nutrition Desk Reference. 3rd ed. New Canaan, Conn; Keats Publishing; 1995:148
4. Schaafsma, G. Bioavailability of calcium and magnesium. Eur J Clin Nutr, 1997;51(Suppl1): S13–S16.
5. Zeigler EE, Filer LJ, eds. Present Knowledge in Nutrition. Washington, DC: ILSI Press; 1996:245.
6. Nguyen UN, Dumloulin G, Henriet MT, Regnard J. Aspartame ingestion increases urinary calcium, but not oxalate excretion, in healthy subjects. J Clin Endocrinol Metab. 1998;83(1): 165–168.
7. Coudray C, Bellanger J, Castiglia-Delavaud, et al. Effect of soluble or partly-soluble dietary fibres supplementation on absorption and balance of calcium, magnesium, iron and zinc in healthy young men. Eur J Clin Nutr. 1997;51:375–380.
8. Garrison R, Somer E. Nutrition Desk Reference. 3rd ed. New Canaan, Conn; Keats Publishing; 1995:151.
9. Garrison R, Somer E. Nutrition Desk Reference. 3rd ed. New Canaan, Conn; Keats Publishing; 1995:150.
10. Murray M. Encyclopedia of Nutritional Supplements. Rocklin, Calif: Prima Publishing: 1996:156.
11. Sanchez M, dela Sierra A, Coca A, et al. Oral calcium supplementation reduces intraplatelet free calcium concentration and insulin resistance in essential hypertensive patients. Hypertension. 1997:29(1Pt 2):531–536.
12. Lind L, Skarfors E, Berglund L, et al. Serum calcium: a new independent, prospective risk factor for myocardial infarction in middle-aged men followed for 18 years. J Clin Epidemiol. 1997: 50:967–973.
13. Garrison R, Somer E. Nutrition Desk Reference. 3rd ed. New Canaan, Conn; Keats Publishing; 1995:150.
14. Murray M. Encyclopedia of Nutritional Supplements. Rocklin, Calif: Prima Publishing:1996:149.
15. Murray M. Encyclopedia of Nutritional Supplements. Rocklin, Calif: Prima Publishing:1996: 154–155.
16. Dawson-Hughes B, Harris SS, Krall EA, Dallal GE. Effect of calcium and vitamin D supplementation on bone density in men and women 65 years of age or older. N Engl J Med. 1997; 337(10):670–676.
17. Zeigler EE, Filer LJ, eds. Present Knowledge in Nutrition. Washington, DC: ILSI Press; 1996:245–246.
18. Garrison R, Somer E. Nutrition Desk Reference. 3rd ed. New Canaan, Conn; Keats Publishing; 1995:166.
19. Garrison R, Somer E. Nutrition Desk Reference. 3rd ed. New Canaan, Conn; Keats Publishing; 1995:166.
20. Garrison R, Somer E. Nutrition Desk Reference. 3rd ed. New Canaan, Conn; Keats Publishing; 1995:166.
21. Zeigler EE, Filer LJ, eds. Present Knowledge in Nutrition. Washington, DC: ILSI Press; 1996:256.
22. Garrison R, Somer E. Nutrition Desk Reference. 3rd ed. New Canaan, Conn; Keats Publishing; 1995:159.
23. Garrison R, Somer E. Nutrition Desk Reference. 3rd ed. New Canaan, Conn; Keats Publishing; 1995:257.
24. Schaafsma, G. Bioavailability of calcium and magnesium. Eur J Clin Nutr. 1997;51(Suppl1): S13–S16.

25. Garrison R, Somer E. Nutrition Desk Reference. 3rd ed. New Canaan, Conn; Keats Publishing; 1995:159.

26. Serebruany VL Herzog WR, Schlossberg ML, Gurbel PA. Bolus magnesium infusion in humans is associated with predominantly unfavorable changes in platelet aggregation and certain homeostatic factors. Pharmacol Res. 1997; 36(1):17–22.

27. Yang CY. Calcium and magnesium in drinking water and risk of death from cerebrovascular disease. Stroke. 1998;29(2):411–414.

28. Murray M. Encyclopedia of Nutritional Supplements. Rocklin, Calif: Prima Publishing: 1996:160.

29. Elamin A, Tuvemo T. Magnesium and insulin-dependent diabetes mellitus. Diabetes Res Clin Pract. 1990;10(3):203–209.

30. Romano TJ. Magnesium deficiency in systemic lupus erythematosus. J Nutr Environ Med. 1997;7:107–111.

31. Paolisso G, Sgambato S, Pizza G, et al. Improved insulin response and action by chronic magnesium administration in aged NIDDM subjects. Diabetes Care. 1989;12(4):265–272.

32. Yang CY. Calcium and magnesium in drinking water and risk of death from cerebrovascular disease. Stroke. 1998;29(2):411–414.

33. Itoh K, Kawasaka T, Nakamura M. The effects of high oral magnesium supplementation on blood pressure, serum lipids and related variables in apparently healthy Japanese subjects. Br J Nutr. 1997;78(5):737–750.

34. Garrison R, Somer E. Nutrition Desk Reference. 3rd ed. New Canaan, Conn; Keats Publishing; 1995:162.

35. Garrison R, Somer E. Nutrition Desk Reference. 3rd ed. New Canaan, Conn; Keats Publishing; 1995:162.

36. Zeigler EE, Filer LJ, eds. Present Knowledge in Nutrition. Washington, DC: ILSI Press; 1996:265.

37. Zeigler EE, Filer LJ, eds. Present Knowledge in Nutrition. Washington, DC: ILSI Press; 1996:266.

38. Zeigler EE, Filer LJ, eds. Present Knowledge in Nutrition. Washington, DC: ILSI Press; 1996: 267–268.

39. Garrison R, Somer E. Nutrition Desk Reference. 3rd ed. New Canaan, Conn; Keats Publishing; 1995:168,172.

40. Garrison R, Somer E. Nutrition Desk Reference. 3rd ed. New Canaan, Conn; Keats Publishing; 1995:169.

41. Garrison R, Somer E. Nutrition Desk Reference. 3rd ed. New Canaan, Conn; Keats Publishing; 1995:169.

42. Garrison R, Somer E. Nutrition Desk Reference. 3rd ed. New Canaan, Conn; Keats Publishing; 1995:173.

43. Whelton PK, He J, Cutler JA, et al. Effects of oral potassium on blood pressure. Meta-analysis of randomized controlled clinical trials. JAMA. 1997;277(20):1624–1632.

44. Zeigler EE, Filer LJ, eds. Present Knowledge in Nutrition. Washington, DC: ILSI Press; 1996:345.

45. Zeigler EE, Filer LJ, eds. Present Knowledge in Nutrition. Washington, DC: ILSI Press; 1996:346.

46. Garrison R, Somer E. Nutrition Desk Reference. 3rd ed. New Canaan, Conn: Keats Publishing; 1995:183.

47. Hasten DL, Hegsted M, Keenan MJ, et al. Damage effects of chromium picolinate on growth and body composition in the rat. Nutr Res. 1997(17):1175-1186.

48. Garrison R, Somer E. Nutrition Desk Reference. 3rd ed. New Canaan, Conn; Keats Publishing; 1995:181.

49. Zeigler EE, Filer LJ, eds. Present Knowledge in Nutrition. Washington, DC: ILSI Press; 1996: 293–296.

50. Garrison R, Somer E. Nutrition Desk Reference. 3rd ed. New Canaan, Conn; Keats Publishing; 1995:217.

51. Murray M. Encyclopedia of Nutritional Supplements. Rocklin, Calif: Prima Publishing: 1996:181.

52. Kremer JM, Bigaouette J. Nutrient intake of patients with rheumatoid arthritis is deficient in pyridoxine, zinc, copper and magnesium. J. Rheumatol. 1996;23(6):990–994.

53. Blostein-Fujii A, DiSilvestro RA, Frid D, Katz C, Malarkey W. Short-term zinc supplementation in women with non-insulin-dependent diabetes mellitus: effects on plasma 5-nucleotidase activities insulin-like growth factor I concentrations and lysoprotein oxidation rates in vitro. Am J Clin Nutr. 1997;66(3):639–642.

54. Zinc lozenges reduce the duration of common cold symptoms. Nutr Rev. 1997;55(3):82–85.

55. Murray M. Encyclopedia of Nutritional Supplements. Rocklin, Calif: Prima Publishing; 1996:189.

56. Garrison R, Somer E. Nutrition Desk Reference. 3rd ed. New Canaan, Conn; Keats Publishing; 1995:221.

57. Zeigler EE, Filer LJ, eds. Present Knowledge in Nutrition. Washington, DC: ILSI Press; 1996:307.

58. Fairweather-Tait SJ. Bioavailability of Copper. Eur J Clin Nutr. 1997;51(Suppl1):S24–S26.

59. Zeigler EE, Filer LJ, eds. Present Knowledge in Nutrition. Washington, DC: ILSI Press; 1996:308.

60. Garrison R, Somer E. Nutrition Desk Reference. 3rd ed. New Canaan, Conn; Keats Publishing; 1995:188.

61. Garrison R, Somer E. Nutrition Desk Reference. 3rd ed. New Canaan, Conn; Keats Publishing; 1995:188.

62. Murray M. Encyclopedia of Nutritional Supplements. Rocklin, Calif: Prima Publishing: 1996:199–200.

63. Garrison R, Somer E. Nutrition Desk Reference. 3rd ed. New Canaan, Conn; Keats Publishing; 1995:189.

64. Murray M. Encyclopedia of Nutritional Supplements. Rocklin, Calif: Prima Publishing:1996:202.

65. Murray M. Encyclopedia of Nutritional Supplements. Rocklin, Calif: Prima Publishing:1996:203.

66. Garrison R, Somer E. Nutrition Desk Reference. 3rd ed. New Canaan, Conn; Keats Publishing; 1995:189.

67. Chandra RK. Micronutrients and Immune Functions: An Overview. In: Bendich A, Chandra RK, eds. Micronutrients and Immune Functions. New York: New York Academy of Sciences; 1990.

68. Garrison R, Somer E. Nutrition Desk Reference. 3rd ed. New Canaan, Conn; Keats Publishing; 1995:194.

69. Murray M. Encyclopedia of Nutritional Supplements. Rocklin, Calif: Prima Publishing: 1996:204.

70. Chandra RK. Micronutrients and Immune Functions: An Overview. In: Bendich A, Chandra RK, eds. Micronutrients and Immune Functions. New York: New York Academy of Sciences; 1990:13.

71. Garrison R, Somer E. Nutrition Desk Reference. 3rd ed. New Canaan, Conn; Keats Publishing; 1995:197.

72. Murray M. Encyclopedia of Nutritional Supplements. Rocklin, Calif: Prima Publishing: 1996:207.

73. Hurrell RF. Bioavailability of iodine. Eur J Clin Nutr. 1997Jan;51(Suppl1):S9-S12.

74. Chandra RK. Micronutrients and Immune Functions: An Overview. In: Bendich A, Chandra RK, eds. Micronutrients and Immune Functions. New York: New York Academy of Sciences; 1990:13.

75. Sherman AR. Influence of iron on immunity and disease resistance in micronutrients and immune functions. In: Bendich A, Chandra RK, eds. Micronutrients and Immune Functions. New York: New York Academy of Sciences; 1990:140–145.

76. Murray M. Encyclopedia of Nutritional Supplements. Rocklin, Calif: Prima Publishing:1996:208-209.

77. Garrison R, Somer E. Nutrition Desk Reference. 3rd ed. New Canaan, Conn; Keats Publishing; 1995:199.

78. Garrison R, Somer E. Nutrition Desk Reference. 3rd ed. New Canaan, Conn; Keats Publishing; 1995:204.

79. Hathcock, JM, Rader JI. Micronutrient Safety in Micronutrients. In: Bendich A, Chandra RK, eds. Micronutrients and Immune Functions.

New York: New York Academy of Sciences; 1990:262.

80. Zeigler EE, Filer LJ, eds. Present Knowledge in Nutrition. Washington, DC: ILSI Press; 1996:334.

81. Zeigler EE, Filer LJ, eds. Present Knowledge in Nutrition. Washington, DC: ILSI Press; 1996:335.

82. Zeigler EE, Filer LJ, eds. Present Knowledge in Nutrition. Washington, DC: ILSI Press; 1996:336.

83. Garrison R, Somer E. Nutrition Desk Reference. 3rd ed. New Canaan, Conn; Keats Publishing; 1995:206.

84. Murray M. Encyclopedia of Nutritional Supplements. Rocklin, Calif: Prima Publishing: 1996:215.

85. Zeigler EE, Filer LJ, eds. Present Knowledge in Nutrition. Washington, DC: ILSI Press; 1996:340.

86. Zeigler EE, Filer LJ, eds. Present Knowledge in Nutrition. Washington, DC: ILSI Press; 1996:358.

87. Murray M. Encyclopedia of Nutritional Supplements. Rocklin, Calif: Prima Publishing: 1996:218.

88. Murray M. Encyclopedia of Nutritional Supplements. Rocklin, Calif: Prima Publishing: 1996:220.

89. Murray M. Encyclopedia of Nutritional Supplements. Rocklin, Calif: Prima Publishing: 1996:221.

90. Zeigler EE, Filer LJ, eds. Present Knowledge in Nutrition. Washington, DC: ILSI Press; 1996:321.

91. Garrison R, Somer E. Nutrition Desk Reference. 3rd ed. New Canaan, Conn; Keats Publishing; 1995:209–210.

92. Heinle K, Adam A, Gradl M, Wiseman M, Adam O. Selenium concentration in erythrocytes of patients with rheumatoid arthritis. Clinical and laboratory chemistry infection markers during administration of selenium. Med Klin. 1997;15;92(suppl3):29–31.

93. Money DFL, Holborow PL. Some aspects of cerebral palsy: a chronic motor dysfunction. NZ Science Rev. 1997:54(1-2);10–15.

94. Spallholz JE, Boylan LM, Larsen HS. Advances in understanding selenium's role in the immune system. In: Bendich A, Chandra RK, eds. Micronutrients and Immune Functions. New York: New York Academy of Sciences; 1990:124.

95. Garrison R, Somer E. Nutrition Desk Reference. 3rd ed. New Canaan, Conn; Keats Publishing; 1995:212.

96. Zeigler EE, Filer LJ, eds. Present Knowledge in Nutrition. Washington, DC: ILSI Press; 1996:365.

97. Garrison R, Somer E. Nutrition Desk Reference. 3rd ed. New Canaan, Conn; Keats Publishing; 1995:327.

98. Goldfine AB, Simonsine DC, Folli F, Patti MC, Kahn, CR. Metabolic effects of sodium metavanadate in humans with insulin-dependent and noninsulin-dependent diabetes mellitus in vivo and in vitro studies. J Clin Endocrinol Metab. 1995;80(11):3311–3320.

99. French RJ, Jones PJ. Role of vanadium in nutrition: metabolism, essentiality and dietary considerations. Life Sci. 1993;52(4):339–346.

100. Murray M. Encyclopedia of Nutritional Supplements. Rocklin, Calif: Prima Publishing: 1996:234.

101. Zeigler EE, Filer LJ, eds. Present Knowledge in Nutrition. Washington, DC: ILSI Press; 1996:357.

102. Murray M. Encyclopedia of Nutritional Supplements. Rocklin, Calif: Prima Publishing: 1996:191.

103. Zeigler EE, Filer LJ, eds. Present Knowledge in Nutrition. Washington, DC: ILSI Press; 1996:358.

104. Zeigler EE, Filer LJ, eds. Present Knowledge in Nutrition. Washington, DC: ILSI Press; 1996:358.

7

Digestion, Absorption, and Gut Ecology

Y OU ARE WHAT YOU EAT" IS ONLY partially true. You are also what you absorb, and separating the nutrients from the food you eat and from the waste products that leave your body involves numerous physiological functions. Among these functions are digestion, assimilation, nutrient distribution, tissue uptake, and use of nutrients at specific cellular sites.

Few practitioners would question the importance of digestion and absorption for optimal health. Yet given the eating patterns and digestive difficulties in the United States, nutritional support of gastrointestinal function is not nearly as widespread in clinical practice as might be expected. U.S. adults frequently list digestive complaints as one of the many reasons for seeing the doctor. U.S. companies compensate millions of dollars in disability wages for employees' digestive disorders. Retail stores carry more than 200 over-the-counter remedies for gastrointestinal problems, many of which actually create additional digestive problems. This portrait of gastrointestinal dysfunction is matched by an equally dysfunctional pattern of food intake. Compared to other countries, U.S. adults consume a disproportionate amount of sweeteners, soda pop, and food additives.

In spite of these patterns, most practitioners have not rigorously addressed digestive and absorptive function in their patients, except when assigning diagnostic codes like peptic ulcer, esophageal reflux, or malabsorption syndrome. Furthermore, when treating chronic conditions not traditionally linked to the GI (for example, dermatological conditions), most practitioners have simply not placed a focus on GI function and its support. Ample research supports the hypothesis that a significant number of patients with chronic dysfunction—even when the dysfunction causes symptoms in body systems with no apparent connection to the GI tract—have digestive and absorptive imbalances that are significantly compromising their health.

This chapter focuses more closely on the functional relationships among digestion, absorption, and dysfunction, and outlines a generic, adaptable system that can address a wide variety of digestive and absorptive problems. What follows first is a brief review of digestion and absorption, with special emphasis given to nutritional components and food-related patterns.

GASTROINTESTINAL FUNCTION

Digestion

The digestive tract is a complex ecological network that must achieve acid/base balance for proper pH, adequate smooth muscle tone for moving materials down the digestive tract, proper acid secretion in the stomach, sufficient pancreatic digestive enzyme secretion into the intestine, sufficient bile secretion for fat absorption, and integrity of the gastrointestinal mucosa for protection and nutrient absorption. Newer research regarding the relationship between lifestyle and digestion illustrates that healthy digestion involves more than simply the physiology of the digestive tract.

Lifestyle Factors Affecting Proper Digestion

In addition to physical behaviors commonly recognized as compromising digestive capacity—e.g., smoking, caffeine, or alcohol consumption—a list of behaviors equally problematic to digestive support is growing. Stressful events in and of themselves may disrupt the digestive process.[1] Reducing stress has successfully ameliorated digestion-related disorders such as abdominal pain, chronic diarrhea, and peptic ulcer in some cases. Relaxation techniques have reduced gastric acid secretion in hyperchlorhydric patients.[2] Balancing digestive function by reducing stress may partially be attributed to a global nervous system shift from a sympathetic to parasympathetic tone.

The Brain and Gut: Cephalic Phase of Digestion

The cephalic phase of the digestive response is critical to healthy digestion. Cephalic (pertaining to the head) is the phase in which a sensory stimulus—any sound, sight, odor, taste, or texture associated with food—provokes a digestion-related response in the body. Some researchers even consider thoughts to be cephalic phase stimuli, since thoughts can alter digestive activity in the absence of external sensory stimuli. Cephalic phase analyses include numerous physiological responses such as thermogenic response, salivary response, heart rate changes, mesenteric flow changes, changes in cardiac output and stroke volume, diuretic changes and natriuresis, digestive enzyme secretions, altered gastric acid secretion, altered intestinal motility, release of GI hormones, and other intestinal process changes.

Although the nature of cephalic phase response appears to be highly transient and limited in duration, the magnitude of the response is dramatic and physiologically significant. Cephalic phase sensory stimuli can increase release of gut peptides like cholecystokinin, somatostatin, and neurotensin by more than 50 percent.[3] Cardiovascular parameters like cardiac output and stroke volumes, release of pancreatic enzymes, and polypeptide hormones like insulin and glucagon receive less impact (ranging from 10 to 15 percent).[4]

To fully support digestion, individuals need to carefully address the circumstances surrounding their eating habits. Practitioners can help patients by recommending simple behavioral changes. For example, practitioners can encourage patients to eat in places that they do not associate with stress (e.g., where they pay their monthly bills). Or practitioners may outline "ritual" steps for patients to follow when they sit down to eat (similar to prayer in religious approaches to eating). For some individuals, such behavioral changes can influence digestion more dramatically than taking pancreatic enzymes, glandulars, bitters, or other digestive aids.

Physiology of Digestion

The 25- to 30-foot digestive tract extends from the mouth to the anus. The tract helps break down the large protein, carbohydrate, and fat molecules in foods into smaller substances that can be absorbed into the blood by the brush border cells of the intestinal mucosa. These small food breakdown products include monosaccharides and disaccharides that originate from carbohydrates, amino acids, dipeptides, tripeptides from proteins, and free fatty acids from fats. In this digestive process, vitamins and minerals are also liberated from food materials, enabling these nutrients to be readily absorbed by the body.

The first physiological aspect of digestion begins with chewing. Macrobiotic approaches to eating suggest that each mouthful of food be chewed 200 times before swallowing. One rule of thumb is that if patients can still identify the food in their mouths based on texture alone, they have not chewed it sufficiently. Whatever chewing does not accomplish mechanically must be completed by the digestive tract chemically through fluid and enzyme secretion. No complete remedy exists for symptoms associated with poorly chewed food. Again, while many practitioners are tempted to prescribe supplements as remedies for poor lifestyle practices, patients can achieve many successful digestive results through cost-free, self-care behaviors.

Digestion in the Mouth

The mouth secretes a variety of fluids essential to digestion. While salivary alpha amylase (also called ptyalin) is the most researched oral digestive enzyme, other important secretions include mucopolysaccharides, ion-containing fluids, and transfer factor (TF)—an important factor in vitamin B12 absorption. Researchers have extensively studied hyposecretion of mouth fluids in older individuals on prescription medications, but even simple factors such as whole body underhydration can reduce salivary secretions and compromise digestion (Table 7.1).

Digestion in the Stomach

Hypochlorhydria—inadequate secretion of gastric acid by the parietal cells in the stomach wall—is an undervalued, under-recognized clinical component of digestion-related health disorders (Table 7.2). Given the excess-calorie, high-fat, animal-based nature of the average US diet, one would not expect hypochlorhydria to be a typical issue. In fact, over-consuming high-fat foods at a single meal typically encourages *oversecretion* of gastric acid. When researchers recognized H2 histamine receptor sites in the nervous system as neurological mediators of gastric secretion in the 1970s, H2 receptor blockers like cimetidine (Tagamet™) and ranitidine (Zantac™) became widely available by prescription. Such supplements have even more widespread use in the 1990s since their status has changed to over-the-counter. Excessive and inappropriate use of these H2-blocking antacids has transformed diet-induced hyperchlorhydria into medication-induced hypochlorhydria in many U.S. adults, while initial instigating dietary causes of indigestion remain unexplored. The introduction of the proton pump inhibitors (hydrogen-potassium adenosine triphosphate

inhibitors like omeprazole) exacerbates the problem.

Research suggests that low gastric acidity may influence the development of diseases such as food allergies, rheumatoid arthritis,[5] acne rosacea,[6] and asthma[7] (Table 7.3). The ability to produce gastric acid decreases with age, and more than half the population over the age of 60 has insufficient secretory abilities.[8]

Chronic inflammation may also play a pivotal role in hypochlorhydria and certain types of hypochlorhydria involve parietal cell antibodies and have a distinct autoimmune component.[9] Overactivity and imbalanced immune system activity in the gut-associated lymphatic tissue (GALT) is connected with a wide variety of gastrointestinal disorders. Chronic inflammation remains a common theme that can be directly addressed through elimination diets to lower immunogenicity.

Chronic reduction of gastric acid secretion has many predictable deleterious effects on the GI tract and digestion. Hypochlorhydria invites bacterial overgrowth in the small intestine since elevated pH values allow greater numbers of small intestine microflora to proliferate. This overgrowth of small intestine bacteria compromises nutrient digestion and absorption, particularly digestion and absorption of the B-complex vitamins and the minerals iron and calcium. Of the B vitamins, folate, B6, and B12 absorption are most compromised. A number of clinical laboratories measure small bowel bacterial overgrowth by a challenge dose of lactulose or glucose with subsequent recapture of hydrogen or methane gases in a breath test. More

TABLE 7.1 *Major Digestive Enzymes*

Enzyme	Source	Substrate	Product
Saliva			
Salivary amylase	Salivary glands	Starches (polysaccharides)	Maltose (disaccharide), maltotriose (trisaccharide), and α-dextrins
Lingual lipase	Glands in the tongue and other lipids	Triglycerides (fats and oils)	Fatty acids and monoglycerides
Gastric Juice			
Pepsin (activated from pepsinogen and HCl)	Stomach chief cells (zymogenetic cells)	Proteins	Peptides
Gastric Lipase	Stomach chief cells (zymogenetic cells)	Short-chain triglycerides (fats and oils) in butterfat and milk	Fatty acids and monoglycerides
Pancreatic Juices			
Pancreatic amylase	Pancreatic acinar cells	Starches (polysaccharides)	Maltose (disaccharide), maltotriose (trisaccharide), and α-dextrins
Trypsin (activated from from trypsinogen by enterokinase)	Pancreatic acinar cells	Proteins	Peptides
Chymotrypsin (activated from chymotrypsinogen by trypsin)	Pancreatic acinar cells	Proteins	Peptides
Elastase (activated from proelastase by trypsin)	Pancreatic acinar cells	Proteins	Peptides
Carboxypeptidase (activated from procarboxypeptidase by trypsin)	Pancreatic acinar cells	Terminal amino acids at carboxyl (acid) ends of peptides	Peptides and amino acids
Pancreatic lipase	Pancreatic acinar cells	Triglycerides (fats and oils) that have been emulsified by bile salts	Fatty acids and monoglycerides
Nucleases			
Ribonuclease	Pancreatic acinar cells	Ribonucleic acid	Nucleotides
Deoxyribonuclease	Pancreatic acinar cells	Deoxyribonucleic acid	
Brush Border			
α-Dextrinase	Small intestine	α-Dextrins	Glucose
Maltase	Small intestine	Maltose	Glucose
Sucrase	Small intestine	Sucrose	Glucose and fructose
Lactase	Small intestine	Lactose	Glucose and galactose
Enterokinase	Small intestine	Trypsinogen	Trypsin
Peptidases			
Aminopeptidase	Small intestine	Terminal amino acids at amino end of peptides	Peptides and amino acids
Dipeptidase	Small intestine	Dipeptides	Amino acids
Nucleosidases and phosphatases	Small intestine	Nucleotides	Nitrogenous bases, pentoses

TABLE 7.2   *Common Signs and Symptoms of Low Gastric Acidity*

Bloating, belching, burning, and flatulence immediately after meals
Chronic candidal infections
Chronic intestinal parasites or abnormal flora
Dilated capillaries in the cheeks and nose (in non-alcoholics)
Indigestion, diarrhea, or constipation
Iron deficiency
Multiple food allergies
Nausea after taking supplements
Post-adolescent acne
Sense of "fullness" after eating
Undigested food in stool
Weak, peeling, and cracked fingernails

traditionally, gastroenterologists have used endoscopy or intestinal fluid cultures to ascertain small bowel overgrowth problems.

Clinical Issues: Gastritis, Ulcers, and Helicobacter pylori *Infection*

Over the past five years, researchers have shown great interest in the relationships among hypochlorhydria, the bacterium *Helicobacter pylori*, and peptic ulcer. *Helicobacter* appears to be a routine colonizer of the human GI tract and uses extensive production of a urease enzyme to break down urea into ammonia and carbon dioxide (e.g., bi-

carbonate). It cloaks itself in this halo of ammonia, which wards off high concentrations of stomach acid. Helicobacter itself does not appear to cause peptic ulcer.[10] For ulcer to occur, the lining of the stomach (or intestine) must first become compromised and initiate a humoral or cellular immune response or both. Because hydrochloric acid (HCl) is a damaging agent for the stomach and intestinal linings, diets promoting excess stomach acid secretion may be doubly problematic in opening the door for *Helicobacter* infection and other GI problems.

The H2-blocking medications that lower stomach acid secretion have an inhibitory effect on Helicobacter growth, but clinicians typically use other regimens to treat Helicobacter infection. These regimens may include bismuth subsalicylate (Pepto-Bismol®), metronidazole (Flagyl®), tetracycline, amoxicillin (Amoxil®), and omeprazole (Prilosec®).

TABLE 7.3   *Diseases Associated with Low Gastric Acidity*

Acne rosacea	Hepatitis
Addison's disease	Hyper- and
Asthma	hypothyroidism
Celiac disease	Lupus erythematosus
Chronic auto-immune	Myasthenia gravis
disorders	Osteoporosis
Chronic urticaria	Pernicious anemia
Dermatitis	Psoriasis
herpetiformis	Rheumatoid arthritis
Diabetes mellitus	Sjögren's syndrome
Eczema	Thyrotoxicosis
Gallbladder disease	Vitiligo
Graves disease	

Digestion in the Small Intestine

Pancreatic enzyme secretion

After food combines with stomach secretions, the resulting mixture, chyme, is pushed through the pyloric sphincter by muscular stomach contractions into the first 18-inch portion of the small intestine, the duodenum. Bicarbonate, secreted by the pancreas, neutralizes the acidic chyme, while the pancreatic enzymes—amylases, proteases, and lipases—break down carbohydrates, proteins, and fats, respectively.

The exocrine pancreas in an average adult secretes approximately 24 ounces of fluid per day into the intestinal tract. This fluid contains an extensive variety of enzymes (Table 7.4).

When such enzymes are not present, normal digestion cannot proceed. Diseases such as chronic pancreatitis or cystic fibrosis compromise pancreatic sufficiency. Less acute pancreatic insufficiencies can also occur. Chronic hyposecretion of pancreatic enzymes not only leads to fat and protein maldigestion and malabsorption but also to micronutrient deficiencies. For example, the pancreatic protease enzymes must separate vitamin B12 from its protein carrier molecule, and pancreatic insufficiency directly causes B12 deficiency.

Bile secretion

Bile, manufactured in the liver and stored in the gallbladder, is also secreted into the duodenum, particularly after high-fat meals. Bile is made of bile salts, cholesterol esters, and lecithin, and acts as an emulsifying agent to

TABLE 7.4 *Enzymatic Secretions of the Pancreas*

Cholesterol esterase
Chymotrypsinogen—Chymotrypsin
Collagenase
Deoxyribonuclease
Lipase & Colipase
Pancreatic alpha amylase
Phospholipase A & B
Procarboxypeptidase—Carboxypeptidase A & B
Proelastase
Retinyl ester hydrolase
Ribonuclease
Trypsinogen—Trypsin

break up fat into smaller globules. This process makes fat more soluble or hydrophilic. Chemists refer to this process as micelle formation and to the tiny droplets of fat as chylomicrons. In this form, fat can be carried to the intestinal mucosa, absorbed into the lymphatic system, and ultimately partitioned to the blood. Not only triglycerides, which are the principal form of dietary fat, but also the fat-soluble vitamins A, D, E, K and, to some degree, beta-carotene, are absorbed in this manner. Absorption of amino acids, monosaccharides, disaccharides, and water-soluble vitamins occurs in the jejunum and ileum of the small intestine.

Clinical Issues: Impaired Digestion and Disease

Intact proteins and other large molecules can cross the intestinal lining to a certain extent, even in healthy individuals.[11] Digestive enzymes break down these proteins and exclude them from crossing this barrier intact. Impaired digestion caused by inadequate enzyme output may be associated with such conditions as food allergies, eczema, steatorrhea, and celiac disease. Experimental studies have shown that the digestive enzyme lipase, critical in fat digestion, can be supplemented to relieve the problems of fat malabsorption.[12,13] In addition, amylase digestive enzymes, which break down carbohydrates, have helped individuals with celiac disease. The carbohydrate fraction in gliadin from grains like wheat and rye is known to contribute to enteropathy.[14] In studies with celiac patients using digestive enzymes baked into wheat bread, results demonstrated that these patients experienced no symptoms associated with gluten intolerance. Those individuals eating untreated bread had symptoms of the disease.[15]

In a similar fashion, digestive enzymes may also help other food allergies. Several factors can trigger food allergies, including increased absorption of poorly digested protein fragments that leak into the systemic circulation across the gut wall.[16] These proteins, recognized as foreign molecules, may stimulate immune responses. By digesting dietary protein, protease enzymes decrease the supply of intact proteins available to leak into the bloodstream. Digestive protease enzymes taken orally may also help digest dietary proteins in the bloodstream. In fact, protease enzymes absorbed intact have a wide range of therapeutic effects.[17]

Lactase is another enzyme important to digestion. This enzyme is secreted by the cells lining the small intestine and required for the disaccharide lactose to be broken into its constituent monosaccharide units, glucose and galactose. Many people suffer from undiagnosed lactose intolerance. Contrary to common belief, lactase is never prolifically manufactured by human intestinal cells. Nursing infants can digest lactose in human milk because the lactase enzyme can be transferred from mother to infant through the milk. By age five, a child's ability to synthesize lactase begins to decrease. It is estimated that by adulthood, approximately 70 percent of the world's population has negligible production of the enzyme, resulting in lactose intolerance (Table 7.5).[18]

Abdominal cramps, gas, nausea, bloating, and diarrhea are common symptoms of lactose intolerance and typically accompany intake of dairy products. Lactase enzyme supplementation has helped individuals unable to digest lactose.[19] Dairy foods are the exclusive dietary source of lactose. In addition, because proteins in dairy products—

TABLE 7.5   *Lactose Intolerance in Ethnic Populations*

Ethnic Group	% Lactose Intolerant
African Blacks	97–100
Asians	90–100
Jewish Descent	60–80
Mediterraneans	60–90
Mexicans	70–80
Middle Europeans	10–20
North American Blacks	70–75
North American Caucasians	7–15
Northern Europeans	1–5

especially milk caseins—are common reactive substances associated with immune-based food allergy, dairy is often high on the list of foods to be eliminated from the diet. Thus dairy may have a "double impact" of lactose intolerance *and* allergenicity. Although lactase, like other enzymes, is available and used supplementally to treat lactose intolerance, the enzyme is most effective when added directly to liquid milk (Table 7.6).

Digestion in the Colon

After being absorbed by active transport across the mucosal cells of the intestine, nutrients are transported by hepatoportal circulation to the liver, where they are processed for use. The remaining material moves through the digestive system to the last three feet of the digestive tract—the colon. In the colon, bacteria act upon the remaining substrate, water is reabsorbed, and stool is formed. Some vitamin synthesis also results from the metabolic activity of bacteria.

In a healthy colon, a rich community of different bacterial organisms exists. These species are generally acid-producing and are a mixture of anaerobic and aerobic bacteria. Infrequently, toxin-producing bacteria, such as *Clostridium* or *Salmonella*, inhabit the colon.

TABLE 7.6   *Common Sources of Dairy*

Obvious Sources	"Hidden" Sources
All cheeses	Artificial sweeteners
Butter, many margarines	Breading on fried foods
Goat's milk	Breads, biscuits and crackers; donuts made with milk
Half-and-half cream	Breakfast and baby cereals containing milk solids
Ice cream and sherbet	Buttered or creamed foods like soups and vegetables
Milk (whole, skim, dry powdered, evaporated)	Cake and pudding mixes, many frostings
Yogurt	Candies made with milk cheese
	Cookies made with milk
	Hot dogs, luncheon meats, sausage, hash, processed and canned meats
	Many "nondairy" creamers
	Many prescription drugs, including birth control pills, thyroid medication, and some medications for gastrointestinal disorders
	Many types of vitamins
	Mayonnaise and salad dressings made with milk
	Pancakes, waffles, toaster tarts
	Pizza
	Weight-reduction formulas
* Plus any food labeled as containing whey, casein, caseinate, sodium caseinate, and lactose	

Usually, the environment of the colon is not fit for these organisms to survive. However, if the pH and water content of the colon change or the digestive and/or absorptive processes further up the gastrointestinal tract are impaired, the colonic environment may encourage these bacteria to grow and disease to flourish.

A FUNCTIONAL APPROACH TO DIGESTION, ABSORPTION, AND INTESTINAL PERMEABILITY

From the mouth to the small intestine, the chemical and mechanical digestive processes are directed toward changing food into forms that can be absorbed through the epithelial cells lining the mucosa into the underlying blood and lymphatic vessels. Essentially all carbohydrates are absorbed as monosaccharides. Proteins are absorbed as single amino acids, dipeptides, and tripeptides. Fats are absorbed as monoglycerides and fatty acids (Figure 7.1).

Food and food constituents have two alternatives for entering the bloodstream. Most commonly, intestinal cells engulf and transfer food molecules into the bloodstream through their basement membranes. This route is referred to as "transcellular." A second route— referred to as "paracellular"—occurs when food molecules pass through spaces between adjacent cells. The extent to which molecules pass into the blood by these routes reflects intestinal permeability.

The 3-mm epithelial cell lining that separates the contents of the lumen from systemic circulation is responsible for absorption and exclusion. It must balance this duty in one of the most metabolically active and diverse areas of the body. When host defenses are overwhelmed and break down, the absorption and systematic distribution of normally excluded substances is enhanced.[20] An increase in the permeability of the intestinal mucosa, often called "leaky gut syndrome," helps to explain the etiology and mechanisms of a wide range of systemic disorders.

Intestinal permeability describes the relative ease with which molecules residing in the interior (lumen) of the intestine are absorbed through the intestinal mucosal cells and released into the general circulation. Because very small molecules like sodium or chloride ions (approximately 100 daltons or less) pass through the intestine regularly by diffusion, the term "intestinal permeability" generally refers to molecules larger than 100-150 daltons. While the walls of the intestine serve as a physical barrier separating food and the bacterial populations of the intestine from the rest of the body, not so obvious are the relatively dynamic biological properties exhibited by this physical barrier. There is a complex array of interlocking and complementary mechanisms, which include tight junctions, a thick mucosal coat, proteolytic enzymes, acidic secretions, intestinal peristalsis, and immunological defenses in the form of secretory Immunoglobulin A (sIgA).

Numerous events alter the permeability of the intestine, including stress,[21] developmental age,[22,23] medication,[24,25] and alcohol.[26] In addition, permeability is disrupted in many health conditions, including rheumatoid arthritis,[27,28] ankylosing spondylitis,[29,30]

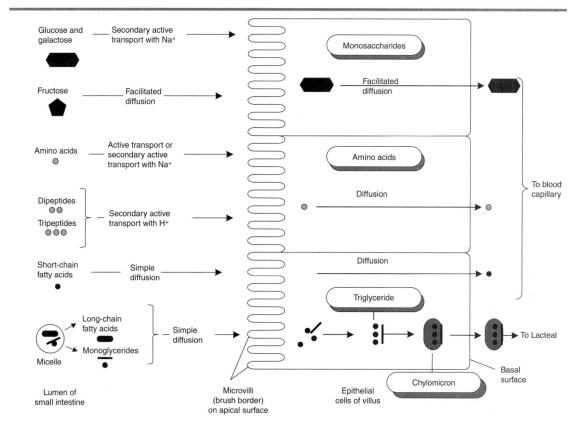

FIGURE 7.1 *Nutrient absorption*

Crohn's disease,[31] burns,[32] pancreatic dysfunction and cystic fibrosis,[33] HIV+,[34,35] celiac disease,[36] marasmus,[37] food allergy,[38,39] and atopic eczema[40] (Tables 7.7 and 7.8).

Permeability in Healthy Individuals: Basic Physiology and Pediatric Gastroenterology

Investigation of permeability in healthy individuals has taken place in two primary research areas: basic physiology, reviewed by Gardner,[41] and pediatric gastroenterology, reviewed by Van Elburg.[42] Gardner has pointed out with respect to protein, the non-diseased intestine appears to sustain an active peptide transport system. Critical to this transport system is the presence of M cells—specialized cells along the intestinal wall whose physical and chemical features appear well designed for peptide transport.[43] Because M cells are not coated with glycocalyx (the protective

TABLE 7.7   *Symptoms Associated with Increased Intestinal Permeability*

Abdominal distention
Abdominal pain
Arthralgias
Cognitive and memory deficits
Diarrhea
Fatigue and malaise
Fevers of unknown origin
Food intolerances
Myalgias
Poor exercise tolerance
Shortness of breath
Skin rashes
Toxic feelings

extension of most intestinal cell membranes), they have less obstructed access to proteins in the gut. The M cells also contain fewer lysosomes—storage structures harboring the enzymes required to break down proteins, carbohydrates, and fats. The reduced number of lysosomes makes the M cells less likely to dismantle proteins. Finally, M cells contain more transfer vesicles—structures designed to carry large molecules in and out of the cell in conjunction with endo- and exocytosis (Figure 7.2).

Increased permeability of the intestine to large macromolecules in healthy, full-term infants has been a consistent finding of research in pediatric gastroenterology. This increased permeability is key to neonatal protection from infection, since immunoglobulins and other anti-infectious factors (including lactoferrin, lactoperoxidase, bifidus factor, antistaphylococcus factor, complement, interferon, lysozyme, B12-binding protein, lymphocytes, and macrophages) are in human milk and must be transferred to breastfeeding infants to maintain proper immunity during neonatal development.[44]

Although secretory IgA is the primary immunoglobulin in human milk, IgM, IgE, IgD, and IgG exist as well. These immunoglobulins range in molecular weight between 146,000 daltons for IgG4 to 970,000 daltons for IgM, making them equivalent or larger in size than

TABLE 7.8   *Diseases Associated with Increased Intestinal Permeability*

Acne	Hepatic dysfunction
AIDS, HIV infection in general	Infectious enterocolitis
Alcoholism	Inflammatory bowel disease
Autism	Irritable bowel syndrome
Celiac disease	Multiple food and chemical sensitivities
CFIDS	NSAIDs
Childhood hyperactivity	Pancreatic insufficiency
Cytotoxic drugs	Psoriasis
Dermatitis herpetiformis	Spondyloarthropathies
Eczema	Urticaria

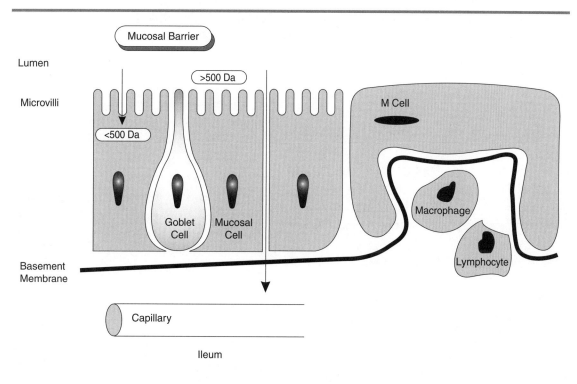

FIGURE 7.2 *Permeability dynamics*

milk proteins like casein (121,700 daltons) or wheat proteins like glutenin (150,000 to 1,000,000 daltons). The permeability of the healthy neonate's intestine to these large immunoglobulin-sized molecules helps explain two phenomena. First, it helps account for lower reports of infection in breastfed infants and decreased allergy-related conditions like atopic eczema. Unfortunately, it also explains the higher degree of allergic reactions in infants prematurely exposed to table foods and their potentially antigenic protein content.

Permeability and Bacterial Imbalance

While the direct causes of disrupted permeability of the intestine are unclear, researchers have found strong connections between events involving dietary intake, eating habits, and bacterial balance/imbalance in the gut.[45,46] Delayed intestinal food transit (poor intestinal motility) and poorly timed intestinal muscle activity (delayed peristalsis) are both connected to excessive permeability. (Compromised motility and peristalsis are also typical features of a low-fiber, high-animal product, and highly processed diet similar to the everyday diet of the average U.S. adult.) Compromised food transit through the gut brings changes in the intestinal bacteria by altering the natural flow of nutrients available to these organisms. Overgrowth of certain species and abnormal bacterial balance can result. Interactions between these abnormal flora (or the substances they produce) and the cells of the intestine result in altered permeability and the absorption of antigenic substances into the bloodstream.

Diet/bacteria relationships make possible two types of unwanted antigen exposure. First, the body may be directly exposed to unwanted food antigens consumed in the diet via disrupted permeability. Second, the body may experience indirect exposure in which the disrupted microfloral balance may produce unwanted endogenous toxins and antigens. Further disruptions in permeability and the release of antigenic molecules into the bloodstream may then result.

Two types of research support this view. First, morbidly obese patients who have undergone intestinal by-pass surgery often exhibit symptoms of immune-related arthritis in which antigens produced by intestinal bacteria have become present in the patients' blood. The second type of evidence stems from studies about the benefits of fasting in rheumatoid arthritis patients.[47] Relatively short periods of fluid/nutrient-supplemented fasting improve symptoms of rheumatoid arthritis and microfloral balance in the intestine.

Bacterial Imbalance and the Development of Chronic Disease

Bacterial imbalance in the gut can also affect other organ systems by altering substances that depend upon bacterial enzymes for chemical processing. For example, blood levels of the hormone estrogen are affected by activity of bacterial enzymes in the intestine and drop significantly when activity is reduced.[48] Since the risks of both breast cancer and osteoporosis have been linked to the levels of circulating estrogen, bacterial imbalance is a possible link between diet and the development of these diseases.

Recent research on intestinal cancers illustrates another possible role of bacterial imbalance. Approximately 90 percent of carcinogenic substances the human body is exposed to require chemical alteration or bioactivation before acting as carcinogens.[49] Imbalances in the gut microflora that alter the type and rate of enzymatic activity in the gut may play a key role in the development of certain cancers, especially those associated with the gastrointestinal tract. Any step that might help restore microfloral balance in the intestine might also potentially reduce the risk of cancer.

Antigenic substances produced by intestinal bacteria also appear related to the development of immune-related disease. For nearly 100 years, research about inflammatory joint diseases has illustrated that immune complexes exist in blood, including peptidoglycans from the cell walls of intestine-inhabiting bacteria. These bacteria have included *Shigella flexneri, Salmonella typhimurium, Yersinia enterocolitica, Campylobacter fetus, Campylobacter jejunii,* and *Chlamydia trachomatis.* Three basic nutritional support strategies have been used in the treatment of these permeability-related health conditions: 1) direct promotion of intestinal bacterial balance through the use of probiotic (bacteria-containing) supplements;[50] 2) indirect promotion of intestinal bacterial balance through the use of prebiotic supplements containing nutrients preferred by under-represented bacteria; and 3) direct support of intestinal cells and their function, through nutritional supplements that target the intestinal mucosa[51] (Figures 7.3 and 7.4).

Direct promotion of bacterial balance through probiotics

To help restore optimal permeability to the intestine, active balancing of bacterial populations in the gut through supplementation with thermophilized (freeze-dried) or living bacteria

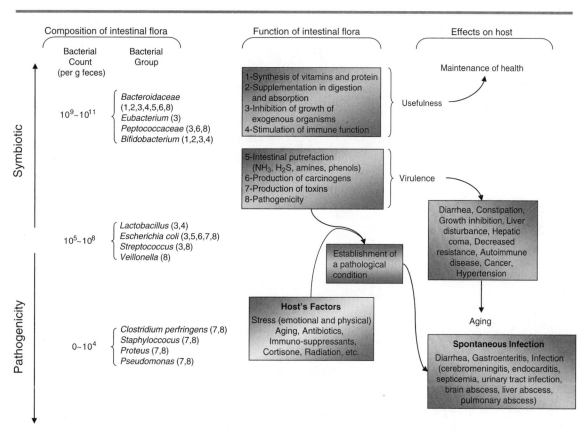

FIGURE 7.3 *Type and activity of intestinal bacteria*

GI Tract Site of Bacteria	Density of Bacteria	Common Bacterial Populations	
Esophagus		Lactobacilli	
Stomach	$[10^3 - 10^5 /g]$		
Small intestine			
Duodenum	$[10^3 - 10^5 /g]$	Lactobacilli	
Jejunum	$[10^3 - 10^5 /g]$	Streptococci	
		Enterobacteria	
Ileum	$[10^3 - 10^{12} /g]$	*Bacteroides spp.*	
Large intestine	$[10^{10} - 10^{12} /g]$	*Bacteroides spp.* *Fusobacterium spp.* *E. Faecalis* Lactobacilli *Staph. Aureis* *Clostridium sp.*	Enterobacteria Klebsiella Eubacteria Bifidobacteria Streptococci Pseudomonas Salmonella
Feces	$[10^9 - 10^{11} /g]$	*Bacteroides spp.* Bifidobacteria Eubacteria	Coliforms *E. Faecalis*

FIGURE 7.4   *Common bacteria in the gastrointestinal tract*

is helpful. Bacteria used in supplementation studies include the bifidobacteria (including the species *bifidum, breve, infantis, longum, adolescentis, angulatum, catenulatum,* and *pseudocatenulatum*), the lactobacilli (including the species *acidophilus, brevis, bulgaricus, casei, delbrueckii, kefir, plantarum, salivarius,* and *yoghurti*), and the streptococci (including the species *thermophilus, faecium, faecalis,* and *lactis*). The bifidobacteria restore microfloral balance in extremely compromised

adults. Favorably altered immune system response and anti-tumor activity have also been reported. Similarly, lactobacillus supplementation improves infantile diarrhea and stabilizes intestinal function, including permeability.

Indirect support of bacterial balance through prebiotic supplementation

Another way to restore bacterial balance and improve permeability disruption involves supplementation with nutrients that serve as preferred fuels for bifidobacteria and lacto-bacilli. This area of research focuses on the carbohydrate subdivision generally referred to as the fructooligosaccharides (FOS). This category of macronutrient includes short chains (3-10 saccharide units) of simple sugars with at least two of the units consisting of the monosaccharide fructose. Fructooligosaccharides have typically been divided into three categories based on the number of fructose units they contain. The GF2s, containing two fructose molecules, include 1-kestose, 6-kestose, and neokestose. Nystose, bifurcose, and neobifurcose constitute the GF3s; and the GF4s include the substances fructosylnystose and a second form of bifurcose. Onion, burdock root, asparagus, and rye are food sources for all three types of fructooligosaccharides. Jerusalem artichoke, banana, sugar maple, and Chinese chive have been recognized as sources of the 2-fructose forms (1-kestose, 6-kestose, and neokestose). (Table 2.4 shows the molecular structures for GF2, GF3, and GF4.)

Studies indicate that fructooligosaccharides are the preferred substrate for all bifidobacteria except the bifidum species. They are ineffective as a substrate for the potentially pathogenic bacterium *Clostridium perfringens*. Supplementation of these nutrients in doses of 1–8 g per day may favorably affect human microfloral balance.[52]

Nutritional support of intestinal mucosal cells

A third type of intervention in health conditions related to altered permeability involves active supplementation of nutrients selectively used by intestinal cells for growth and function. These nutrients include the following: 1) glutamine, a nonessential amino acid; 2) butyric acid, a short-chain fatty acid; 3) fibers that intestinal bacteria can convert to short-chain fatty acids; 4) EPA and GLA, the omega 3 and omega 6 fatty acids; and 5) gamma-oryzanol.

L-glutamine. L-glutamine is a nonessential amino acid that can be formed from the essential amino acids leucine, isoleucine, and valine, or by transformation of alpha ketoglutarate, a breakdown product of the simple sugar glucose. In the small intestine, L-glutamine is the preferred fuel for intestinal cells. Supplementation with glutamine has become increasingly widespread for hospitalized patients with severely compromised intestinal function. When added to enteral (tube) feedings, glutamine increases the number of cells in the small intestine, the number of villi (absorptive spaces) on those cells, and the height of the villi.[53] Glutamine supplementation in parenteral (intravenous) feedings decreases the spread of infection from the intestine to other tissue. Glutamine also helps prevent intestinal tissue loss after surgery and improves immune function. Doses of glutamine range from 300 to 500 mg of glutamine per kg of body weight.

Butyric acid. Butyric acid, a small, 4-carbon nonessential short-chain fatty acid, functions in the large intestine similarly to glutamine in the small intestine—as fuel of choice. Like glutamine, butyric acid can form in the body from alpha ketoglutarate, a breakdown product of simple sugar. Surprisingly, 75 percent of all dietary carbohydrate that reaches the colon (mostly in the form of undigested fiber) can be converted by colonic bacteria into short-chain fatty acids, including butyrate. For persons on a high fiber-containing diet, between 5 and 10 percent of the body's energy needs may be met by short-chain fatty acid generation and metabolism by bacteria in the large intestine.

Support for butyric acid production, like supplementation of glutamine, may improve intestinal function and integrity[54] and act as an anti-cancer agent. Butyrate may provide a key to the link between dietary fiber and colorectal cancer. Because bacteria in the large intestine can convert dietary fibers into butyrate, and because butyrate has anti-cancer properties, diets high in fiber may protect against colorectal cancer. Diets higher in vegetable and leguminous fiber may protect against colorectal cancer better than diets high in grain fiber. Bacteria in the large intestine may be better able to convert these vegetable and leguminous fibers into butyrate than fibers derived from whole grains.

EPA and GLA. EPA (eicosapentaenoic acid) and GLA (gamma linolenic acid) are nonessential fatty acids belonging to the omega 3 and omega 6 families, respectively. Because EPA and GLA stand at the chemical gateways for the body's manufacturing of many key immune-related substances, each has been extensively investigated relative to

inflammatory disease, including intestinal diseases. For example, EPA decreased inflammation, improved intestinal function in animals, and improved symptoms in a group of patients with Crohn's disease.[55]

Gamma-oryzanol. Gamma-oryzanol, a naturally occurring component of rice bran oil, is a well-documented antioxidant that provides intestinal support for permeability-related conditions like irritable bowel syndrome and ulceration of the gastric and intestinal linings.[56,57] Several components of gamma-oryzanol, including its ferulic acid esters of triterpenoid compounds (cycloartenol, 24-methyl cycloartenol) and its phytosterols (beta sitosterol, campestrol), have become the subjects of increasing research in relationship to intestinal health. Protective intestinal support by gamma-oryzanol includes free radical scavenging activity, metal chelating activity, and autonomic nervous system mediated normalization of gastric secretions.[58]

Permeability and the 4R Gastrointestinal Support Program

A comprehensive approach to normalization of gastrointestinal function, commonly referred to as the "4R" approach, comprises four basic clinical steps: Remove, Replace, Reinoculate, and Repair. Although intestinal permeability is connected most closely to "Repair," it is indirectly connected to the other steps as well (Figure 7.5).

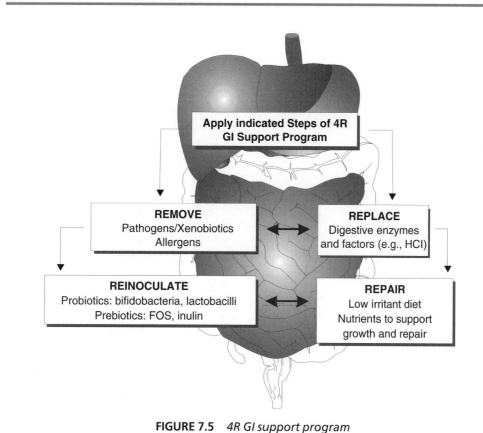

FIGURE 7.5 *4R GI support program*

Remove

"Remove" focuses on eliminating pathogenic bacteria, viruses, fungi, parasites, allergens, and toxins from the gastrointestinal tract. Laboratory tests involving digestive microbiology and parasitology are often needed to verify the presence of unwanted microbial organisms in the intestine. Removing these organisms may require prescription medicines, and knowledge of the sensitivity and resistance of specific or-

ganisms to therapeutic agents. Dietary alterations, including removal of toxins and allergens from an individual's food intake, are also vital. Oligoantigenic diets, containing only those foods that are known to pose very little risk of an allergic reaction, are typically part of the "Remove" phase of 4R. Failure to remove pathogens, toxins, and allergens from the gastrointestinal environment can make proper intestinal permeability virtually impossible to attain. Intestinal support nutrients intended for the enterocytes and colonocytes lining the intestinal wall may never reach their cellular destination. Instead, they may fuel unwanted microbial pathogens. Dietary allergens and toxins may also provoke intestinal immune responses and further damage intestinal integrity.

Replace

The second clinical step in the 4R program, "Replace" replenishes enzymes and other digestive factors lacking or insufficient in an individual's gastrointestinal environment. Gastrointestinal enzymes needing to be replaced include pancreatic enzymes and the proteases, lipases, cellulases, and saccharidases that are normally secreted into the intestine. Other digestive factors that may require replenishment include hydrochloric acid (HCl) and intrinsic factor (IF), normally secreted by cells in the stomach wall, and bile, synthesized in the liver. As in step one, laboratory tests may be required to verify the need for replacement enzymes and digestive factors. Failing to replace these critical components of the digestive process can also greatly compromise any attempts to establish proper intestinal permeability. Without appropriate breakdown of food, intestinal support nutrients may never be available to the intestinal cells. Instead, they may be lost from the body in the fecal stream. In addition, insufficient enzymatic processes may decrease the availability of fuels to desirable microbial populations.

Reinoculate

"Reinoculate" is the third step in 4R gastrointestinal support. Reinoculate refers to the reintroduction of desirable bacteria into the intestine to establish microfloral balance. A variety of supplemental sources may be considered helpful in this phase, including cultured and fermented foods containing live bacteria, refrigerated liquid supplements containing live bacteria, or freeze-dried bacteria packaged in powder, tablet, or capsule form. Frequently supplemented species include *Lactobacillus acidophilus, Lactobacillus bulgaricus, Lactobacillus thermophilus, Bifidobacterium bifidus, Bifidobacterium longum,* and *Bifidobacterium breve.* In addition to directly reintroducing bacteria, this step may also involve indirectly bolstering the reinoculation process through foods or food products that enhance lactobacilli or bifidobacteria growth without simultaneously enhancing pathogenic bacteria growth. Supplementing with fructooligosaccharides (FOS) derived from foods like Jerusalem artichoke illustrates this indirect bolstering process. In the absence of bacterial balance in the intestine, proper intestinal permeability is unlikely. On the one hand, a lack of beneficial nutrients exists, often resulting from a lack of desirable bacteria populations available to produce such nutrients. For example, a lack of *Bifidobacteria* species able to convert various types of dietary fiber into butyric acid often means a lack of this short-chain fatty acid preferred by the colonocytes as an energy substrate. On the other hand, excess endo-toxic substances produced by overgrowth of unwanted bacteria in an imbalanced mi-crofloral environment exist. Along with im-mune activation, these substances can disrupt intestinal permeability.

Repair

The fourth and final step in a 4R approach, "Repair," is the step most closely associated with the intestinal permeability concept. This step involves direct nutritional support of the intestinal cells through the use of supplements containing nutrients known to be critical in in-testinal wall structure and function. In this group of nutrients are many of the antioxi-dants, including vitamins C, E, and A/beta-carotene, the minerals zinc and manganese, the amino acids cysteine, N-acetylcysteine, and glutamine, the tripeptide glutathione, and the carbohydrates inulin and/or FOS. Supplemen-tation of other nutrients closely involved with collagen formation, including the vitamin pan-tothenic acid, is also practiced. As previously discussed, pre- and post-testing using lactu-lose/mannitol is typically conducted to evalu-ate and monitor the repair process.

When considered together, the four steps of the 4R gastrointestinal support program appropriately address, from a clinical stand-point, many of the critical factors underlying GI dysfunction. Each of these factors can contribute to increasing and self-generating pathophysiology. It is therefore imperative to establish a comprehensive therapeutic regi-men that addresses them effectively.

SUMMARY

The barrier function of the intestine—now measured with reasonably reliable and nonin-vasive laboratory techniques—can be com-promised by a wide variety of commonly occurring life events. These events include stress, toxic exposure, poor dietary habits, and medications. Altered intestinal perma-bility is not a localized, organ-specific dis-order but a root level bodily imbalance in which whole-body function is compromised. Disrupted permeability functionally links in-testinal dysbiosis and neuroendocrine, muscu-loskeletal, and immunological problems. According to functional medicine, altered per-meability serves as a landmark in pattern iden-tification. This finding enhances understanding and nutritional support for a wide variety of diagnostic conditions, including food allergy, irritable bowel syndrome, Crohn's disease, pancreatic disease, rheumatoid arthritis, anky-losing spondylitis, cystic fibrosis, celiac dis-ease, atopic eczema, failure to thrive, and general malnutrition. The failure to address altered permeability and practice aggressive nutritional support of intestinal integrity may compromise long-term treatment of the listed health conditions.

CHAPTER 7 REFERENCES

1. Hill P. It is not what you eat, but how you eat it—digestion, lifestyle, and nutrition. Nutr. 1991;7:385–395.

2. Schuster MM. Biofeedback control of gastrointestinal motility. In: Basmajian JV, ed. Biofeedback—Principles and Practice for Clinicians. New York: Williams and Wilkins. 1979;217–229.

3. Mattes RD. Physiologic responses to sensory stimulation by food: nutritional implications. J Am Diet Assoc. 1997;97:406–413.

4. Mattes RD. Physiologic responses to sensory stimulation by food: nutritional implications. J Am Diet Assoc. 1997;97:408–409.

5. Henriksson K, Uvnas-Moberg K, Nord CE, Johansson, C, Gullberg R. Gastrin, gastric acid secretion, and gastric microflora in patients with rheumatoid arthritis. Ann Rheumatic Dis. 1986; 45:475–483.

6. Ryle J, Barber H. Gastric analysis in acne rosacea. Lancet. 1920;2:1195–1196.

7. Bray G. The hypochlorhydria of asthma in childhood. Quart J Med. 1931;24:181–197.

8. Vellas B, Balas D, Albarede JL. Effects of aging process on digestive functions. Comprehensive Therapy. 1991;17(80):46–52.

9. Kassarjian Z, Russell RM. Hypochlorhydria: a factor in nutrition. Annu Rev Nutr. 1989; 9:271–285.

10. Anderson ML. Helicobacter pylori infection when and whom is treatment important? Postgrad Med. 1994; 96(6):40–50.

11. Gardner ML. Gastrointestinal absorption of intact proteins. Annu Rev Nutr. 1988;8: 329–350.

12. Griffin SM, Alderson D, Farndon JR, et al. Acid resistant lipase replacement therapy in chronic exocrine insufficiency: a study in dogs. Gut. 1989;30:1012–1015.

13. Schneider MU, Knoll-Ruzicka ML, Domschke S, Heptner G, Domschre W. Pancreatic enzyme replacement therapy: comparative effects of conventional and enteric-coated microspheric pancreatin and acid-stable fungal enzyme preparations on steatorrhea in chronic pancreatitis. Hepatogastroenterol. 1985;32:97–102.

14. Phelan J. The nature of gliadin toxicity in coeliac disease. Biochem Soc Trans. 1974;2:1368–1370.

15. Phelan JI, Stevens FM, NcNicholl B, Fottrell PF, McCarthy CF. Coeliac disease: the abolition of gliadin toxicity by enzymes from Aspergillus niger. Clin Sci Molec Med. 1977;53:35–43.

16. Gardner ML. Intestinal assimilation of intact peptides and proteins from the diet—a neglected field? Biol Rev.1984;59:289–331.

17. Taussig ST, Yoloyama MM, Chignon A, Onari K, Yamokidom M. Bromelain, a proteolytic enzyme and its clinical application. A review. Hiroshima J Med Sci. 1975;24:185–193.

18. Mahan LK, Escott-Stump S. Food Nutrition and Diet Therapy. Philadelphia, Pa: W.B. Saunders. 1996:625–626.

19. Barillas C, Solomons NW. Effective reduction of lactose maldigestion in preschool children by direct addition of beta-galactosidases to milk at mealtime. Pediatrics. 1987;79:766–772.

20. Olaison G, Sjodahl R, Tagesson C. Abnormal intestinal permeability in Crohn's disease. A possible pathogenic factor. Scand J Gastroenterol. 1990;25(4):321–328.

21. Menzies IS. Alimentary disacchariduria in adults related to the osmolality of ingested solutions. Biocem J. 1972;126:19–20.

22. Hollander D, Taranawski H. Aging-associated increase in intestinal absorption of macromolecules. Gerontol. 1985;31:133-137.

23. Grusky FL. Gastrointestinal absorption of unaltered proteins in normal infants. Pediatr. 1955; 16: 763.

24. Bjarnason I, Williams P, Smethurst P, Peters TJ, Levi AJ. Effect of non-steroidal anti-inflammatory drugs and prostaglandins on the permeability of the human small intestine. Gut. 1986; 27:1292–1297.

25. Jenkins AP, Trew DR, Crump BJ, et al. Do nonsteroidal anti-inflammatory drugs increase colonic permeability? Gut. 1991;32(1):66–69.

26. Bjarnason I, Wise RJ, Peters TJ. The leaky gut of alcoholism: possible route of entry for toxic compounds. Lancet. 1984;1:179–182.

27. Rooney PJ, Jenkins RT, Buchanan WW. A short review of the relationship between intestinal permeability and inflammatory joint disease. Clin Exper Rheum. 1990;8:75–83.

28. Skoldstam L, Magnusson KE. Fasting, intestinal permeability and rheumatoid arthritis. Rheum Dis Clin N Amer. 1991;17(2):363–371.

29. Martinez-Gonzalez O, Cantero-Hinojosa J, Paule-Sastre P, Gomez-Magan, JC, Salvatierra-Rios D. Intestinal permeability in patients with ankylosing spondylitis and their healthy relatives. Br J Rheum. 1993;33:644–647.

30. Smith MD, Gibson RA, Brooks PM. Abnormal bowel permeability in ankylosing spondylitis and rheumatoid arthritis. J Rheum. 1985;12:299–305.

31. Olaison G, Sjodahl R, Tagesson C. Abnormal intestinal permeability in Crohn's disease. Scand J Gastroenterol. 1990;25: 321–328.

32. Shippee RL, Johnson AA, Cioffi WG. Simultaneous determination of lactulose and mannitol in urine of burn patients by gas-liquid chromatography. Clin Chem. 1990;38(3):343–345.

33. Shippee RL, Johnson AA, Cioffi WG. Simultaneous determination of lactulose and mannitol in urine of burn patients by gas-liquid chromatography. Clin Chem. 1992;38(3):343–345.

34. Lim SG, Menzies IS, Lee CA, Johnson MA, Pounder RE. Intestinal permeability and function in patients infected with human immunodeficiency virus. Scand J Gastroenterol. 1993;28: 573–580.

35. Tepper RE, Simon D, Brandt, LJ, Nutovits R, Lee JM. Intestinal permeability in patients infected with the human immunodeficiency virus. Am J Gastroenterol. 1994;89(6):878–882.

36. Cobden I, Rothwell J, Axon AT. Intestinal permeability and screening tests for coeliac disease. Gut. 1980;21:512-518.

37. Behrens RH, Lunn PG, Northrop CA, Hanlon PW, Neale G. Factors affecting the integrity of the intestinal mucosa of Gambian children. Am J Clin Nutr. 1987;45:1433–1441.

38. Andre C, Andre F, Colin L, Cavagna S. Measurement of intestinal permeability to mannitol lactulose as a means of diagnosing food allergy and evaluating therapeutic effectiveness of disodium cromoglycate. Ann Allerg. 1987;59: 127–129.

39. Troncone R, Caputo N, Florio G, Finelli E. Increased intestinal sugar permeability after challenge in children with cow's milk allergy or intolerance. Allerg. 1994;49:142–146.

40. Caffarelli C, Cavagni G, Menzies IS, Bertolini P, Atherton DJ. Elimination diet and intestinal permeability in atopic eczema: a preliminary study. Clin Exp Allergy. 1993;23:28–31.

41. Gardner ML. Gastrointestinal absorption of intact protein. Annu Rev Nutr. 1998;8:329–350.

42. Van Elburg RM, Uil JJ, De Monchy JG, Heymans HS. Intestinal permeability in pediatric gastroenterology. Scand J Gastroenterol. 27 Suppl 1992;194:19–24.

43. Wolf JL, Bye WA. The membranous epithelial (M) cell and the mucosal immune system. Ann Rev Med. 1984;35:95–112.

44. Worthington-Roberts BS, Veermerch J, Williams SR, eds. Nutrition in pregnancy and lactation. St. Louis, MO: Times Mirror/Mosby; 1985:277.

45. Hollander D, Taranawski H. Aging-associated increase in intestinal absorption of macromolecules. Gerontol. 1985;31:133–137.

46. Hollander D, Taranawski H. Aging-associated increase in intestinal absorption of macromolecules. Gerontol. 1985;31:133–137.

47. Skoldstam L, Magnusson KE. Fasting, intestinal permeability and rheumatoid arthritis. Rheum Dis Clin N Amer. 1991;17(2):363–371.

48. Gorbach SL, Goldin BR. Nutrition and the gastrointestinal microflora. Nutr Revs. 1992; 50(12):378–381.

49. Chadwick RW, George SE, Claxton LD. Role of the gastrointestinal mucosa and microflora in the bioactivation of dietary and environmental

mutagens or carcinogens. Drug Metab Revs. 1992;24(4):425–492.

50. Hollander D, Taranawski H. Aging-associated increase in intestinal absorption of macromolecules. Gerontol. 1985;31:133–137.

51. Grusky FL. Gastrointestinal absorption of unaltered proteins in normal infants. Pediatr. 1955; 16:763.

52. Hidaka H, Hirayama M, Tokunaga T, Eida T. The effects of undigestible fructo-oligosaccharides on intestinal microflora and various physiological functions on human health. In: Furda I, Brine CJ, eds. New Developments in Dietary Fiber. New York: Plenum; 1990.

53. Evans MA, Shronts EP. Intestinal fuels: glutamine, short-chain fatty acids, and dietary fiber. J Amer Diet Assoc. 1992;92:1239–1246.

54. Evans MA, Shronts EP. (1992). Intestinal fuels: glutamine, short-chain fatty acids, and dietary fiber. J Amer Diet Assoc. 92:1239–1246.

55. Belluzi A, Brignola C, Campleri M, Pera A, Boschi S, Miglioli M. Fish oil reduced relapse and maintained remission in Crohn's disease. NEJM. 1996;334(24):1557–1560.

56. Chuma Y. Effectiveness of gamma-oryzanol (Hi-Z fine granules) on chronic gastritis, gastric ulcer scar tissue, and irritable colon syndrome. Shinyaku to Rinsho. 1976;25(10):2.

57. Inove T. Therapeutic effectiveness of gamma-oryzanol on chronic gastritis. Shinyaku to Rinsho. 1976;25(5):3.

58. Okada T, Yamaguchi N. Antioxidative effect and pharmacology of oryzanol. J Jap Org Chem Soc. 1983;32(6):305.

8

Energy

TRADITIONAL RESEARCH ABOUT THE ROLE of energy in clinical nutrition has focused mainly on macronutrients as primary substrates for metabolic activity. Such studies have explored human energy needs in many ways, including basal metabolic rate, thermogenesis, physical activity, regulation of energy intake, and calculation of energy needs.[1,2,3] While these issues should be the core of our understanding about how the body uses nutrients, recent discoveries are forging new visions about the role of nutrition and human energy.

Most notably, research has linked mitochondrial dysfunction to a variety of clinical conditions related to major organ systems and functions (Table 8.1).[4] One study discovered that individuals with fatigue and accelerated age conditions had a significant decline in skeletal muscle mitochondrial respiration.[5] Such findings indicate that the loss of mitochondrial respiratory chain function may influence factors associated with aging. Studies like this are only the beginning of an exciting investigation of the relationship between mitochondria and illness. The list of clinical conditions related to mitochondria will no doubt expand as research into mitochondrial function continues.

In this chapter, we examine how nutrition influences mitochondrial activity and energy production. According to a functional approach, nutritional therapeutics can help regulate energy processes related to disease. This chapter provides a general overview of the basic biochemical pathways producing body energy, discusses the role of nutrition in support of energy production, and introduces

TABLE 8.1   *Clinical Conditions Related to Mitochondrial Dysfunction*

Mitochondrial dysfunction has been noted in the following diseases:	
Diseases of the heart	Wolff-Parkinson-White syndrome, cardiomyopathies
Diseases of the eye	optic neuropathies, ophthalmoplegias
Diseases of the musculoskeletal system	lipid myopathies, chronic fatigue, fibromyalgia syndrome
Diseases of the pancreas	diabetes mellitus
Diseases of the kidney	Fanconi's syndrome, glomerulonephropathies
Diseases of the blood	Pearson's syndrome
Diseases of the brain	Alzheimer's disease, Parkinson's disease, migraines, seizures, strokes

a functional approach to nutritionally supported energy production.

ENERGY

Mitochondria and Energy Production

Known as the power plants of the cell, mitochondria contain enzymes important for cell metabolism, including those that convert food to usable energy (Figure 8.1). Mitochondria exist in the cytoplasm of all cells except erythrocytes. Each cell contains about 2,500 mitochondria, which means that over one quadrillion mitochondria exist in the adult human body—more than three times the number of adult human cells and twice the number of microorganisms found in the gut. Cells can even increase their mitochondrial number through fission of the mitochondrion.

Mitochondria are the sites of cellular respiration, the catabolic process that uses oxygen to generate the energy-containing molecule adenosine triphosphate (ATP). Essentially, the energy released when proteins, lipids, and polysaccharides are oxidized is coupled with a reaction that allows the energy to be repackaged into ATP. ATP functions as the common currency of energy within a cell (roughly 10^9 molecules of ATP are present in the intracellular space of the average cell at any given time).[6]

ATP contains a high-energy phosphate bond that stores energy to be transferred and released based on body need. This stored energy is released when ATP is converted to adenosine diphosphate (ADP) and inorganic phosphate (P_i). In turn, the ADP and P_i produce ATP in the mitochondrion when combined with energy-releasing catabolic reactions. This process allows the body to maintain energy through the regeneration of ATP from ADP and P_i (Figure 8.1).

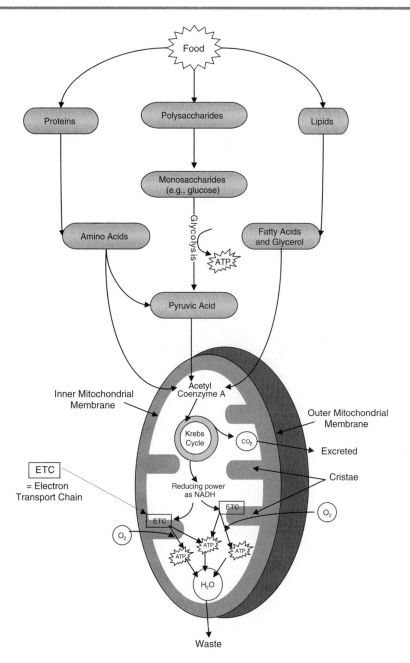

FIGURE 8.1 *Mitochondrial energy production (from food)*

The process of regenerating ATP from ADP and P_i is similar to recharging a battery. In this analogy, ATP acts as the battery and the mitochondrion as the recharger. When the battery (ATP) runs down (and becomes ADP and P_i), it must be placed in the battery recharger (the mitochondrion) for recharging (phosphorylation). The fully charged battery (ATP) can then return to the body for use. However, the process is not quite as simple as recharging a battery. Unlike a standard battery, ATP is unable to maintain a charge at length. A single ATP molecule must be recycled within a mitochondrion approximately 1,000 times per day for the body to maintain its energy supply.

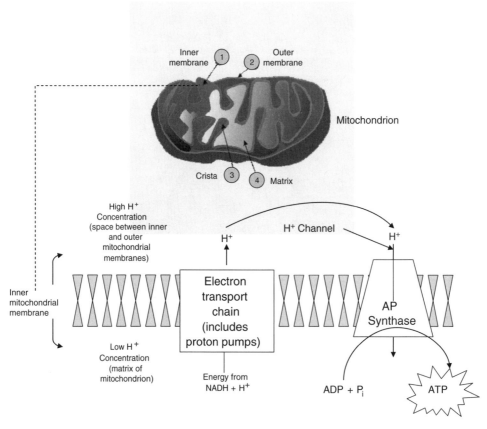

FIGURE 8.2   *Mitochondria and energy production*

Structure Influences Function

Mitochondria vary in shape: spherical or elongated, cylindrical, or threadlike. Tissue environment determines their cell position. For example, mitochondria are relatively free moving and almost spheroid in shape in the liver. In muscle, they are bound tightly to the fibers of the contractile system. In the kidney, they are cylindrical.

Mitochondria consist of two membranes: an *outer* membrane that is permeable to most small molecules and an *inner* membrane that does not readily allow molecules to pass through it. The inner membrane is arranged to form invaginations, or cristae, which increase the surface area of the membrane. The larger surface area allows a greater quantity of enzymes to exist in the inner membrane. This mitochondrial *matrix* contains enzymes involved with the citric acid cycle and fatty acid oxidation as well as the enzymes responsible for ATP production. In contrast to the outer membrane, the inner membrane also uses an elaborate, energy-driven transport system to usher most nutrients. Examples of molecules permeating the inner layer include ATP, ADP, P_i, pyruvate, succinate, malate, citrate, and alpha-ketoglutarate.

Anaerobic vs. Aerobic Metabolism

Eukaryotic cells produce ATP through two basic metabolic processes: *aerobic metabolism* and *anaerobic metabolism*. Aerobic metabolism requires oxygen for the production of energy, while anaerobic metabolism produces energy in the absence of oxygen.

When the body produces energy by anaerobic metabolism (Figure 8.3), a molecule of glucose is separated into two molecules of pyruvate by a process called glycolysis. These pyruvate molecules remain in the cytosol of the cell where they are converted to ethanol and lactate by fermentation. The energy released during the breakdown of pyruvate forms ATP from ADP and P_i. Without mitochondria, all cells would be anaerobic and depend entirely on glycolysis for their production of energy.

Anaerobic metabolism is relatively inefficient, as fermentation provides only about two molecules of ATP per molecule of glucose. Yet tissues in the body, such as skeletal muscle, function anaerobically when oxygen is scarce.

Aerobic metabolism, on the other hand, serves as the predominant means of human energy production. Over 90 percent of cellular oxygen consumed by the body fuels this mitochondrial process. In addition to pyruvate, aerobic metabolism uses a variety of molecules to yield energy. Amino acids, organic acids, and fatty acids can all be metabolically transformed to create a series of energy-producing enzymatic reactions known as the *Krebs cycle*.

The Krebs Cycle

The Krebs cycle (Figure 8.4) is the first of two sequential processes aerobically producing

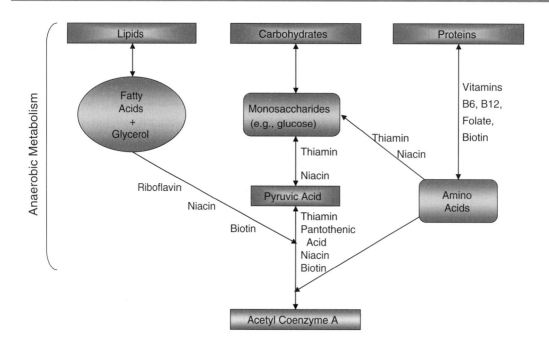

FIGURE 8.3   *The role of vitamins in early energy production (pre-mitochondria)*

energy in mitochondria. The Krebs cycle, followed by *oxidative phosphorylation,* takes the two molecules of pyruvate produced by glycolysis and converts them into CO_2 and H_2O. This process yields a large amount of energy, as one molecule of glucose can produce 36 molecules of ATP.

The Krebs cycle, named after its 1953 Nobel Prize-winning discoverer, Hans Krebs, involves oxidative metabolism of acetyl units and produces high-energy phosphate compounds. This process, also called the tricarboxylic acid cycle, or TCA, occurs in the outer compartment of mitochondria. Once an or-

ganic molecule such as pyruvate crosses the outer mitochondrial membrane, a series of four dehydrogenase enzymes strip the electrons from the molecule (in the form of hydrogen atoms). One passage through the Krebs cycle is sufficient to strip off four pairs of hydrogen atoms containing four pairs of transferable electrons. After these electron-containing hydrogen atoms are removed from the organic substrate, they are added to the vitamin B3- and vitamin B2-containing cofactors, NAD^+ and FAD. They form NADH and $FADH_2$ respectively. These hydrogen-receiving cofactors transport the electrons to their last stop within

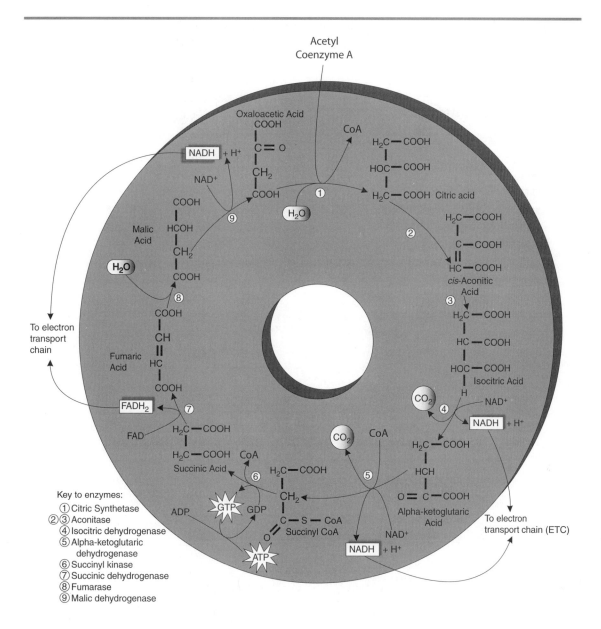

FIGURE 8.4 *Krebs cycle*

the mitochondrion, the electron transport chain (ETC), where they prepare for oxidative phosphorylation.

Oxidative Phosphorylation

Oxidative phosphorylation produces ATP using energy derived from the redox reactions of the electron transport chain (Figure 8.5). Although considered part of aerobic metabolism, the reactions in the Krebs cycle do not actually use oxygen. Instead, they produce cofactors NADH and $FADH_2$. In oxidative phosphorylation, NADH and $FADH_2$ combine with molecular oxygen through a series of electron transfers in the electron transport chain to form water (H_2O). The cofactor NADH is recycled to NAD^+ during the electron transfers or *oxidation* stage.

An electrochemical proton gradient performs the second step of the process as it crosses the mitochondrial membrane. In this

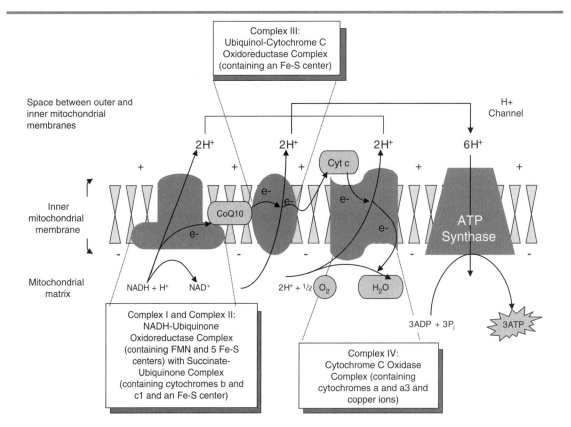

FIGURE 8.5 *Proton pumps in oxidative phosphorylation [Electron transport chain]*

step, the backflow of protons produced from this gradient activates the membrane-bound enzyme ATP synthase. *Phosphorylation* occurs when ATP synthase uses the energy from the proton flow to form ATP from ADP and P_i (Figure 8.5).

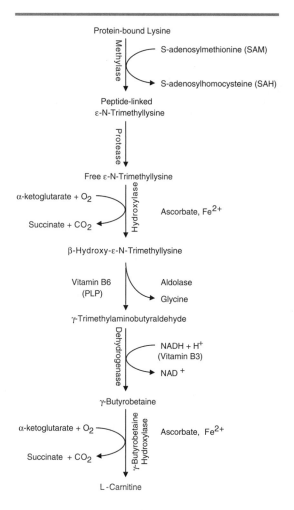

FIGURE 8.6 *Carnitine biosynthetic pathway in mammals*

ENERGY AND NUTRITION

Mitochondria and Nutrition

Mitochondrial production of aerobic energy begins with the successful transport of substrate into the mitochondrial matrix. Passage of fatty acids across the inner mitochondrial membrane and into the matrix is an active process that is dependent upon the fatty acid transport molecule L-carnitine (Figure 8.6). To function as a fatty acid transport shuttle, L-carnitine must be in its acyl-carnitine form and exit from the matrix during the transport.[7] Carnitine is synthesized by the amino acid lysine. During synthesis, three methyl groups donated by the amino acid methionine are attached to the lysine molecule to form trimethyllysine. Four subsequent steps are required for final synthesis of L-carnitine; they depend upon enzymatic cofactors vitamin C, vitamin B3, vitamin B6, and iron. (The carnitine molecule is pictured in Figure 8.7.)

Cells commanding immediate high energy, like muscle cells, need creatine for energy storage. Produced by the liver, kidneys, and pancreas, creatine is converted to a

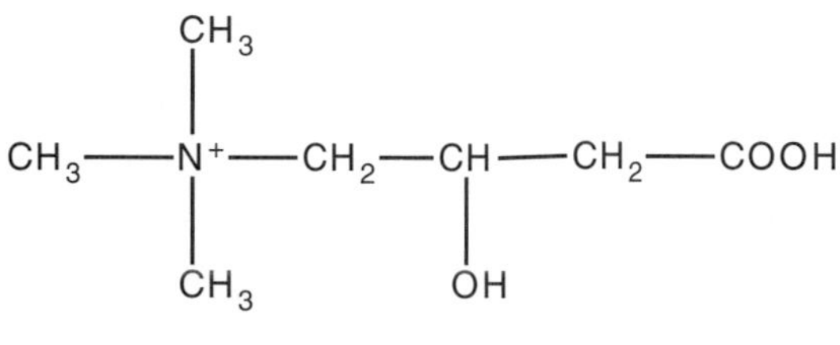

$$CH_3-N^+(CH_3)(CH_3)-CH_2-CH(OH)-CH_2-COOH$$

FIGURE 8.7 *Structural formula of carnitine*

high-energy, phosphorylated derivative called phosphocreatine (Figure 8.8). Phosphocreatine converts ADP to ATP by transferring its high-energy phosphate via creatine kinase. Carbohydrate intake and insulin secretion increase muscle cell use of creatine.[8] Gerbitz et al. propose that creatine shuttled through mitochondria may signal glucokinase to bind glucose and pancreas beta cells to secrete insulin.[9] Creatine is excreted by the kidneys as creatinine.

Energy and Absorption of Nutrients

Mitochondria are central to the body's general energy needs, especially bringing dietary nutrients into the body. While some nutrients diffuse across the intestinal membrane, car-

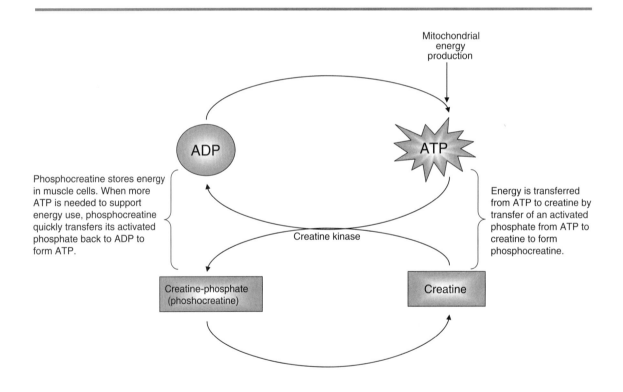

Mitochondrial energy production

ADP

ATP

Phosphocreatine stores energy in muscle cells. When more ATP is needed to support energy use, phosphocreatine quickly transfers its activated phosphate back to ADP to form ATP.

Creatine kinase

Energy is transferred from ATP to creatine by transfer of an activated phosphate from ATP to creatine to form phosphocreatine.

Creatine-phosphate (phoshocreatine)

Creatine

FIGURE 8.8   *The creatine-phosphate energy shuttle*

rier substances transport other nutrients across the intestinal border to the blood. This process is called *active transport*. Active transport requires energy in the form of ATP generated by the mitochondria. Digestion and transport of nutrients into the bloodstream use approximately one-fourth of the body's metabolic energy.

In active transport, a molecule or element, such as uric acid or calcium, is bound to a carrier on the outside of the intestinal cell. The carrier transports its nutrient cargo to the inner membrane of the cell and returns to the outer membrane to repeat the process. This movement is central in absorbing nutrients such as glucose, amino acids, iron, calcium, sodium, potassium, magnesium, and uric acid.[10]

KEY COFACTORS IN MITOCHONDRIAL METABOLISM

Once shuttled into the matrix, organic substrates travel through the Krebs cycle (Figure 8.4) where they undergo a series of nine enzymatic steps involving eight enzymes. This complex series of reactions requires several nutrients at different stages, including vitamins B1, B2, B3, B5, lipoic acid, iron, magnesium, sulfur, and phosphorus. Magnesium and vitamin B3 are present in three of the steps. Key organic acid intermediary compounds formed during the Krebs cycle include citrate, succinate, malate, fumarate, oxaloacetate, alpha-ketoglutarate, isocitrate, and cis-aconitate.

Embedded within the inner mitochondrial membrane are five enzyme complexes and two carrier systems collectively referred to as the electron transport chain (ETC). Embedded in the membrane, ATP-synthase enzyme, or complex V, can be found at the end of the ETC. Each mitochondrion contains approximately 17,000 ETCs. The key enzyme and transport structures within the ETC include flavoproteins, iron-sulfur proteins, and cytochromes. The ETC proteins require vitamins B2, B3, C, K, magnesium, and zinc as cofactors.[11]

A carrier system between enzyme Complexes II and III that involves ubiquinone, or coenzyme Q10, facilitates the ETC. Not only is coenzyme Q10 the only nonprotein component of the electron transport system, it is the only component capable of simultaneously transporting two electrons in the process. Cells rich in mitochondria also have a high concentration of the critical carrier molecule coenzyme Q10.[12] For example, cardiocytes contain more than 10 times the amount of coenzyme Q10 than do intestinal cells.

Mitochondrial Free Radicals and Oxidative Stress

Mitochondria derive their uniqueness from their individualized, circular DNA. This structure is similar to the structure of bacterial DNA. Mitochondrial genes primarily code for the proteins necessary to produce ATP. However, unlike nuclear DNA, mitochondria inherit DNA exclusively from the female of a species. At least in energy production, we owe our roots to our mothers.

More than 90 percent of all cellular oxygen consumption fuels mitochondrial processes. This means that mitochondria must transfer tremendous numbers of electrons to produce energy. Both free oxygen and free electrons may contribute to oxidative stress by forming reactive oxygen species. Under normal conditions, roughly four to five percent of the oxygen processed in the mitochondria generates reactive oxygen species such as superoxide, hydrogen peroxide, and hydroxyl radical. While an efficiently operating mitochondrial system has the capacity to minimize the adverse effects of this "low-level" oxidant leakage, an inefficient system may not. In the latter case, mitochondrial damage may result.[13]

When oxidative stress occurs, mitochondrial function can be compromised or lost long before other cellular functions. Two factors increasing mitochondrial DNA's susceptibility to damage include proximity to the production site of oxygen radicals in the inner membranes and lack of protective histones, which normally protect nuclear DNA. A mutation in mitochondrial DNA creates a mixture of normal and mutant molecules that pass to daughter cells during subsequent replications. Mitochondrial bioenergetic capacity drops as a consequence, ultimately falling below a minimum threshold value necessary for tissues to function normally. Tissues that rely on mitochondrial bioenergetics, like those in the central nervous system, heart, skeletal muscle, kidney, liver, and endocrine system, suffer first from this process. Such changes may accelerate biological aging and the onset of various disease-related conditions.

Uncoupling

The transfer of electrons through the electron transport chain coordinates the production of water and the recycling of cofactors NAD^+ and FADH. The "coupling" of these events yields high energy, efficient conversion of oxygen to water, and low amounts of harmful reactive oxygen species. However, if this coupling is impaired, so too is ATP formation (energy production). Such results are becoming increasingly linked to a number of clinical conditions.

Some drugs, xenobiotics, and other substances appear to uncouple electron transport and oxidative phosphorylation. These exogenous influences may lead to disease by altering mitochondrial function. For example, exposure to toxins, such as 3-nitropropionate, a fungal toxin found on sugar cane, can cause oxidative phosphorylation to uncouple, thus initiating mitochondrial oxidative stress, and ultimately leading to neuronal death. Certain antibiotic drugs such as doxycycline, imipenem, and leucinostatins A and B may also uncouple mitochondrial oxidative phosphorylation and increase oxidative stress.[14,15,16]

Clinical Issues: Mitochondrial Dysfunction

The integral role of mitochondria in energy production and cellular support illustrates how mitochondrial dysfunction can affect nearly all organ systems (Figure 8.9).[17] Studies have found that mutations in mitochondrial DNA are associated with a variety of diseases. For example, since mitochondrial DNA changes often occur over a long period of time, researchers suggest that such mutations affect the aging process. In 1993, Wallace and colleagues compared the mitochondrial DNA of non-Alzheimer's patients to that of Alzheimer's patients. Alzheimer's patients exhibited significantly higher levels of DNA mutation than those without the disease. Such changes may result from induced factors related to long-term exposure to mutagenic agents (xenobiotics, radiation, etc.). Dr. Flint Beal of Massachusetts General Hospital argues that neuronal mitochondrial defects

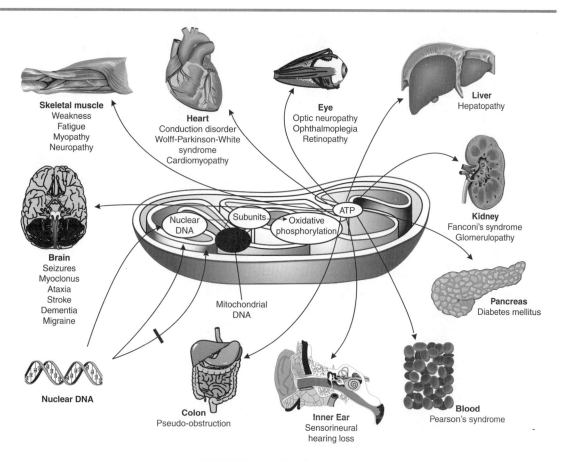

FIGURE 8.9 *Mitochondrion*

may predispose people to neurodegenerative diseases such as amyotrophic lateral sclerosis, Huntington's, Parkinson's, and Alzheimer's diseases later in life.[18]

In the evolving understanding of genetic susceptibility, there are known mitochondrial disorders that relate to polymorphism of the mitochondrial DNA.[19] Individuals with these genetic characteristics, which range from mild to severe mitochondrial dysfunction, may have increasing degrees of risk to neurotoxins and brain inflammatory conditions. The relationship of mitochondrial DNA polymorphism to ApoE characteristics and the risk of beta amyloid-related toxicity have not been outlined fully, but literature suggests relationships among different genetic factors that give rise to individual risks of neurodegenerative and cardiovascular disease beyond the presently accepted risk factors.

Until recently, scholars believed that most disorders involving compromised mitochondrial function were created by mutated mitochondrial DNA. They argued that the mutation contributed to a nonfunctional protein and disrupted oxidative phosphorylation. The diagnosis of mitochondrial myopathy in world-renowned, long-distance cyclist Greg LeMond challenged this view. His disorder, characterized by debilitating fatigue, muscle impairment, and other symptoms that forced him to retire, marked the first defined case for a healthy, athletic, middle-aged individual to have such symptoms unrelated to a recognized genetic mitochondrial disorder.[20] LeMond's case suggests that mitochondrial

abnormalities may be induced, leading to disorders that may express themselves as energy deficiency accompanied by fatigue, sleep disturbance, cognitive dysfunction, immune dysregulation, or pain (Table 8.2).

Clinical Issues: Mitochondrial Energy Crisis and Parkinson's Disease

Scholars have recently noted a meaningful relationship among mitochondrial dysfunction, oxidative stress, and Parkinson's disease.[21] They cite oxidative stress as an important contributor to nigral cell death in Parkinson's disease, which is also a secondary phenomenon in uncoupling of mitochondrial function. Studies have not uncovered the primary cause of mitochondrial respiratory failure, but investigators suggest that the additive effect of environmental neurotoxins in genetically predisposed individuals may play a key role.[22] Birkmayer proposed that NADH can have a significant effect in modulating mitochondrial energy deficits in Parkinson's disease. In one open trial, 71 percent of patients responded positively to daily intravenous administration of 50 mg of NADH.[23] Further studies suggest that younger Parkinson's patients and those with shorter duration of the disease may benefit most from this approach.[24] This treatment regime is still considered controversial, and similar results have not been reported by other investigators, but Birkmayer noted success with Alzheimer's patients as well as individuals experiencing depression and energy deficit.[25,26]

TABLE 8.2 *Mitochondrial-related Symptoms and Dysfunction*

The range of mitochondrial-related symptoms and dysfunction may include:
Cardiac problems (e.g., conduction disorders, cardiomyopathies)
Central nervous system problems associated with seizures, ataxia, stroke, dementia, and migraine
Colonic dysfunction associated with pseudo-obstruction
Fatigue
Inner ear dysfunction (e.g., some cases of sensorineural hearing loss)
Liver dysfunction
Neuropathies
Ocular disorders (e.g., optical neuropathies, retinopathies)
Pancreatic dysfunction (e.g., secondary effects of diabetes mellitus)
Renal dysfunction (e.g., glomerulonephropathy)
Weakness

A FUNCTIONAL APPROACH TO ENERGY

Mitochondrial Resuscitation

A functional medicine approach to health maintains that intervention into clinical conditions must occur at root levels of metabolic imbalance in order to be effective. Mitochondrial dysfunction is a good example of metabolic imbalance at root level—a level that has been shown to cut across all organ systems and to underlie a variety of symptom patterns and clinical conditions.

According to a functional medicine perspective, support of mitochondrial function must involve restoration or "resuscitation" of the mitochondrial vitality through in- creased intake of metabolites concentrated in mitochondrion. Functional medicine also aims to reduce and eliminate endogenous and exogenous circumstances that contribute to mitochondrial oxidative stress.

A nutritional support program for mitochondria should include cofactors, transport molecules, intermediary metabolites, and antioxidants essential to mitochondrial activities. A functional medicine approach recommends the following guidelines:

- key cofactors and antioxidants specific for mitochondrial function, including lipoic acid, coenzyme Q10, and carnitine;
- a balance of antioxidant factors and cofactors, including glutathione,

cysteine, vitamin E, vitamin C, carotenoids, flavonoids, and the minerals zinc, copper, selenium, and manganese;

- cofactors appearing in the Krebs cycle and the ETC, such as vitamins B1, B2, B3, B5, and K, and the minerals magnesium, phosphorus, and sulfur; and

- direct provision of Krebs cycle intermediates, including the organic acids citrate, succinate, malate, fumarate, oxaloacetate, alpha-ketoglutarate, isocitrate, and cis-aconitate.

Reducing Mitochondrial Oxidative Stress

Maintaining a mitochondrial environment free from oxidative stress is a difficult and complex task. While humans have built-in protective mechanisms to minimize the effects of oxidative stress, the very nature of mitochondrial activity (especially its oxygen use and electron transfer) creates a state of oxidative stress. Functional medicine recommends nutrition as an effective way to control oxidative stress. Ensuring adequate nutrient status can promote efficient electron transport and oxidative phosphorylation and maintain redox balance.

Three molecules found in the mitochondrion protect the membrane and other components from oxidant damage: 1) *lipoic acid*, a sulfur-containing organic acid, 2) *coenzyme Q10*, the nonprotein component of the

ETC, and 3) *glutathione*, a tripeptide formed from glutamate, glycine, and cysteine. (The glutathione redox cycle is depicted in Figure 8.10.) Insufficient amounts of these molecules increase oxidative stress and may compromise mitochondrial function. The interaction of these factors may alter oxidative stress and mitochondrial energy production—states associated with disorders of accelerated aging.

Specific Nutrient Substances Useful in Improving Mitochondrial Efficiency

A number of nutrient-derived substances can improve mitochondrial function in oxidative stress or cellular toxicity (Table 8.3). This approach balances the redox potential of the cell by improving mitochondrial oxidative phosphorylation and reducing expression of oxidant stress factors. McCord explains that the oxidant/antioxidant balance is crucial to reduce the risk of many age-related diseases.[27] Mechanisms may exist by which nutrient pharmacology can improve the metabolism of oxygen-rich tissues, including the brain and cardiovascular system.

Nutrient intervention that improves mitochondrial function, "mitochondrial resuscitation," includes strengthening the Krebs cycle function, stabilizing the electron transport chain, protecting mitochondrial membranes against oxidative damage, re-establishing proper glutathione cycle function, and reducing oxidation-related gene expression. What

TABLE 8.3   *Nutritional Modulators of Mitochondrial Oxidative Phosphorylation*

Nutritional Agent	Daily Range	Influence
Ascorbate	500–6000 mg	Part of glutathione—lipoate redox activity
Catechin	50–1000 mg	Hydroxyl radical and peroxynitrite quencher
Copper	1–3 mg	Necessary for Zn-CuSOD
CoQ10 (ubiquinone)	20–1000 mg	Maintenance of electron transport chain function
Ferulic acid	100–300 mg	Hydroxyl radical quencher
Glutathione	100–1000 mg	Antioxidant and Phase II mercapturate formation
Lipoic acid	50–1000 mg	Multiple roles in mitochondrial protection
Magnesium	50–1000 mg	Mitochondrial Krebs Cycle activator
Manganese	2–5 mg	Necessary for MnSOD
N-3 fatty acids (EPA/DHA)	500–3000 mg	Mitochondrial membrane and blocking action of cytokines
N-acetyl-carnitine	50–1000 mg	Fatty acid transport into the mitochondrion
N-acetyl-cysteine (NAC)	50–1500 mg	Stimulates mitochondrial glutathione synthesis
Niacin	10–50 mg	NADH and NADPH production
Niacinamide	200–2000 mg	NADH and NADPH production
Riboflavin	10–200 mg	$FADH_2$ activator and Krebs Cycle nutrient
Selenium	100–500 mcg	Activator of GSH peroxidase
Sodium succinate	100–4000 mg	Mitochondrial Krebs Cycle activator
Thiamin	10–200 mg	Transketolase activator for hexose monophosphate shunt
Vitamin E (tocopherols)	100–1000 mg	Mitochondrial membrane protection
Vitamin K	100–1000 mcg	Electron transport chain protector
Zinc	10–50 mg	Necessary for Zn-CuSOD

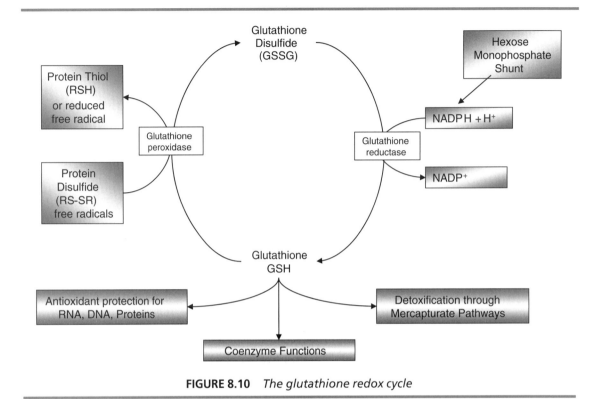

FIGURE 8.10   *The glutathione redox cycle*

follows are key factors to consider in nutritional support.

Coenzyme Q10

Intervention with coenzyme Q10, either alone or as one component of therapy, in individuals with mitochondrial myopathies or encephalomyopathies, results in decreased muscle weakness, improved central and peripheral nerve conductance, and reduced serum levels of lactate and pyruvate.[28,29,30,31,32] Intervention with coenzyme Q10, sodium succinate, and the Krebs cycle intermediate demon-strates the same effect in the mitochondrial disorder called Kearns-Sayre syndrome.[33,34]

Lipoic acid

Lipoic acid is an important antioxidant and has an essential role in mitochondrial dehydrogenase reactions. It also protects membranes by interacting with vitamin C and glutathione to aid in the recycling of vitamin E. Lipoate is tolerated well by individuals and protects against a number of oxidative stress-associated conditions and symptoms including neurotoxicity, neurodegeneration, radiation injury, ischemia-reperfusion injury, and NMDA and malonate-induced striatal lesions.[35,36]

Vitamin E

Vitamin E is an important antioxidant that helps improve mitochondrial function. A notable case example using an aggressive vitamin E therapy was published in *The Lancet* in 1993. A young, normally developing boy began to experience muscle weakness that confined him to a wheelchair by age two. Analysis revealed he suffered from a mitochondrial myopathy that resulted in significant free radical production. Physicians reasoned that antioxidant nutrition might reduce the damaging effect of the mitochondrial oxidant activity. After several weeks on a regimen of 2000 IU daily vitamin E, there was notable improvement in ATP production as well as improvement in muscle tone. Eventually, he was able to walk.[37]

L-carnitine

Carnitine serves two major roles in energy metabolism: shuttling fatty acids into the mitochondrial matrix for oxidation and modulating the intramitochondrial levels of acetyl Coenzyme A, an important cofactor in the Krebs cycle reactions. The main consequences of carnitine deficiency are symptoms associated with impaired energy production. Studies illustrate that acetyl-L-carnitine improves mitochondrial energy production.[38] The majority of carnitine is derived from the diet. Estimated safe, non-therapeutic levels of carnitine intake range from 150 to 500 micro-

moles per day. Therapeutic levels of carnitine may be much higher.[39]

B-complex vitamins

Thiamin (vitamin B1) is a cofactor for pyruvate dehydrogenase and has been used to stimulate production of NADH.[40] Riboflavin (vitamin B2) is converted to flavin monophosphate or flavin adenine dinucleotide (FAD) and functions as a cofactor for electron transport in the ETC. High doses of thiamin (300 mg three times daily) have been reported to normalize plasma pyruvate and lactate levels and improve fatigue in patients with Kearns-Sayre syndrome and mitochondrial myopathy.[41,42] As a precursor to NADH, nicotinamide (vitamin B3) is also essential to the full functioning of both the Krebs cycle and the ETC and has shown clinical benefit. Biotin and vitamin B6 are also important cofactors.[43] The B-complex vitamins, including high-dose thiamin and niacinamide, should be administered at doses as high as 300 mg per day to get clinical benefit in cases of genetically related mitochondrial dysfunction.[44,45]

Vitamin K

Menadione (vitamin K3) and phylloquinone (vitamin K1) are two vitamin K compounds that have both been used in conjunction with vitamin C in nutritional support approaches to mitochondrial disorders. Vitamin K administration has been shown to enhance energy production in cultured cells and improve cellular phosphate metabolism in a patient with mitochondrial myopathy.[46] High doses of vitamin

K have also improved Complex I activity and Complex III activity in the electron transport chain of mitochondria in cultured cells.[47] Oral vitamin K helps alleviate symptoms associated with defects in Complex III.[48]

N-acetylcysteine and/or glutathione

Glutathione has been shown to decrease during the aging process. Mitochondria appear to be especially susceptible to this decrease.[49] Glutathione is particularly low in neurons, and neuronal levels may be compromised during aging even when plasma levels of glutathione appear to be adequate. N-acetylcysteine can serve as a precursor to glutathione. In addition to their function(s) in the glutathione antioxidant cascade, N-acetylcysteine and glutathione can also serve as inhibitors of pro-inflammatory cytokines such as tumor necrosis factor.[50]

Creatine

Oral creatine supplementation has been shown to increase creatine supplies in skeletal muscle[51] and phosphocreatine resynthesis following intense exercise.[52] It also sustains high ATP rates during strenuous exercise.[53]

SUMMARY

This chapter introduces what will undoubtedly become an exciting point of intervention in the field of clinical nutrition. Given today's knowledge, each of these components alone may be a beneficial, but rudimentary, approach to solving problems of mitochondrial metabolism. Our expanding understanding suggests that a complex mixture of vitamins, minerals, cofactors, amino acids, fatty acids, and accessory nutrients may be needed to address the unique factors involved in mitochondrial metabolism.

The variety of nutrients that influence mitochondrial function will likely expand considerably. Additional nutrients to consider (presently undergoing clinical experimentation in patient care) include vitamin C, vitamin E, magnesium, succinate, and anthocyanidins. Nutrients of import to consider include unsaturated fatty acids (including GLA, ALA, EPA, DHA) and selected amino acids (depending upon individual need).

CHAPTER 8 REFERENCES

1. Linder MC. Nutritional Biochemistry and Metabolism with Clinical Applications. 2nd ed. Norwalk, Conn; Appleton & Lange; 1991.
2. Groff JL, Gropper SS, Hunt, SM. Advanced Nutrition and Human Metabolism. Minneapolis, Minn: West Publishing Co.; 1995.
3. Ziegler EE, Filer LJ, Jr, eds. Present Knowledge in Nutrition. Washington, D.C.: International Life Sciences Institute Press; 1996.
4. Johns DR. Mitochondrial DNA and disease. N Engl J Med. 1995;333(10):638–644.
5. Trounce I, Byrne E, Marzuki S. Decline in skeletal muscle mitochondrial respiratory chain function: possible factor in aging. Lancet. 1989;1(8639): 637–639.
6. Alberts B, Bray D, Lewis J, et al. Molecular Biology of the Cell. New York: Garland Publ., Inc; 1983:67–75.
7. Tanphaichitr V, Leelahagul P. Carnitine metabolism and carnitine deficiency. Nutr. 1993;9: 246–254.

8. Green AL, Sewell DA, Simpson L, et al. Carbohydrate ingestion stimulates creatine uptake in human skeletal muscle. J Physiol. 1995;489: 27P–28P.

9. Gerbitz KD, Gempel K, Brdiczka D. Mitochondria and diabetes. Genetic, biochemical, and clinical implications of the cellular energy circuit. Diabetes. 1996;45:113–126.

10. Guyton, AC. Textbook of Medical Physiology. 8th ed. Philadelphia, Pa: W.B. Saunders Co.; 1991:46–50.

11. Aw TY, Jones DP. Nutrient supply and mitochondrial function. Annu Rev Nutr. 1989;9: 229–251.

12. Levin B. Coenzyme Q10: clinical monograph. Qrtly Rev Nat Med. 1994; Fall:235–250.

13. Ames BN, Shigenaga MK, Hagen TM. Mitochondrial decay in aging. Biochem Biophys Acta. 1995;1271:165–170.

14. Riesbeck K, Bredberg A, Forsgren A. Ciprofloxacin does not inhibit mitochondrial functions but other antibiotics do. Antimicrobial Agents Chemother. 1990;34(1):167–169.

15. Tune BM, Hsu CY. The renal mitochondrial toxicity of beta-lactam antibiotics: in vitro effects of cephaloglycin and imipenem. J Am Soc Nephrol. 1990;1(5):815–821.

16. Shima A, Fukushima K, Arai T, et al. Dual inhibitory effects of the peptide antibiotics leucinostatins on oxidative phosphorylation in mitochondria. Cell Struc Func. 1990;15:53–58.

17. Johns DR. Mitochondrial DNA and disease. N Engl J Med. 1995;333(10):638-644.

18. Beal MF. Aging, energy, and oxidative stress in neurodegenerative diseases. Ann Neurol. 1995; 38(3):357–366.

19. Larsson NG, Clayton DA. Molecular genetic aspects of human mitochondrial disorders. Ann Rev Genetics. 1995;29:151–178.

20. LeMond steps down: rare muscular disease forces LeMond to retire. USA Today. 1994; December 5:1B.

21. Mizuno Y, Ikebe S, Hattori N, et al. Mitochondrial energy crisis in Parkinson's disease. Adv Neurol. 1993;60:282–287.

22. Mizuno Y, Ikebe S, Hattorik N, et al. Role of mitochondria in the etiology and pathogenesis of Parkinson's disease. Biochem Biophys. 1995; 1271:265–274.

23. Birkmayer GJ, Birkmayer W. Stimulation of endogenous L-dopa biosynthesis—a new principle for the therapy of Parkinson's disease. Acta Neurol Scand. 1989;126:183–187.

24. Birkmayer JG, Vrecko C, Volc D, Birkmayer W. Nicotinamide adenine dinucleotide (NADH)—a new therapeutic approach to Parkinson's disease. Acta Neurol Scand. 1993;87(Suppl 146): 32–35.

25. Birkmayer JGD. Coenzyme nicotinamide adenine dinucleotide—new therapeutic approach for improving dementia of the Alzheimer type. Annals Clin Lab Sci.1996;26:1–9.

26. Birkmayer JGD, Birkmayer W. The coenzyme nicotinamide adenine dinucleotide (NADH) as biological antidepressive agent—experience with 205 patients. New Trends Clin Neuropharmacol. 1991;3/4:75-86.

27. McCord JM. Human disease, free radicals, and the oxidant/antioxidant balance. Clin Biochem. 1993;26:351–357.

28. Ihara Y, Namba R, Kuroda S, Sato T, Shirabe T. Mitochondrial encephalomyopathy (MELAS): pathological study and successful therapy with coenzyme Q10 and idebenone. J Neurol Sci. 1989;90:263–271.

29. Nishikawa Y, Takahashi M, Yorifuji S, et al. Long-term coenzyme Q10 therapy for a mitochondrial encephalomyopathy with cytochrome C oxidase deficiency: a 31P NMR study. Neurol. 1989;39:399–403.

30. Yamamoto M, Sato T, Anno M, Ujike H, Takemoto M. Mitochondrial myopathy, encephalopathy, lactic acidosis, and strokelike episodes with recurrent abdominal symptoms and coenzyme Q10 administration. J Neurol Neurosurg Psychiatry. 1987;50:1475–1481.

31. Goda S, Hamada T, Ishimoto S, Kobayashi T, Goto I, Kuroiwa Y. Clinical improvement after administration of coenzyme Q10 in a patient

with mitochondrial encephalomyopathy. J Neurol. 1987;234:62–63.

32. Bresolin N, Bet L, Binda A, et al. Clinical and biochemical correlations in mitochondrial myopathies treated with coenzyme Q10. Neurol. 1988;38:892–899.

33. Ogasahara S, Nishikawa Y, Yorifuji S, et al. Treatment of Kearns-Sayre syndrome with coenzyme Q10. Neurol. 1986;36:45–53.

34. Ogasahara S, Yorifuji S, Nishikawa, et al. Improvement of abnormal pyruvate metabolism and cardiac conduction defect with coenzyme Q10 in Kearns-Sayre syndrome. Neurol. 1985; 35:372–377.

35. Packer L, Witt EH, Tritschler HJ. Alpha-lipoic acid as a biological antioxidant. Free Rad Biol Med. 1995;19:227–250.

36. Beal MF. Aging, energy, and oxidative stress in neurodegenerative diseases. Ann Neurol. 1995; 38:357–366.

37. Bakker HD, Sholte HR, Jeneson JA. Vitamin E in a mitochondrial myopathy with proliferating mitochondria. Lancet. 1993;342(8864):175–176.

38. Gadaleta MN, Petruzzella V, Daddabbo L, et al. Mitochondrial DNA transcription and translation in aged rat: effect of acetyl-L-carnitine. Ann NY Acad Sci. 1994;717:150-160.

39. Tanphaichitr V, Leelahagul P. Carnitine metabolism and carnitine deficiency. Nutr. 1993; 9:246–254.

40. Shoffner JM, Wallace DC. Oxidative phosphorylation diseases and mitochondrial DNA mutations: diagnosis and treatment. Annu Rev Nutr. 1994;14:535–568.

41. Lou HC. Correction of increased plasma pyruvate and plasma lactate levels using large doses of thiamin in patients with Kearns-Sayre syndrome. Arch Neurol. 1981;38:459.

42. Mastaglia FL, Thompson PL, Papadimitriou JM. Mitochondrial myopathy with cardiomyopathy, lactic acidosis and response to prednisone and thiamine. Aust N Z J Med. 1980; 10:660–664.

43. Aw TY, Jones DP. Nutrient supply and mitochondrial function. Annu Rev Nutr. 1989;9: 229–251.

44. Shoffner JM, Wallace DC. Oxidative phosphorylation diseases and mitochondrial DNA mutations: diagnosis and treatment. Annu Rev Nutr. 1994;14:535–568.

45. Aw TY, Jones DP. Nutrient supply and mitochondrial function. Annu Rev Nutr. 1989;9: 229–251.

46. Shoffner JM, Wallace DC. Oxidative phosphorylation diseases and mitochondrial DNA mutations: diagnosis and treatment. Annu Rev Nutr. 1994;14:535–568.

47. Wijburg FA, de Groot CJ, Feller N, Wanders RJ. Restoration of NADH-oxidation in complex I and complex III deficient fibroblasts by menadione. J Inher Metab Dis.1991;14: 293–296.

48. Aw TY, Jones DP. Nutrient supply and mitochondrial function. Annu Rev Nutr. 1989;9: 229–251.

49. Benzi G, Moretti A. Age and peroxidative stress-related modifications of the cerebral enzymatic activities linked to mitochondria and the glutathione system. Free Rad Biol Med. 1995; 19:77–101.

50. Peristeris P, Clark BD, Gatti S, et al. N-acetylcysteine and glutathione as inhibitors of tumor necrosis factor production. Cell Immunol. 1992; 140:(2)390–399.

51. Hultman E, Soderlund K, Timmons JA, et al. Muscle creatine loading in men. J Appl Physiol. 1996;81:232–237.

52. Greenhaff PL, Bodin K, Soderlund K, Cedarblad G, Greenhaff PL. Effect of oral creatine supplementation on skeletal muscle phosphocreatine resynthesis. Am J Physiol. 1994;266:E725–E730.

53. Volek JS, Kraiemer WJ. Creatine supplementation: its effect on human muscular performance and body composition. J Strength Conditioning Res. 1996;10:200–210.

9

Environment and Toxicity

ESTERN SCIENCE AND MEDICINE tend to view illness as a cause-and-effect phenomenon. According to this approach, disease happens to a person, and a clinician's task is to determine the cause of the disease. Illness is typically explained in terms of events or agents that develop outside of an individual, a concept that dates back to the early stages of medicine. The discovery of microorganisms that directly cause disease—microbes—has strengthened this perspective in Western practice, encouraging nearly every area of modern medicine to embrace it. Practitioners must realize that viewing illness as having solely external causes overlooks the powerful effect of the host response. However, considering the magnitude of chemical compounds in the environment and their effect on human physiology, it is difficult to ignore the profound power these external agents exert over health. Indeed, the combination of four million synthetic compounds coupled with thousands of natural compounds must be taken as a serious potential threat to human health.

How do clinicians assess the impact of these external compounds? How do they distinguish external factors from internal responses? How can they intervene to restore their patients' health? Answers to questions like these lie in basic understanding about xenobiotics, their sources, and the metabolic resources required to transform these substances. *Xenobiotic* describes chemicals or molecules foreign to living organisms. More specifically, the action of toxic agents, or toxicants, on the organism (on the structure and function of molecules) may occur at or within multiple sites, including the functional cellular components (e.g., active transport mechanisms), enzymes, receptors, and nucleic acids. The toxicant may make it difficult for the organism to properly carry out essential functions, including absorption, distribution/solubility, metabolism, and excretion of the toxicant. Collectively, these factors contribute to *end effects* of the toxicant.

For example, a toxic agent that diminishes the functional capacity of the liver or the kidneys to metabolize and excrete that substance may become increasingly "toxic" as functional capacity decreases. In addition, the rate of distribution and tissue accumulation of a substance affects the toxicity of that substance relative to specific organ/tissue structure and function. The adage, "There are no harmless substances, only 'harmless' ways of using them," underscores the relative complexity of toxicity.

This chapter focuses on chemical substances and the role of nutrients in the body's protection against and elimination of these substances. Both roles are critical since the impact of a xenobiotic is inherently dependent upon an individual's response mechanisms. Specifically, this chapter reviews the basic xenobiotics to which humans are exposed and explores some of the nutrient-dependent processes that transform xenobiotics.

TOTAL LOAD

Understanding how xenobiotics affect human health is germane to the concept of total load.

Total load describes the total of all exposures and influences that bear on human physiology. Since these factors often determine the efficiency of the body's detoxification system, nutrient status and organ reserve, they are central to any question of how xenobiotics affect humans. The concept of total load suggests that the sum of the factors may overwhelm an individual's system of metabolic management.

For many years, efforts to understand how xenobiotics affect human health focused on determining whether or not a substance produced cancer in laboratory animals. Once studies confirmed this finding for animals, researchers applied these studies to humans. While these efforts provided much insight into detoxification, metabolism, and cell biology, in many ways they now detract from more pertinent questions: What is the capacity of xenobiotics to alter the *function* of biological systems, and how does this contribute to illness? According to the latter perspective, cancer, as an end-stage manifestation of chemical exposure, seems to be only a second-order issue, since so many physiological events precede its development.

In the early 1990s, two seminal volumes published by the National Academy of Sciences raised concerns about the *functional* changes induced by exposure to low levels of xenobiotics. These volumes, *Environmental Neurotoxicology*[1] and *Biologic Markers in Immunotoxicology*,[2] highlight two important issues—functional changes result from low-level chemical exposure, and their effects can multiply when an individual is exposed to more than one agent.

An animal study about the lethal dose of lead and mercury dramatically illustrates this latter point—the multiplicity of toxic effects. In this study, scientists administered LD1 of mercury *combined* with the LD1 of lead to animals. (LD1 is the acute dose leading to death of 1 percent of a test population. LD50 refers to the dose that produces a fatal response in 50 percent of the animals and is a typical measure used in toxicology.) Remarkably, the LD1 of mercury + LD1 of lead resulted in LD100, or 100 percent mortality, within five days.[3] This study demonstrated a profound difference in outcome between low-toxicity substances administered in combination and low-toxicity substances administered alone.

Given the ubiquitous nature of chemicals in the environment, it is likely that *single* exposure is more the exception than the rule. As such, it is likely that we know very little about the true extent of chemicals on human function, since so little study is done on chemical synergy. More important, considering the little we know about factors that influence physiologic function and their synergistic effect on chemical function, determining the effect of chemicals on human function is extremely difficult.

However, working within the concept of total load, it is clear that assessing both the sources of foreign substances and the patient's ability to deal with and process those foreign substances is central to the question of how toxicants and xenobiotics differen-

tially affect humans. Rea[4] has succinctly outlined the following factors that influence the total load phenomenon:

- Xenobiotics (insecticides, herbicides, drugs, solvents, metals, etc.)
- Infections (streptococcus, pseudomonas, parasites, etc.)
- Toxicants (aflatoxin, fumosine, penicillium toxins, ergot toxins, etc.)
- Biological inhalants (molds, algae, pollens, foods, etc.)
- Physical phenomena (electromagnetic fields, ionizing radiation)
- Lifestyle (drinking, smoking, etc.)
- Mechanical problems (biomechanical dysfunction, such as nasal, intestinal, or other obstruction)
- Hormonal aberration (DHEA, cortisol, estrogen, progesterone, testosterone, etc.)
- Psychosocial factors (stress, coping skills, belief systems, psychological trauma)

While nutritional status is not a direct part of the total load, the factors noted above are widespread and influenced by nutritional status. Rea, who has followed more than 20,000 patients with chemical sensitivity, reported laboratory evidence that nutrient abnormalities are widespread among these patients. He noted that nutrient supplementation was central to restoring physiologic balance; however, reducing total load was also essential to patient recovery. His findings suggest that total load *and* nutrient metabolism are inseparable components of any program designed to manage the physiological alteration associated with chemicals.

ENDOGENOUS TOXICANTS

In addition to exposure from external substances, toxic agents may be produced internally as well. In many ways, internally generated toxicants may be as harmful as xenobiotics from the environment.

Inborn Errors of Metabolism

Some cases of toxicant accumulation are due to mild inborn errors of metabolism. Inborn errors of metabolism are characterized by genetic mutations that result in the accumulation of an intermediate compound that deleteriously, if not lethally, affects patients. These metabolites act as endogenously created toxic substances.

Where metabolites accumulate because of a genetic defect, the altered gene often results in impairment in enzyme function. In the classically defined inborn errors of metabolism, the consequence can sometimes be counteracted by restricting dietary precursors. An example of this is phenylketonuria with a phenylalanine hydroxylase deficiency. Patients experiencing this disorder can obtain fair to good results by adopting a low-phenylalanine diet. Individuals with galactosemia function well on a galactose-free diet. Individuals who suffer from pyruvate dehydrogenase deficiency may do well on a

ketogenic diet that is enriched with thiamin, aspartic acid, and glutamate.[5] Table 9.1 outlines some of the more common diseases associated with inborn errors of metabolism.

Imbalanced Metabolism

By definition, endogenous toxicants are generated within the body and therefore may contribute to the total toxic load. Toxicity may occur when the body's normal metabolic mechanisms function inefficiently. For example, it typically takes several steps to convert the amino acid methionine into cysteine. If one step is sluggish, an intermediate called homocysteine accumulates in tissues. Accumulation of homocysteine leads to homocysteine thiolactone that can damage the vascular system and contribute to cardiovascular disease.[6] A condition called homocysteinemia results from one or more of the genetic enzymatic abnormalities. However, folic acid, vitamin B12, vitamin B6 and betaine can reduce accumulating homocysteine.

Polymorphisms, Biochemical Individuality, and Toxicity

Inborn errors of metabolism are extreme examples of genetic individuality. However, we all have a unique combination of genes and environment that makes us very different from one another. Every enzyme in the body is generated from two genes, one from the mother and one from the father. The combination of two genes, then, is one of the main factors in how well an enzyme functions.

TABLE 9.1 *Diseases Attributable to One or More Mutations in a Single Case*

Disease	Mutated Gene Product	Characteristics
Albinism	Tyrosinase	Lack of melanin (skin pigment) formation; increased sensitivity to sunlight, lack of eye pigment
Alcaptonuria	Homogentisate oxidase	Elevated urine levels of homogentisate; slow deposits of homogentisate in bones, connective tissue, and internal organs, resulting in gradual darkening of these structures; increased susceptibility to arthritis.
Fabry's	α Galactosidase A	Skin rash, kidney failure, pain in legs and feet, ceramide trihexoside accumulates
Fucosidosis	α-1-Fucosidosis	Cerebral degeneration, spastic muscles, thick skin
Gaucher's	Glucocerebrosidase	Enlarged liver and spleen, erosion of long bones and pelvis, mental retardation
Generalized gangliodosis	Gmi, gangliodosis: β galactosidase	Mental retardation, enlarged liver
Histidinemia	Histidase	Elevated levels of histidine in blood and urine; can give false positive results in tests for phenylketonuria; elevated urocanase levels in sweat
Krabbe's (Globoid leukodystrophy)	Galactocerebrosidase	Mental retardation, sulfatides accumulate
Maple syrup urine	Branched chain keto acid dehydrogenase (several variants) ketoacidosis, early death	Elevated levels of ketoacids and their metabolites in blood and urine; mental retardation
Metachromatic leukodystrophy	Arylsulfatase A	Mental retardation, sulfatides accumulate
Niemann-Pick	Sphingomyelinase	Enlarged liver and spleen, mental retardation, sphingomyelin accumulates
Parkinson's	Enzyme not identified	Decreased dopamine production by certain brain areas resulting in muscle tremors
Refsum's	α Hydroxylating enzyme	Neurological problems: deafness, blindness, cerebellar ataxia, phytanic acid accumulates
Sandhoff-Jatzkewitz	Hexosaminidase A and B	Same as Tay-Sachs but develops more quickly
Tay-Sachs	Hexosaminidase A	Early death, CNS, ganglioside GM2 accumulates

During the 1990s the concept of polymorphism entered clinical medicine. This concept was particularly present in discussions of how nutrition affects each person, and a leading example of a clinically relevant polymorphism is seen with the homocysteine cycle. As discussed above, homocysteinemia can result from a deficiency of folic acid, vitamin B12, or vitamin B6. However, studies have shown that some people with adequate (RDA) levels of folate and vitamin B12 show elevated homocysteine.

Investigation into this phenomenon led to the discovery that one of the enzymes in the folate/homocysteine cycle exists in several forms in the population, and one of these forms is a "sluggish" enzyme. The gene for this "sluggish enzyme" occurs in about 30% of the population, and about 10% of the population will have two copies of this gene. The result is that these individuals are more likely to have elevated homocysteine and may require more than the RDA level of folate to overcome, or push, this sluggish enzyme. Because the gene encoding this sluggish enzyme occurs in a small percentage of people, and is not the most common gene, it is called a "polymorphism."

As knowledge of biochemical pathways merges with our understanding of biochemical individuality through the interaction of environment and genetic uniqueness (polymorphisms), many more clinically relevant metabolic conditions will be discovered. Many of these conditions will lead to imbalanced metabolism, and be considered disorders of metabolic toxicity, since they relate to accumulation of a toxic substance as a result of inadequate processing. In these cases, the toxic substance must be handled properly for optimal health and functioning of an individual.

Gastrointestinal Microbial Metabolism

The human large intestine hosts at least 50 genera of bacteria comprised of nearly 400 species. There are roughly 10^{12} gut bacteria for every gram of gut contents. The rich diversity of intestinal microbes originates when a newborn is inoculated with the mother's vaginal and fecal flora during birth.[7] As a child develops and matures, this bacterial population is modified but still very important to optimum health (Chapter 7).

Intestinal microbial activity accounts for a large part of metabolic activity. Each species uses substrate in the form of diet-derived molecules for metabolic maintenance. The 400 different species are not equally beneficial. The salutary ones synthesize vitamins such as B12, biotin, and vitamin K, degrade toxicants, prevent colonization by pathogens, crowd out other less beneficial species, stimulate the immune system, and produce short-chain fatty acids (SCFAs) from fiber.[8]

The bacteria in the gut lumen constitute a continuous source of gut-derived metabolites that reach the systemic circulation. When colonic microbes become imbalanced, species that produce unfavorable metabolites may emerge. At Children's Mercy Hospital in Kansas City, Missouri, Dr. William Shaw dramatically illustrated this phenomenon when he determined that elevated metabolites in the urine of two autistic children were of fungal origin. Since the children did not have systemic fungal infections, the source was believed to be the colon.[9] Further work by Shaw and others has revealed that administering antifungal agents (in the case of fungal overgrowth) can reduce such metabolites.[10]

Shaw has since discovered metabolites of fungi and bacteria in the urine of patients with various neurological conditions such as multiple sclerosis, depression, and psychosis.[11] These findings suggest that microbes in the intestinal tract produce metabolites that are absorbed into systemic circulation. The term *dysbiosis* refers to a state of imbalance in the beneficial organisms in the colon. Among the organisms which may be associated with dysbiosis are:

> *Klebsiella pneumoniae*
> *Citrobacter freundii*
> *Bacteroides fragilis*
> *Proteus vulgaris*
> *Enterotoxigenic Escherichia coli*
> *Clostridium difficile*
> *Campylobacter jejunii*
> *Candida albicans*
> *Candida tropicalis*
> *Geotrichum spp.*

Metabolites associated with microbial overgrowth of the bowel may include:

> Arabinose
> Benzoate
> Hippurate
> p-Hydroxybenzoate
> p-Hydroxyphenylacetate
> p-Hydroxyphenyllactate
> beta-Ketoglutarate
> Hydrocaffeate
> Tartarate
> Citramalate

EXOGENOUS TOXICANTS

Xenobiotics are molecules that are foreign to a living organism. Xenobiotics that influence human function include the following general groups:

- Prescription and over-the-counter (OTC) drugs, such as cimetidine and acetaminophen
- Restricted and/or illegal drugs, such as cocaine, amphetamines, and barbiturates
- Food additives, dyes, and coloring agents
- Pesticides, such as diazinon, chlordane, and heptachlor
- Pediculicides, such as lindane, found in over-the-counter anti-lice preparations
- Herbicides, such as atrazine
- Fungicides, such as dithiocarbamates, thiocarbamates, copper arsenates
- Natural food components
- Alcohols, such as ethanol from beverages; other alcohols in paint remover, solvents, etc.
- Volatile organic compounds (VOCs), such as vinyl chloride, toluene, trichloromethane, and formaldehyde

(which are found in building materials, finishing materials, and furnishings)
- Toxic or heavy metals, including lead, mercury, cadmium, arsenic, nickel, and aluminum
(Note: This list is significantly abbreviated since more than four million chemical compounds have been identified.)

Although it is beyond the scope of this chapter to explore each of these factors at length, we will review a few groups from the list to provide insight into the research underlying the concept of environmental toxicants.

Heavy Metals

Interest in toxic elements has increased with enhanced understanding of the debilitating effects that chronic, low-level exposure can have on human function. While environmental exposure to toxic metals may be highly variable, evidence illustrates that toxic elements directly influence behavior by impairing brain function, influencing neurotransmitter production and utilization, and altering metabolic processes. Gastrointestinal, neurological, cardiovascular, and urological systems are areas in which heavy metals can likely induce impairment and dysfunction. One way researchers can garner meaningful information about the toxic load in a patient who may be experiencing cumulative toxic intake and exposure over time is through hair element analysis.[12,13,14]

Even minute levels of toxic elements can detrimentally affect the body. Such effects typically vary with mode, degree of exposure, and individual capabilities for metabolism and detoxification. The multiple mechanisms of toxicity include enzyme or cofactor inhibition, enzyme potentiation, disruption of membrane and other transport processes, and weakened neuronal functioning or nerve conduction processes. Some of these effects may be synergistic among elements or toxic chemicals.

The level of toxicity of these elements and associated adverse effects varies among individuals (see discussion of biochemical individuality in Chapter 1). Chronic, subacute exposures may lead to subtle or overt long-term problems in certain individuals. The concept of biochemical individuality, a term coined by Roger Williams in 1956,[15] helps explain different reactions to toxic element exposure. A tragic and stark example of biochemical individuality is the mercury toxicity episode known as Minamata disease (named for the bay in Japan where it was first observed in the mid-1950s). The disease was originally called congenital Minamata disease until researchers observed that the offspring of symptom-free parents suffered paralyzing neurological effects. Because every individual is biologically unique, not every victim of toxic element poisoning experiences all symptoms and deviations to the same extent. In fact, as little as 5 parts per million (ppm) may be associated with mercury toxicity.[16] (By comparison, victims of Minamata disease have a concentration of 183 ppm.)

The most common metals that cause toxic illness are mercury, lead, cadmium, arsenic, aluminum, and nickel. Table 9.2 identifies symptoms associated with excess amounts of some of these toxic elements. Consider the following examples that illustrate how excessive exposure can lead to significant symptomatology:

First, the toxicity of mercury involves both tissue destruction and enzyme inactivation. Not only does excess mercury result in pronounced toxicity, as in Minamata, intriguing evidence connects increased mercury levels to certain chronic insidious disease conditions. For instance, chronic mercury ingestion may be a risk factor for cardiovascular disease. Recent data suggest that a high intake of mercury from nonfatty freshwater fish and the accumulation of mercury in the body may indicate an increased risk of acute myocardial infarction (MI) as well as death from cardio-

vascular disease in general. Researchers suggest that promoting lipid peroxidation by mercury increases this risk.[17] A Finnish case-controlled study illustrating that higher numbers of dental fillings in individuals increased the risk of acute MI further supports these findings.[18] Chronic low level exposure can result in increased body burden. For example, scalp hair of British dentists and dental hygienists had two to three times higher mercury levels than the hair of support staff.[19] Both hair and urinary mercury have been strongly connected to elevated titers of immune complexes containing oxidized LDL.[20] Such studies illustrate mercury's power to induce autoimmune disease in humans and experimental animals.[21] Considering the complexity

TABLE 9.2 *Signs and Symptoms Associated with Toxic Element Exposure*

Element	Associated Signs and Symptoms
Arsenic	Fatigue, headaches, dermatitis, increased salivation, muscular weakness, loss of hair and nails, hypopigmentation of skin, anemia, skin Jashes
Cadmium	Loss of sense of smell, anemia, dried scaly skin, hair loss, hypertension, kidney problems
Lead	In children: delayed mental development, hyperactivity, delayed learning, behavioral problems. In children and adults: fatigue, anemia, metallic taste, loss of appetite, weight loss, headaches, insomnia, nervousness, decreased nerve conduction and possibly motor neuron disorders
Mercury	Reduced sensory abilities (taste, touch, vision, and hearing), metallic taste with increased salivation, fatigue, anorexia, irritability and excitability, psychoses, mania, anemia, paresthesias, tremors and incoordination, increased risk for cardiovascular disease, hypertension with renal dysfunction

of the immune system, it is likely that a combination of genetic and environmental factors rather than a single mechanism is responsible for the induction of autoimmune responses and disease by toxic metals such as mercury. It is interesting to note that the level of hair mercury was shown to be significantly higher in patients with multiple sclerosis than in non-MS controls.[22]

Lead is another example of a problem associated with long-term, chronic, low-level toxic exposure. Lead can have a significant effect on cognition and mental development. Hair lead (and cadmium) was significantly correlated with reduced intelligence scores and lowered school achievement scores.[23] One study noted a seven-fold increase in failure to graduate from high school in students who experienced lead toxicity.[24] The acceptable threshold for lead-engendered neurotoxicity in children has declined steadily over the past decade as more sophisticated population studies have been conducted with larger samples, better designs, and superior analysis.

While the elements listed in Table 9.2 play no known role in the body, minerals with known, important roles in the body can also become toxic in high levels. For example, when excess copper accumulates, a condition called Wilson's disease results. Excess iron accumulates in individuals with hemochromatosis. In this common genetic condition, iron is eliminated from the body by frequent blood removal. Excess manganese can accumulate in the substantia nigra of the human brain, causing a condition similar to Parkinson's disease. Along with the elements

in the table, other elements exhibiting toxicity at elevated levels are antimony, barium, beryllium, bismuth, boron, lithium, strontium, and thallium.

Food Additives

Food additives are substances added to food during processing. They are not natural to the food itself. In the United States, nearly 4,000 additives are allowed in foods and are commonly divided into the following categories:

- Preservatives (BHT, BHA, benzoate, sulfite, nitrogen oxide, etc.)
- Food colorings (FD & C yellow #5, 6, etc.)
- Sweeteners (aspartame, sorbitol, etc.)
- Stimulants (caffeine, theophylline, etc.)
- Flavor enhancers (monosodium glutamate, more commonly known as *MSG*)

Researchers have tried to link certain food additives to various health complaints. However, this has been difficult since the goal of double-blind, placebo-controlled crossover trials is to measure the effect of the additive against a placebo. Individuals rarely encounter additives this way in the food supply, making such trials an unrealistic reflection of the additive's effect.

In addition, because humans are diverse biochemically, a given additive may not produce the same response in all individuals. In assessing the safety of a given additive, the FDA reviews population data for minimum risk. Clinicians working with individual patients are in a decidedly different position. They must evaluate the effect of an additive on a single individual with unique medical history, unique dietary habits, unique nutritional status, unique environmental history, and unique psychological profile. While a given additive may present a low risk in the population, it may be a significant risk for a particular individual.

The Excitotoxin Concept

Dr. Russell L. Blaylock, assistant professor at the University of Mississippi Medical Center, outlined the excitotoxin concept in his book, *Excitotoxins*. He defines *excitotoxins* as substances added to foods and beverages that cause neuronal hyperexcitability. Glutamate and aspartate, two of the most common neurotransmitters found in the brain and spinal cord, are known as excitatory neurotransmitters. They are pervasive molecules and central to brain function; however, in excess, these molecules may lead to overstimulation of neurons. Blaylock suggests that excess excitatory neurotransmitters may be associated with amyotrophic lateral sclerosis, Alzheimer's, and Parkinson's diseases.[25]

Both of these molecules are naturally occurring and found in protein. However, they are also found in food additives. For example, monosodium glutamate (MSG) is the sodium salt of glutamic acid. Ingested MSG has led to substantial increase in blood levels of MSG.

Blaylock cites an extensive body of literature describing the way these excitotoxins deplete neuronal adenosine triphosphate (ATP), cause influx of calcium ions into neurons, and lead to neuronal degeneration. He also notes that the adverse effect of ingested MSG is enhanced by inadequate amounts of nutrients such as magnesium, vitamin C, and vitamin E. MSG is an example of a naturally occurring compound being consumed in high, "unnatural" levels when consumed as an additive. The sweetener, aspartame, is also noted as providing an "unnatural" level of an excitotoxin. Aspartame is composed of phenylalanine and aspartate, and has been linked to various forms of brain tumors.[26]

The reported link between ingestion of naturally occurring compounds that are important for brain function and neuronal degradation has raised controversy in consumer and medical communities. The issue may not be one of a "good" or "bad" molecule, but rather how much is too much and for whom. While the FDA has identified MSG and aspartame as safe for human consumption, clinicians may wish to review the data compiled by investigators such as Blaylock,[27] Roberts,[28] and Schwartz.[29]

Prescription Drugs

Modern pharmacology has fostered a vast development of drugs with potent effects on physiologic function. While therapeutic drugs are designed for a particular clinical outcome, they must always be viewed as agents of potential toxicity. Drug/nutrient interaction should be considered when studying the effects of drugs in individuals. While some data about how drugs and nutrients interact exist, most relationships remain poorly understood. Drug/nutrient interactions can be classified according to the following criteria:[30]

- Location (stomach, gallbladder, etc.)
- Mechanism (chelation, precipitation, etc.)
- Pharmacologic or nutritional outcomes (drug variables, diet variables)
- Drug or drug group (antibiotic, antacids)
- Nutrient (folic acid, pyridoxine, etc.)
- Temporal relationship to food or nutrient ingestion (effect of drug/food/nutrient interaction over time)
- Patient group affected (asthmatic, arthritic, diabetic, epileptic)
- Risk factors (laxative abuse, fasting, drug excess, etc.)

A few examples illustrate the many dynamic drug/nutrient interactions at work in humans today. Cimetidine may impair vitamin B12 absorption by influencing acid secretion. Bicarbonate may increase pH and decrease folate absorption. In drug, diet, and patient variables, there are many considerations such as drug dose and duration, dietary fat intake, age, sex, and genetics. For example, drug type classification reveals that tetracycline impairs absorption of calcium, magnesium, iron, and zinc. Simultaneous ingestion of cholestyramine and vitamin A hinders vitamin A absorption. Simultaneous ingestion of tetracycline and milk lowers drug bioavailability.

While this chapter only introduces questions about the relationship between drugs and nutrients, practitioners should consider the potential of drugs to contribute to the total toxic load and be aware of how drugs and nutrients interact to influence the metabolic status of the patient. In addition, because of the critical relationship between nutrient adequacy and drug detoxification, nutrient adequacy must always be considered in light of drug therapy. It is possible to find many internet sites (and books and journal articles) providing extensive information about drug interactions—with nutrients, with botanicals, and with other drugs. Clinicians are strongly urged to become informed and to regularly update their knowledge.

A FUNCTIONAL APPROACH TO TOXICITY

The idea that toxicants accumulate in the body and cause various health problems has long been recognized by traditional healthcare systems around the world. For centuries, various cultures have valued therapies that promote the idea of cleansing and detoxifying. From the simple water fast to the elaborate detoxifying regimes of spas, saunas, enemas, hydrotherapy treatments, and dietary modifications, detoxification has been a valued therapeutic goal.

As our society becomes increasingly exposed to toxic compounds in air, water, and food, an individual's ability to detoxify substances becomes increasingly important to health. From a functional perspective, assessing relationships among toxicants, toxic load, and clinical manifestations is critical. At the core, patient management must focus on successfully decreasing toxic exposure and increasing toxicant removal.

Decrease Toxic Load

Decreasing toxic load should be an immediate consideration when dealing with toxicity. Toxic load can come from both endogenous and exogenous sources. Exogenous sources should be assessed by questionnaire and/or interview with the patient, and lifestyle approaches to minimizing exposure should be pursued. Food allergens are toxic to the allergic individual, and so food allergy assessment should be considered (see Chapter 10). However, in addition to the toxic load created by environmental exposure and lifestyle, a clinician should also consider the toxic load from endogenous sources.

Promote Bacterial Balance

In Chapter 7, we suggested that bacterial flora imbalance and increased intestinal permeability might increase toxic load (Figure 9.1). Not only is a strong barrier from a healthy gastrointestinal tract important in keeping out toxic substances, but the healthy, beneficial microflora of the gut also help to decrease toxic load. Evidence suggests that beneficial intestinal microflora protect against a broad range of pathogens, including pathogenic *E.*

coli, salmonella, shigella, and yeast such as *Candida albicans*.[31] Supplementation with probiotics and prebiotics (described in Chapter 7) may be indicated for a specific patient to promote bacterial balance and decrease endogenous toxic load. Antimicrobials may also be indicated. For a discussion of assessment of gastrointestinal function, see Chapter 10.

Promote Healthy Detoxification

Detoxification refers to a broad spectrum of bodily processes that help maintain the body's health when exposed to harmful substances (endo- or exogenous substances).[32] The body's primary detoxification system converts lipid-soluble substances to water-soluble substances that can be excreted through urine. This is important since lipid-soluble substances can be sequestered in the fatty tissues and accumulate if they are not converted to water-soluble metabolites. Converting toxic substances to nontoxic metabolites and excreting them takes place in many tissues, but is primarily the function of the intestinal mucosal wall and the liver.

The biochemistry of detoxification

Two distinct phases exist in the biochemical process called detoxification. These two phases, traditionally known as Phase I and Phase II, chemically biotransform lipid- (fat-) soluble substances into progressively more water-soluble substances (rendering them excretable) through a series of chemical reactions (Figure 9.2).

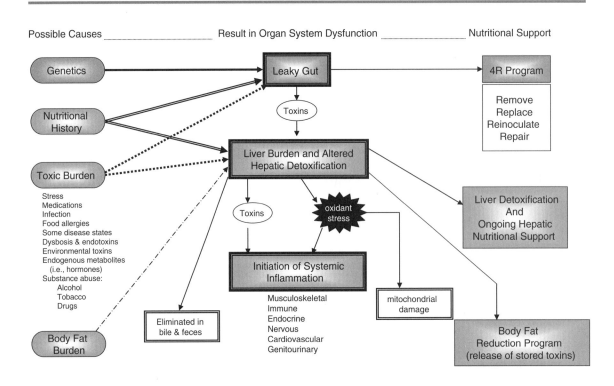

FIGURE 9.1   *Managing problems of altered GI permeability, hepatic detoxification, and oxidative stress*

Phase I reactions usually involve oxidation, reduction, or hydrolysis. A family of enzymes commonly referred to as cytochrome P450 mixed-function oxidases (CYP P450s) begins the process of detoxifying xenobiotics and endogenous substances.[33] This system is actually a group of many isoenzymes that have specific affinity for differing substrates. In Phase I, the biochemical reaction involves adding or exposing a functional group, most commonly a hydroxyl (OH), to the toxic molecule. In most cases, this biotransformation allows the Phase I compound to undergo Phase II conjugation reactions. In some cases, the compound may be eliminated directly after the Phase I reaction.[34]

In the more common scenario, the Phase I reaction produces an intermediate that must undergo further transformation. These intermediates can be highly reactive and are often more toxic than the original compound. This intermediate step in the transformation of toxic substances to excretable, harmless metabolites is called *bioactivation*.

One consequence of this biotransformation is an increase in free radical molecules. As

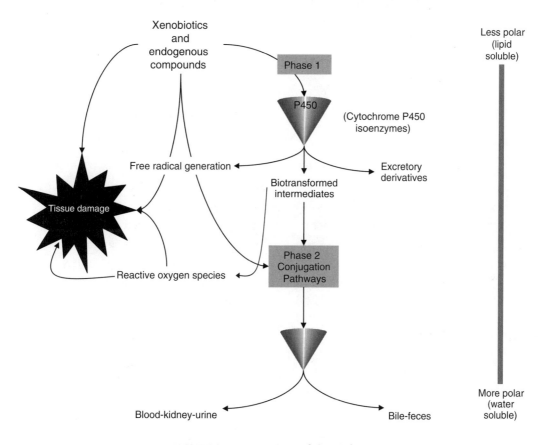

FIGURE 9.2   *Overview of detoxification*

a result, the more efficiently Phase II reactions act on these intermediates, the less likely it is that tissue damage will occur from excess reactive molecules. Therefore, the balance of activities between Phase I and Phase II is critical to detoxification. If Phase II reactions are inhibited in any way, or if Phase I has been upregulated without a concomitant increase in Phase II, optimal balance is compromised.

Whereas the primary Phase I reactions involve a family of isoenzymes, Phase II reactions, in which various biotransformed molecules are conjugated, involve distinct reactions. The main conjugation reactions are glucuronidation, amino acid conjugation, sulfation, glutathione conjugation, acetylation, and methylation.[35] These conjugation reactions add a water-soluble molecule to the intermediate metabolite to further increase its hydrophilic (water-loving) qualities. This process prepares the metabolite for urine or bile elimination.[36] Many different metabolites are conjugated through these various pathways (Table 9.3).

Clinical Relationships

Over the past 10 years, extensive research in detoxification has enhanced our understanding about how toxic substances affect individuals and how clinicians can help patients overcome toxicity.[37,38] Sluggish, imbalanced, or impaired detoxification systems can result in the accumulation and deposition of metabolic toxicants, increased free radical production and its ensuing pathology, impaired oxidative phosphorylation, and reduced energy. Various nutrients are necessary for proper detoxification function (Figure 9.3). Substances that upregulate Phase I, such as alcohol, smoking, and certain medications can deleteriously affect this balance because the Phase II pathways may be unable to keep up with the increased demand. Conversely, various medications such as fluoxetine and H2 blockers (cimetidine) may inhibit Phase I (Table 9.4).

Drugs and detoxification pathways

Researchers have known for many years that the body's detoxification system is strongly influenced by drugs. They have also known that the detoxification system influences the way drugs act and are metabolized. The relationship between drugs and the detoxification system has important implications for individuals exposed to other chemical insults, since drugs may either block one phase or deplete nutrients from another phase of the detoxification pathway.

A case example was reported of a male in Dallas, Texas, who was exposed to low levels of lawn chemicals while taking the prescription drug cimetidine. This exposure critically damaged his central and peripheral nervous system. He responded so severely to low levels of a toxic agent (the lawn herbicide) that investigators concluded cimetidine, a cytochrome P450 inhibitor, impaired his liver's ability to detoxify the compounds in the lawn treatment. He was unable to metabolize these compounds properly; instead, their toxicity was seemingly enhanced, which led to permanent neurological damage.[39]

This example emphasizes that the relative detoxification ability of an individual plays an important role in the toxicity or carcinogenicity of a specific substance. Upregulation of various P450 isoenzymes may be detrimental, as most chemical carcinogens do not cause genetic damage by themselves. Instead, they require electrophilic species activation.[40] For instance, the risk for hepatic carcinoma is associated with the activity of a particular isoenzyme of the cytochrome P450 system.[41]

Studies also illustrate that evaluation of detoxification rates can stratify risk for bladder cancer when other factors are constant.[42] Individuals with a high inducibility phenotype for P4501A1 appear to have a higher risk for cancer, regardless of exposure to smoking or other known carcinogens.[43] As

TABLE 9.3   *Detoxification: Bio-Reactive Mechanisms*

Glutathione conjugation ↓	Sulfation ↓	Peptide conjugation		Glucuronidation ↓	Acetylation ↓	Methylation ↓
		Glycine ↓	Taurine ↓			
Drugs						
Acetaminophen	Acetaminophen	Salicylates		Salicylates	Clonazepam	Thiouracil
Penicillin	Methyl dopa	Nicotinic acid		Morphine	Dapsone	Isoetharine
Ethacrynic acid	Minoxidil	Chlorpheniramine		Acetaminophen	Mescaline	Rimiterol
Tetracycline	Metaraminol	Brompheniramine		Benzodiazepines	Isoniazid	Dobutamine
	Phenylephrine			Meprobamate	Hydralazine	Butanephrine
				Clofibric acid	Procainamide	Eluophed
				Naproxen	Benzidine	Morphine
				Digoxin	Sulfonamides	Levorphanol
				Phenylbutazone	Promizole	Nalorphine
				Valproic acid		
				Steroids		
			Propionic acid	Lorazepam		
			Caprylic acid	Ciramadol		
				Propranolol		
				Oxazepam		
Xenobiotics						
Styrene	Aniline	Benzoic acid		Carbamates	2 Aminofluorine	Paraquat
Acrolein	Pentachbrophenol	Phenylacetic acid		Phenols	Anilines	Beta Carbolines
Ethylene Oxide	Terpenes	Naphthylacetic		Thiophenol		Isoquinolines
Benzopyrenes	Amines	acid		Aniline		Mercury
Methylparathion	Hydroxylamines	Aliphatic amines		Butanol		Lead
Chlorobenzene	Phenols	Organic acid		N-hydroxy-2-		Arsenic
Anthracene				napthylamine		Thallium
Tetrachlorvinphos						Tin
Toxic metals						Pyridine
Petroleum						
distillates						
Naphthalene						
Dietary/Endogenous						
Bacterial toxins	DHEA	Bile acids	Bile acids	Bilirubin	Serotonin	Dopamine
Aflatoxin	Quercetin	Cinnamic acid	Stearic acid	Estrogens	PABA	Epinephrine
Lipid peroxides	Bile acids	PABA	Palmitic acid	Melatonin	Histamine	Histamine
Ethyl alcohol	Safrole	Plant acids	Myristic acid	Bile acids	Tryptamine	Norepinephrine
Quercetin	Tyramine		Lauric acid	Vitamin E	Caffeine	L-dopa
N-acetylcysteine	Thyroxine		Decanoic acid	Vitamin A	Choline	Apomorphine
Prostaglandins	Estrogens		Butyric acid	Vitamin K	Tyramine	Hydroxyestradiols
Bilirubin	Testosterone			Vitamin D	Coenzyme A	
Leukotriene A4	Cortisol			Other steroid		
	Catecholamines			hormones		
	Melatonin					
	3-hydroxy					
	coumarin					
	25 hydroxy					
	vitamin D					
	Ethyl alcohol					
	CCK					
	Cerebrosides					

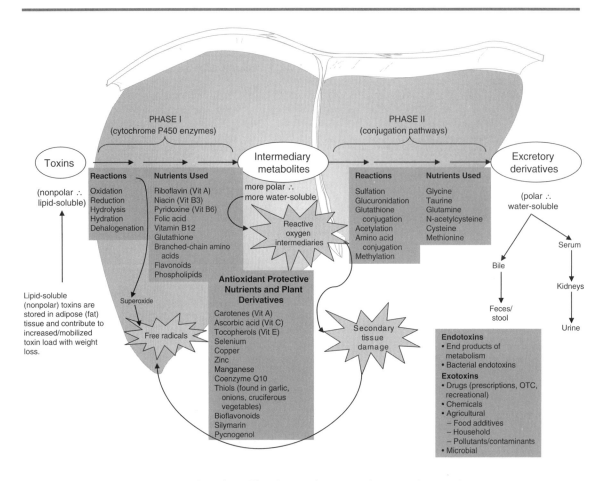

FIGURE 9.3   *Liver detoxification pathways and supportive nutrients*

the majority of cancers relate to environmental exposure or dietary intake, individual detoxification ability can be important for their development.[44]

As noted, various drugs or chemicals may have an inhibitory or stimulatory effect on detoxification capacity. Because of this, other molecules involved in the same pathway may be detoxified at a quicker or slower rate. For example, cigarette smoking upregulates certain Phase I P450 isoenzymes. These same enzymes are involved in the detoxification of estrogen. As a consequence, estrogen is detoxified faster, and therefore serum estrogen levels are lower in women who smoke. This may in part explain the increased osteoporosis and

TABLE 9.4   *Inhibitors and Substrates of P450 Enzymes*

Inhibitors of P450 Enzymes		Substrates of P450 Enzymes			
Drug	P450 Family Inhibited	Drug	P450 Family involved in Metabolism	Drug	P450 Family involved in Metabolism
Antiarrhythmics		*Antiarrhythmics*		*Neuroleptics*	
Quinidine	2D6	Encainide	2D6	Clozapine	2D6, 1A2
Propafenone	2D6	Mexiletine	2D6	Haloperidol	2D6, 1A2
Antibiotics		Propafenone	2D6	Molindone	2D6
Macrolides		Quinidine	3A4	Perphenazine	2D6
Erythromycin	3A4	*Anticonvulsants*		Risperidone	2D6
Clarithromycin	3A4	Phenytoin	2C19	Thioridazine	2D6
Troleandomycin	3A4	Carbamazepine	3A4	*Opiates*	
Fluoroquinolones	1A2	*Antihistamines*		Codeine	2D6
Antidepressants		Astemizole	3A4	Methadone	1A2
Nefazodone	3A4	Terfenadine	3A4	Oxycodone	2D6
SSRIs*		*Antidepressants*		Pentazocine	2D6
Fluoxetine	2D6, 2C19, 3A	Bupropion	2D6	*Other*	
Fluvoxamine	2D6, 1A2	SSRIs*		Cisapride	3A4
Norfluoxetine	2D6	Paroxetine	2D6	Cyclosporine	3A4
Paroxetine	2D6	Fluoxetine	2D6,3A4	Dextromethorphan	2D6
Sertraline	2D6	*Tricyclics*		Lidocaine	3A4
Antifungals		Amitriptyline	2D6, 2C19	Lovastatin	3A4
Itraconazole	3A4	Clomipramine	2C19	mCPP#	2D6
Fluconazole	3A4	Desipramine	3A4	Phenacetin	1A2
Ketoconazole	3A4	Imipramine	2D6, 1A2, 2C19	Tacrine	1A2
Other		Nortriptyline	2D6, 3A4	Tamoxifen	3A4
Cimetidine	3A4	*Venlafaxine*	2D6	Testosterone	3A4
		Benzodiazepines		Tolbutamide	2C19
		Alprazolam	3A4, 1A2	*Steroids*	
		Desmethyldiazepam	2C19	Hydrocortisone	3A4
		Diazepam	3A4, 1A2, 2C19	Dexamethasone	3A4
		Midazolam	3A4	Exogenous steroids	1A2
		Triazolam	3A4	*Xanthines*	
		β-Blockers		Caffeine	1A2
		Metoprolol	2D6	Theophylline	1A2
		Propranolol	1A2, 2C19		
		Calcium channel blockers			
		Diltiazem	3A4		
		Nifedipine	3A4		

* Selective Serotonin Reuptake Inhibitors   # m-chlorophenylpiperazine

menopausal symptoms in women smokers as compared to nonsmokers.[45]

Idiopathic disease and detoxification

Variability of detoxification may influence diseases thought to be benign. Gilbert's syndrome (GS), thought to be a condition with little morbidity, is a genetically induced, nutritionally exacerbated metabolic disorder caused by a glucuronosyl transferase enzyme deficiency. This enzyme catalyzes the Phase II conjugation step of glucuronidation.[46] Recent studies suggest that GS can predispose individuals to the bioactivation, and potentially the toxicity, of drugs for which glucuronidation constitutes a major, alternate pathway of elimination.[47] Some evidence suggests that nutritional support in GS patients improves a wide variety of symptomatology that had not been associated with this disorder.[48] Although research continues, this line of inquiry may initiate exploring how other detoxification "defects" impinge upon health.

Current research on the etiology of chronic fatigue immune deficiency syndrome (CFIDS) suggests that, in some patients, a relationship may exist between impaired detoxifying pathways and symptomatology,[49] and that toxic exposure may influence CFIDS.[50] Correcting these imbalances and deficiencies significantly alleviates some patients' symptoms.[51] In a trial using nutritional modulation to support detoxifying pathways and a food elimination diet, a significant improvement was observed in subjective symptom evaluation as well as objective Phase I and Phase II balance in people suffering from a variety of chronic illnesses.[52]

Neurologic disease and detoxification

Detoxification may also clinically impact chronic degenerative diseases. Research on the etiology of Parkinson's disease suggests that such patients cannot adequately metabolize sulfur-containing xenobiotics.[53] Altered detoxification may render higher-risk individuals susceptible to neurotoxicity when exposed to sulfur-containing compounds.[54] A combination of genetic susceptibility, reduced detoxification capacity, and increased exposure to neurotoxicants may lead to clinical disease over time. Similar connections have been made between Alzheimer's and other motor neuron diseases.[55] Other research suggests relationships among altered hepatic detoxification ability, lupus erythematosus, and rheumatoid arthritis.[56] Inheritability of disease is only one factor that must be considered in light of the strong nutritional and environmental factors.[57]

Nutritional Support for Detoxification

Regulation of Phase I and Phase II activity levels has a dietary component.[58,59,60,61,62,63,64,65] Nutritional support of Phase I and Phase II activity involves administering increased amounts of enzymatic cofactors and other nutrients involved in cytochrome P450 enzymes. Detoxification support nutrients include vitamins B2 (riboflavin), B3 (niacin), B6 (pyridoxine), B12 (cobalamin), and folic acid. The tripeptide glutathione and the branched-chain amino acids leucine, glycine, isoleucine, and valine are also required. Flavonoids and phospholipids are supportive as well.

Protective antioxidant support is required for handling reactive oxygen intermediates produced during Phase I activity. Antioxidant support involves the carotenoids, including beta-carotene (pro-vitamin A), ascorbic acid (vitamin C), the tocopherols (vitamin E), and coenzyme Q10 (ubiquinone). The antioxidant minerals selenium, zinc, copper, and manganese are also required.

Thiol compounds found in garlic, onions, and cruciferous vegetables, flavonoids, silymarin, and anthocyanidins also provide antioxidant support. Nutritional Phase II activity support also includes a wide variety of sulfur-containing compounds that serve as sulfur donors in the sulfate conjugation process. These compounds include the amino acids cysteine, N-acetyl cysteine, methionine, and taurine. Inorganic sulfates can also support sulfation. Other amino acid conjugation pathways require supplementation of glycine, glutamine, ornithine, and arginine. Glucuronic acid and glutathione are necessary in their respective conjugation pathways (Figure 9.3).

Assessment of Detoxification

The body's detoxification systems are highly complex, show a great amount of variability, and are extremely responsive to an individual's environment, lifestyle, and genetic uniqueness. For example, more than 10 families of enzymes,

including over 35 genes, compose the Phase I CYP P450 system alone. Only a limited number of these activities (such as CYP P450 2D6) are determined by genetics alone. In such cases, a genetic test can indicate whether someone is a "fast" or "slow" metabolizer. In most cases, however, assessment of detoxification status is not so straightforward, and a full discussion is beyond the scope of this book. A few considerations are addressed below and the reader is encouraged to consult laboratories performing detoxification assessments to obtain the most recent, detailed information available on detoxification assessment. Often, laboratories will provide a profile of the tests they offer to assess detoxification, which can be helpful in understanding this complex system. Clinicians may request to see the research upon which the test and its interpretation are based.

Several types of genetic tests are available for assessment of Phase I detoxification enzymes and are becoming more commonly used in association with specific narrow-spectrum drugs or to assess propensity for certain cancers. Since this is an active field, accessibility and ease of use of these tests can change rapidly. The reader is urged to consult the internet for a list of active laboratories and available tests.

Another common approach to assessing general detoxification is a challenge test (a concept that is discussed in more detail in Chapter 10). Briefly, a challenge test for detoxification would involve giving a patient a known amount of a substance not normally in their body (for example a drug like acetaminophen), obtaining urine over a specified time period, and then assessing how much of the different metabolites of that substance have been excreted. Using this type of test, the clinician can often get a fairly thorough picture of how well a person is detoxifying exogenous substances.

Detoxification reserve may be assessed by looking at specific metabolites necessary for detoxification. For example, sulfur-bearing compounds are critical to adequate functioning of many of the Phase II conjugation pathways. Humans are particularly susceptible to inhibition of Phase II detoxification due to compromised sulfate cofactor status. Errors in sulfur metabolism, such as seen with homocysteinemia, and inadequate reserves of sulfur-bearing compounds can pose considerable obstacles to efficient detoxification. For this reason, many laboratories offer an assessment of sulfate status as part of a detoxification profile.

SUMMARY

As we are increasingly exposed to higher levels of xenobiotics in the food we eat, the water we drink, the air we breathe, and the increased endogenous load from faulty digestion, detoxification and our unique "detoxification personalities" will play an increasingly vital role in our health. Detoxification studies suggest that the enzymes that control Phase I and Phase II processes may vary significantly from person to person, even among seemingly healthy people.[66,67,68] These findings raise many questions concerning how to identify people who need detoxification, properly counsel them, and prescribe appropriate dietary, environmental, or supplemental modification for biochemically diverse individuals.

Our understanding about detoxification enhances our appreciation for Roger Williams's work and his concept of "biochemical individuality."[69] Differences among individual detoxification capacities based upon individual genetic disposition, environmental exposure, and nutritional insufficiencies indeed have a profound effect upon disease susceptibility. Xenobiotics may act as immunotoxic agents, suggesting biochemical connections among the immune, nervous, and hepatic detoxification systems.[70]

Many intriguing questions about detoxification remain. How many diseases considered idiopathic (of unknown origin), are connected to atypical detoxification reactions? Disordered detoxification may have wide-ranging impact upon hepatic, renal, cardiovascular, neurological, endocrine, and immune system function. Certainly, the complicated relationships involving exposure to various substances, genetically determined detoxification pathways, alteration of the pathways by foods, drugs, and chemicals, and sensitivity of tissues to secondary metabolites from toxic substances profoundly contribute to many health problems.

CHAPTER 9 REFERENCES

1. Environmental Neurotoxicology. National Research Council. Washington, D.C.: National Academy Press; 1992.

2. Biologic Markers in Immunotoxicology. National Research Council. Washington, D.C.: National Academy Press; 1992.

3. Schubert J, Riley EJ, Tyler SA. Combined effects of toxicology—a rapid systematic testing procedure: cadmium, mercury, and lead. J Toxicol Environ Health. 1978;4:763–776.

4. Rea WJ. Chemical Sensitivity. Vol. 4. Boca Raton, Fla: CRC Press, Inc.; 1997:1011–1067.

5. Scriver CR, Beaudet AL, Sly WS, Valle D, eds. The Metabolic Basis of Inherited Disease. Vol. I & II. 6th ed. New York, NY: McGraw-Hill Information Services Company; 1989.

6. Graham I, Daly L, Refsum H, et al. Plasma homocysteine as a risk factor for vascular disease. JAMA. 1997:277;1775–1781.

7. Mevissen-Verhage EA, Marcelis JH, de Vos MN, Harmsen-van Amerongen WC, Verhoff J. Bifidobacterium, Bacteroides and Clostridium spp. in fecal samples from breast-fed and bottle-fed infants with and without iron supplement. J Clin Microbiol. 1987;25:285–289.

8. Galland L. Effects of intestinal microbes on systemic immunity. In: Mowbray P, Jenkins R, eds. Post Viral Fatigue Syndrome. London: John Wiley and Sons; 1991:405–430.

9. Shaw W, Kassen E, Chaves E. Increased urinary excretion of analogs of Krebs cycle metabolites and arabinose in two brothers with autistic features. Clin Chem. 1995;41(8):1094–1104.

10. Shaw W, Chaves E, Luxem M. Abnormal urine organic acids associated with fungal metabolism in urine samples of children with autism: Preliminary results of a clinical trial with antifungal drugs. Unpublished monograph. Kansas City, Missouri, 1994.

11. Shaw W. Personal communication. Developmental Delay Registry Symposium. San Diego, Calif; 1996.

12. Foo SC, Khoo NY, Heng A, et al. Metals in hair as biological indices for exposure. Intl Arch Occup Environ Health. 1993;65:S83–S86.

13. Petering HO, Yeager DW, and Witherup SO. Trace element content of hair: cadmium and lead of human hair. Arch Environ Health. 1973; 27:327–333.

14. Clemente G. Trace element composition of hair in the Italian population. Conference on Nuclear Activation Techniques in the Life Sciences. Vienna: May 1978.

15. Williams RJ. Biochemical individuality: The basis of the genetotrophic concept. New York, NY: John Wiley; 1956.

16. Katz SA, Katz RS. Use of hair analysis for evaluating mercury intoxication of the human body: A Review. J Applied Toxicology. 1992;12(2): 9–84.

17. Salonen JT, Seppanen K, Nyyssonen K, et al. Intake of mercury from fish, lipid peroxidation, and the risk of myocardial infarction and coronary, cardiovascular, and any death in eastern Finnish men. Circulation. 1995;91(3);645-655.

18. Mattila KJ, Nieminen MS, Valtonen VV, et. al. Association between dental health and acute myocardial infarction. Br Med J. 1989;298:779–781.

19. Lenihan JM, Smith H, Harvey W. Mercury hazards in dental practice. Br Dent J. 135:1973; 365–396.

20. Salonen JT, Seppanen K,Nyyssonen K, et al. Intake of mercury from fish, lipid peroxidation, and the risk of myocardial infarction and coronary, cardiovascular, and any death in eastern Finnish men. Circulation. 1995;91(3);645–655.

21. Bigazzi P. Autoimmunity and heavy metals. Lupus. 1994;3:449–453.

22. Siblerod RL, Kienholz E. Evidence that mercury from silver dental fillings may be an etiological

factor in multiple sclerosis. Sci Total Environ. 1994:142(3);191–205.

23. Thatcher RW, Lester ML, McAlaster R, Horst R. Effects of low levels of cadmium and lead on cognitive functioning in children. Arch Environ Health. 1982:37(3);159–166.

24. Needleman HL, Schell A, Bellinger D, Leviton A, Allved EN. The long-term effects of exposure to low doses of lead in childhood. N Engl J Med. 1990:322(2);83–88.

25. Blaylock RL. Excitotoxicants: The Taste That Kills. Santa Fe, NM: Health Press; 1997.

26. Blaylock RL. Excitotoxicants: The Taste That Kills. Santa Fe, NM: Health Press; 1997.

27. Blaylock RL. Excitotoxicants: The Taste That Kills. Santa Fe, NM: Health Press; 1997.

28. Roberts HJ. Aspartame: Is it Safe? Philadelphia, Penn.: The Charles Press; 1990.

29. Schwartz, GR. In Bad Taste: The MSG Syndrome. Santa Fe, NM: Health Press; 1988.

30. Linder MC, ed. Nutritional Biochemistry and Metabolism with Clinical Applications. Norwalk, Conn.: Appleton & Lange; 1991:59–71.

31. Salminen S, Isolauri E, Onnela T. Gut flora in normal and disordered states. Chemotherapy. 1995:41(suppl 1):5–15.

32. Reeves AL. The metabolism of foreign compounds. In: Reeves AL, ed. Toxicology: Principles and Practice. Vol 1. New York, NY: John Wiley & Sons; 1981.

33. Grant DM. Detoxification pathways in the liver. J Inher Metab Dis. 1991:14;421–30.

34. Timbrell J. Principles of Biochemical Toxicology. 2nd ed. London: Taylor and Francis; 1991.

35. Murray R, Granner D, Mayes P, Rodwell V. Harper's Biochemistry. Norwalk Conn.: Appleton & Lange; 1990.

36. Grant DM. Detoxification pathways in the liver. J Inher Metab Dis. 1991:14;421–430.

37. Davies MH, Gough A, Sorhi RS, Hassell A, Warning R, Emery P. Sulphoxidation and sulphation capacity in patients with primary biliary cirrhosis. J Hepatol. May 1995;22(5):551–560.

38. Bradley H. Sulfate metabolism is abnormal in patients with rheumatoid arthritis. Confirmation by in vivo biochemical findings. J Rheumatol. Jul 1994;21(7):1192–1196.

39. Allen FE. One man's suffering spurs doctors to probe pesticide-drug link. The Wall Street Journal. October 14, 1992.

40. Miller EL, Miller JA. Searches for ultimate chemical carcinogens and their reactions with cellular macromolecules. Cancer. 1981:47;2327.

41. Agundez JA, Ledisma MC, Benitiz J, et al. CYP2D6 genes and risk of liver cancer. Lancet. 1995;345(8953):830-831.

42. Talaska G, Tannenbaum SR, Vineis P, et al. Genetically based N-acetyltransferase metabolic polymorphism and low-level environmental exposure to carcinogens. Nature. 1994:369:154–156.

43. Kawajiri K, Nakaji K, Imai K, Yoshi A, Shinoda N, Watanabe J. Identification of genetically high risk individuals to lung cancer by DNA polymorphisms of the cytochrome P4501A1 gene. FEBS Lett. 1990:263;131.

44. Ketterer B, Harris JM, Talaska G, et al. The human glutathione S-transferase supergene family, its polymorphism, and low level environmental exposure to carcinogens. Nature. 1994;369:154–156.

45. Michnovicz J. Environmental modulation of oestrogen metabolism in humans. Intl Clin Nutr Rev. 1987;7(4):169–173.

46. Black M, Billings BH. Hepatic bilirubin UDP-glucuronyl transferase activity in liver disease and Gilbert's syndrome. New Engl J Med. 1969:280;1266–1271.

47. De Morais SM, Uetecht JP, Wells PG. Decreased glucuronidation and increased bioactivation of acetaminophen in Gilbert's syndrome. Gastroenterology. 1992:102;577–586.

48. Lonsdale D. Gilbert's disease: symptomatic response to nutritional supplementation in ten patients. J Nutr Med. 1992:3;319–324.

49. Rigden DS, Bralley JA, Bland JS. Nutritional upregulation of hepatic detoxification enzymes. J Appl Nutr. 1992;44(3&4):2–15.

50. Buist RA. Chronic fatigue syndrome and chemical overload. Intl Clin Nutr Rev. 1988;8(4):173–175.

51. Rigden DS. Entero-hepatic resuscitation program for CFIDS. The CFIDS Chronicle. Spring, 1995;46–49.

52. Bland JS, Barrager E, Reedy RG, Bland K. A medical food supplemented detoxification program in the management of chronic health problems. Alt Therapies. Nov 1995;1:562–571.

53. Steventon GB, Heafield MT, Waring RH, Williams AC. Xenobiotic metabolism in Parkinson's disease. Neurology. 1989;39:883–887.

54. Heafield MT, Fearn S, Steventon GB, et al. Plasma cysteine and sulphate levels in patients with motor neurone, Parkinson's and Alzheimer's disease. Neuroscience Letters. 1990; 110:216–220.

55. Steventon GB, Heafield MT, Waring RH, Williams AC. Xenobiotic metabolism in Alzheimer's disease. Neurology. 1990;40: 1095–1098.

56. McKinnon RA, Nebert DW. Possible role of cytochromes P450 in lupus erythematosus and related disorders. Lupus. 1994;3:473-478.

57. Wy JM. Carcinogen hemoglobin adducts, urinary mutagenicity, and metabolic phenotype in active and passive cigarette smokers. J Natl Cancer Inst. 1991;83(13):963.

58. Anderson KE, Kappas A. Dietary regulation of cytochrome P-450. Annu Rev Nutr. 1991;11: 141–167.

59. Bland JS, Bralley JA. Nutritional upregulation of hepatic detoxification enzymes. J Appl Nutr. 1992;44(3&4):2–15.

60. Earl-Salotti AGL, Charland SL. The effect of parenteral nutrition on hepatic cytochrome P-450. JPEN. 1994;18:458–465.

61. Guengerich FP. Effects of nutritive factors on metabolic processes involving bioactivation and detoxification of chemicals. Annu Rev Nutr. 1984;4:207–231.

62. Guengerich FP, Kim DH. In vitro inhibition of dihydropyridine oxidation and aflatoxin B-1 activation in human liver microsomes by naringenin and other flavonoids. Carcinog. 1990; 11(12):2275–2279.

63. McIntosh MK, Goldfarb AH, Cutris LN, Cote PS. Vitamin E alters hepatic antioxidant enzymes in rats treated with dehydroepiandrosterone (DHEA). J Nutr. 1993;123:216–224.

64. Zhang Y, Tallalay P, Cho C. Anticarcinogenic protective enzymes from broccoli: isolation and elucidation of structure. Proc Natl Acad Sci. 1992;89:2399–2403.

65. Halpert JR, Guengerich FP, Bend JR, Correia MA. Selective inhibitors of cytochromes P450. Toxicol Appl Pharmacol. 1994;125:163–175.

66. Temellini A, Mogavero S, Giulianotti PC, Pietrabissa A, Mosca F, Pacifici GM. Conjugation of benzoic acid with glycine in human liver and kidney: a study on the interindividual variability. Xenobiotica. 1993;23(12):1427–1433.

67. Meyer U, Zanger U, Grant D, et al. Genetic polymorphisms of drug metabolism. Adv Drug Res. 1990:19;197–241.

68. Meyer U, Zanger U, Grant D, et al. Genetic polymorphisms of drug metabolism. Adv Drug Res. 1990:19;197–241.

69. Williams RJ. Biochemical individuality: The basis of the genetotrophic concept. New York, NY: John Wiley; 1956.

70. Goldin FE, Tatnayaka ID. Acetaminophen and macrophage activation. Intl Hepato Comms. 1995;4:16–18.

10

Assessment of Nutritional Status

Clinical nutrition has evolved from preventing deficiency diseases to using food to optimize health by assuring nutrient precursors, cofactors, structural molecules, and accessory nutrients are present at optimal levels. Signs and symptoms of frank nutrient deficiency diseases are well documented, and most of those cases can be identified on clinical assessments alone. Understanding what is "optimal" for a patient, however, is a challenge because of the interconnected way nutrients function as well as the difficulty of identifying subclinical deficiencies. For example, fatigue may result from:

- a subclinical deficiency of a B vitamin resulting in compromised ATP synthesis (see Chapters 5 and 8),

- a mitochondrial myopathy or genetic defect in mitochondrial function (see Chapter 8), or
- an under-functioning detoxification pathway resulting in increased oxidative stress that can influence several biochemical pathways (see Chapter 9).

Therefore, assessment of nutritional status involves collecting the clues that are available through patient history, clinical observation, and laboratory tests, and then using good clinical judgment in interpreting those clues.

While clinical observation remains an important initial step in patient assessment, laboratory tests enable clinicians to consider areas of metabolism that just a few years ago were difficult to assess in daily practice. With advancements in laboratory testing, clinicians may also be able to ask specific questions about absolute levels of specific nutrients and metabolic efficiency. However, no single test or approach provides a complete understanding of a patient's nutrient dynamics and functional status. Each method usually involves collecting and interpreting data in relation to another parameter to create a meaningful picture of an individual's health from a nutritional perspective. Emerging data on the genetic polymorphisms that are relevant to nutriture are just beginning to enter the clinical realm as well, and this information will improve our understanding of individual nutrient needs for optimal health.

While it is beyond the scope of this textbook to discuss every means by which a clinician may evaluate a patient's nutritional status, this final chapter provides a general overview and some tools to begin the process of incorporating nutritional assessment from a functional perspective. In addition, this chapter will introduce some commonly used nutritional assessments and provide examples of some key areas for consideration in developing nutrition-based interventions. Since laboratory testing is a dynamic field, clinicians interested in specific areas of nutritional support should obtain the most up-to-date information on testing from reputable laboratories that are active in the field. In addition, resources that provide a more thorough discussion of laboratory testing can also be consulted.[1]

CLINICAL ASSESSMENT OF NUTRITIONAL STATUS

Clinical assessment is commonly the first place to begin the evaluation of an individ-

$$BMI = \frac{(\text{Weight in kg}^2)}{(\text{Height in m}^2)}$$

Notes:
- Healthy BMI is generally between 18 and 25.
- BMI between 25 and 30 is considered overweight.
- BMI of 30 or greater is considered obese.
- BMI may not be accurate in assessing body composition for people who are very short, very tall, muscular, or who suffer from certain medical conditions that involve edema.

FIGURE 10.1   *Body mass index (BMI) calculation*

ual's nutritional status. Such assessments might include individual case history and physical exam to evaluate weight changes, anthropometric measurements, and body mass index (BMI) assessment (Figure 10.1) for signs of malnutrition, unusual energy needs, or vitamin and mineral deficiencies. Diet diaries and lifestyle or diet recall questionnaires can also help a clinician determine a patient's nutrient intake and environmental influences. (These common clinical approaches to nutritional assessment are discussed in detail in many nutritional textbooks.[2])

Clinical assessment approaches are useful for developing a broad picture of an individual's daily food intake, obvious signs or symptoms of dietary insufficiencies, and environmental exposure. In fact, a detailed description of dietary intake, anthropometrics, and growth parameters, coupled with accurate clinical examination, may provide the quickest, most cost-effective assessment for gross nutritional deficiencies in need of immediate attention (Table 10.1).

However, clinical assessment relies on the more obvious signs of nutritional inadequacy, which may not enable clinicians to determine a patient's full scope of nutrient inadequacies. In many cases, individuals may show deficiencies in only one nutrient but require supplementation with several nutrients to maintain healthy nutrient levels. In addition, clinicians using clinical assessment may not notice hourly or daily metabolic or biochemical changes that signify a patient's insufficient nutrient intake, because changes indicating nutritional defi-

ciency in anthropometric or other physical parameters may take longer to develop.[2]

Recognizing such limits of clinical assessment is important, particularly with increasing interest in the potential consequences of subclinical deficiencies. In subclinical nutrient deficiencies, poor nutrient status with depleted reserves or localized tissue deficiencies may develop, while classical deficiency signs are unnoticed (Figure 10.2).[3] Undetected subclinical deficiencies may affect an individual's ability to manage stress or heal wounds and maintain adequate immune system function. For such reasons, clinical assessment alone may be less reliable for diagnosis of a nutrition problem than other methods of assessment, unless the deficiency is severe.

A FUNCTIONAL APPROACH TO LABORATORY ASSESSMENT OF NUTRIENT STATUS

Laboratory tests that assess nutritional status are particularly useful when approached from a functional perspective. While a functional approach to laboratory assessment involves thinking about the tests differently, it doesn't always mean doing different tests than would be used in a conventional approach. For example, standard laboratory analyses of static nutrient levels can be interpreted in different ways. A conventional interpretation would mean if a nutrient is low, provide that nutrient and things should resolve. A functional perspective would look at

TABLE 10.1   *Common Features of Nutritional Deficiencies*

Deficiency	Feature
Biotin	Dermatitis, hyperesthesia
Calcium	Poor bone and teeth mineralization, tetany, rickets
Carbohydrate	Hypoglycemia, especially after minimal starvation; seizures
Chromium	Altered glucose tolerance
Cobalamin	Anemia, irritability, glossitis, ataxia, peripheral neuropathy, paresthesia
Copper	Anemia, osteoporosis
Energy	Reduced weight for height
Fat	Reduced subcutaneous fat as evidenced by well-demarcated bony prominence and veins, loss of gluteal and perianal fat; dry, scaly skin with desquamation in essential fatty acid deficiency
Fluorine	Dental caries
Folate	Anemia, irritability
Iodine	Goiter, hypothyroidism
Iron	Anemia, behavior disturbances, platyonychia of koilonychia
Magnesium	Tetany
Niacin	Dermatitis in exposed areas such as hands, feet, legs, and neck; stomatitis; glossitis, loss of papillae
Phosphorus	Rickets, muscle weakness
Protein	Muscle wasting; muscle weakness, peripheral edema; dry, dull, sparse, depigmented hair
Pyridoxine	Irritability, seizures, peripheral neuropathy, cheilosis, glossitis
Riboflavin	Cheilosis, glossitis, angular stomatitis, loss of papillae
Selenium	Cardiomyopathy, myopathy
Thiamin	Peripheral neuropathy, paresthesia, loss of proprioception, muscle weakness, cardiac failure
Vitamin A	Night blindness, conjunctival xerosis, corneal xerosis, Bitot's spots, keratomalacia, follicular hyperkeratosis
Vitamin C	Bony tenderness, pseudoparalysis, petechiae, bleeding gums, follicular hyperkeratosis
Vitamin D	Craniotabes, prominent costochondral junctions, widening of wrist and ankle, wide open anterior fontanelle, frontal bossing, delayed eruption of teeth, bony deformities, delayed motor milestones
Vitamin E	Muscle weakness, anemia, peripheral neuropathy
Vitamin K	Ecchymosis, hemorrhagic disorder

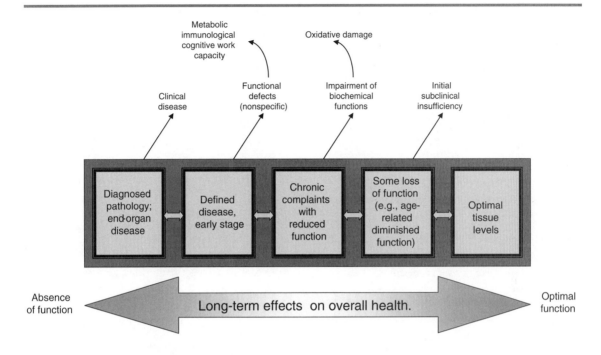

FIGURE 10.2   *Continuum of nutrient sufficiency / insufficiency*

the same laboratory test but instead of immediately correcting the direct deficiency, the functional perspective would first consider questions such as these:

- How is this nutrient used in the body?
- What other nutrients interact with this nutrient?
- Can this nutrient be deficient for reasons other than intake, such as decreased absorption because of an unhealthy GI environment?
- Is there a problem in transport or storage of this nutrient?

- Does this person's history suggest others in the family have similar issues and may that suggest a genetic sensitivity where this nutrient is concerned?

In a functional medicine approach, it is important to keep in mind the principle of biochemical individuality, and consider laboratory tests within the perspective of the individual patient, not take them entirely at face value.

While laboratory tests may be effective in detecting signs of deficiencies before a classic deficiency state appears, interpretation of such data can be extremely complex. For example, many factors can influence a laboratory test result: nutrient levels may reflect recent rather than long-term intakes; non-nutrient conditions may influence metabolite results; or clinical signs of a primary deficiency may conceal signs of a secondary deficiency. In addition, clinicians may find themselves inundated and confused about the many types of laboratory tests available today. Thus, since no single test can reveal absolute nutritional status, it is important to understand the general types of tests and their limitations to help create an overall meaningful picture of an individual's nutritional status. The most common types of tests fit into one of these three categories:

1. *Static level determination* of a nutrient or a metabolite, in which the level of the nutrient or metabolite is directly determined in a sample of tissue;

2. *Challenge tests*, in which the ability of the body to manage the challenge is monitored after an individual receives a challenge (either a substance or activity/situation); and

3. *Indirect nutrient assessment*, which includes tests for *nutrient-dependent activity* in which the activity of an enzyme or other function that is dependent on that nutrient is determined, as well as *surrogate markers* of a nutrient imbalance, which include metabolites that reflect a nutrient deficiency.

Static Level Determination of a Nutrient or Metabolite

In assessing a patient's nutrient status, the most common laboratory analyses involve tests that determine the static level of a nutrient or metabolite. Many vitamin and mineral levels can be identified from a variety of tissue samples including serum, plasma, erythrocytes, lymphocytes, whole blood, hair, and urine. Stool and saliva are also used for assessment of hormones and other bioactive molecules.

When assessing vitamin or mineral status by static level determination, clinicians should bear in mind that these nutrients are concentrated in various tissue compartments. Thus, some compartments (e.g., tissues, blood) may poorly represent the nutrient status for a particular vitamin or mineral, which makes it impossible to recommend one tissue as the source by which to assess all micronutrients. For example, a person may show signs of a nutrient deficiency when blood levels appear to be adequate, but the deficiency may be inside the cell, not in the blood. Therefore, the *intake* of the nutrient may not be in question, but the ability of the cell to receive that nutrient may be the issue.

Another issue is that the nutrient may be present but not in the exact form that is being assayed. For example, if the nutrient is bound to a protein for transport, it is important to know what is being assayed—only the free nutrient, or the bound as well? In addition, some minerals can be present in different valence forms, which may influence whether they are functional or not.

Clinicians should also consider that these tests reflect nutrient status at one particular time and may not reflect most recent changes. Assays in blood cells for some nutrients may also be more sensitive to dietary changes as well. Laboratories performing these tests

BOX A

Clinical and Laboratory Assessment of Fatty Acid Insufficiencies

Dietary intake, digestion, absorption, genetic factors, and metabolic activity can influence a patient's fatty acid levels. Dietary intake is critical, as essential fatty acids (EFA) must be ingested (or infused) or they will ultimately become deficient. Therefore, impairment of digestion and/or absorption may lead to EFA insufficiency despite what may seem to be adequate intake. Genetic factors may also affect metabolic activity, and can lead to changes such as the excessive long chain saturated fatty acid accumulation seen in adrenoleukodystrophy. Metabolic activity may also be affected by exogenous factors such as smoking and intake of *trans*-fatty acids with resultant inhibition of delta-6-dehydrogenase activity and reduction of conversion of precursors to longer chain fatty acid metabolites.

Laboratory Assessment

Adipose tissue biopsies reflect linoleic and α-linolenic acid stores but not derivative fatty acids; therefore, assessment of fatty acids is generally performed on plasma or erythrocytes after a 14-hour fast. Analysis of plasma fatty acids is generally preferred because all the fatty acids can be measured, which provides clues to fatty acid metabolism and body utilization of fatty acids. *Fasting plasma fatty acids* reflect body stores, but this is easily influenced by the patient's last meal. The subfraction analysis of fatty acids in lipoproteins, triglycerides, cholesterol esters and phospholipids is difficult to measure and generally not practical. *Fasting red blood cell (rbc) fatty acid analysis* measures phospholipids in the rbc membranes with results fairly independent of total cholesterol and triglyceride levels. Results are probably reflective of body stores but may change in response to diet. Recent meals influence the composition far more than older meals and results, therefore, may not reflect eating over the average rbc life expectancy of 120 days.

When EFA levels are low, the following levels increase: $\omega 7$, $\omega 9$, $16{:}1\omega 7$ and $20{:}3\omega 9/20{:}4\omega 6$ (triene/tetraene ratio).

Clinical Assessment

Given the challenges of laboratory analysis for EFA deficiency, clinical assessment plays a primary role in indications for exogenous fatty acid support. Clinical features of EFA deficiencies include:

dermatitis	polydipsia
dry hair and/or dandruff	polyuria
brittle nails	fatty liver
thirst	

Findings that suggest omega-3 deficiencies include neuropathy, reduced visual acuity, decreased memory and mental abilities, cardiac arrhythmias, and psychological disturbances.

Inflammatory conditions may be associated with increased arachidonic acid levels.

When fatty acid abnormalities exist, it is often necessary to determine the adequacy of other nutrients as well. Oxidative stress may contribute to fatty acid inadequacy by participating in the degradation of membrane fatty acids. If fatty acid imbalance exists, clinicians should also consider the potential influence of oxidative events and antioxidant adequacy (see Box B).

Further Reading

http://www.essentialfats.com/goodlab.htm#Differences

Siguel EN: Essential Fatty Acids in Health and Disease, Nutrek Press, Brookline, MA, 1994.

Siguel EN, Lerman RH: Altered fatty acid metabolism in patients with angiographically documented coronary artery disease. Am J Cardiol 1993;916–920.

	Omega-3 Deficiency	**Omega-6 Deficiency**
Laboratory Markers	Decreased α-linolenic acid	Decreased linoleic acid
	Decreased eicosapentaenoic acid	Decreased arachidonic acid
	Decreased docosahexaenoic acid	

should have specifics on the variables and limitations related to each test. An example of the types of limitations and benefits of these types of tests is shown in the analysis of fatty acids (see Box A).

Because it is not always practical or economical to order a single test for each nutrient, a clinician often uses a panel of tests that analyzes a group of nutrients. This compromise can work well if the clinician is aware of the drawbacks of this approach—namely, a limited nutrient picture and differences in reliability of specific laboratory assessment for specific nutrients. Therefore, interpreting these tests requires an understanding of the nutrient compartments, tissues, or fluids most representative of that particular nutrient. In addition, the nutrient may be present but may not be in its active form, or it may be unavailable for use in a specific tissue because of constraints on transport.

Challenge Tests

A challenge test is a direct assessment of the functioning of an organ or system. A challenge test is generally performed by loading the body with a challenge substance and measuring either the excretion of the nutrient or a product of the nutrient's metabolism. The first challenge test of this type was reported by Keller in 1842, in which he took a dose of a xenobiotic, benzoic acid, collected his urine, and showed a direct relationship between ingestion of the benzoic acid and the hippuric acid that was subsequently excreted (Figure 10.3).[4] In doing so, Keller illustrated that generation of hippuric acid in urine depends on the body's ability to metabolically convert ingested benzoic acid, or detoxify the xenobiotic to the end product, hippuric acid.

A particularly useful challenge test is the 2-hour postprandial glucose/insulin test, which uses a challenge of a glucose load (usually a drink providing a specific amount of glucose) provided to the patient 2 hours before obtaining a blood sample. The 2-hour postprandial blood is then analyzed for presence of insulin and/or glucose. Often, a change in blood insulin or glucose in response to a glucose load is noticeable prior to changes in fasting blood insulin or glucose and can identify a person at high risk of developing type II diabetes.

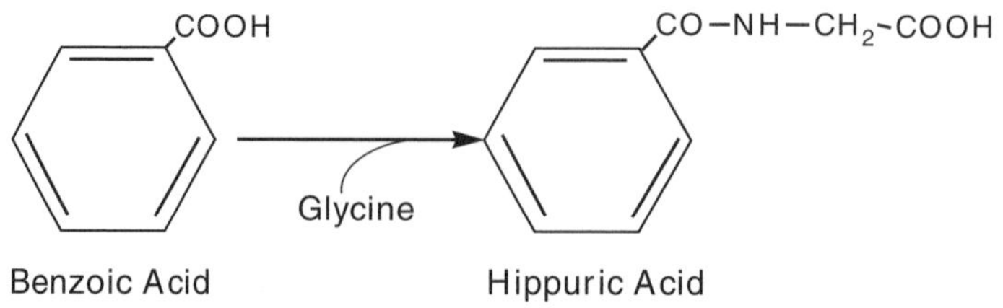

FIGURE 10.3   *Glycination of benzoic acid*

Stress tests can be considered challenge tests because they measure the body's ability to respond to a performance challenge. Some challenge tests are direct measures of nutrient status. For example, one test of magnesium status is a loading test in which administration of magnesium is followed by a urine test to determine the quantity of magnesium excreted. Low magnesium excretion implies that the body had insufficient magnesium and thus retained the oral loading dose.

Challenge tests also provide an effective means for testing function. For example, a test that measures muscle power seems to predict surgical complications better than anthropometric measurements such as weight loss or muscle circumference.[5] The caveat with challenge tests is that, although they test overall function, they generally do not lead to an understanding of the individual nutrients or interventions that might be most helpful to a specific patient. However, the magnesium load test illustrates that, when dealing with laboratory tests, no rule is set in stone, because that type of challenge test determines the helpful nutrient.

Indirect Nutrient Assessment

Many tests provide an indirect indication of nutrient deficiency. This approach determines nutriture by considering the function of that nutrient and the related metabolic events that influence it. These tests can be very helpful when reviewed in the context of a clinical assessment and can identify the areas in which a clinician may want to obtain more detailed

tests or perform a trial of nutritional supplementation with reassessment after a specified intervention time.

The most common indirect measure of nutrient assessment is conducted by measuring the activity of an enzyme that depends upon a particular nutrient for its function—a *nutrient-dependent activity* assessment. For example, glutathione reductase is an enzyme that requires riboflavin for its function. Glutathione reductase activity may, therefore, help measure functional riboflavin status. Another indirect assessment of nutrient is determination of a metabolite or a surrogate marker. For example, research has shown that elevated homocysteine (HCys), a risk factor for CVD, is attenuated by supplemental folate and vitamin B12. Therefore, elevated HCys is highly suggestive of a folate deficiency.

Another example of metabolite or surrogate marker assessment is seen in evaluation for oxidative stress. For example, oxidative stress occurs when the production of reactive oxygen species (ROS) exceeds the ability of the antioxidant nutrients in the body to quench these reactive molecules. Therefore, excessive ROS production suggests a need for higher levels of antioxidant nutrients, such as vitamin C, vitamin E, and the carotenoids. Direct assay for ROS is not generally possibly, however, since ROS are highly reactive and readily attack protein, DNA, RNA, and the lipids in cell membranes. Therefore, assay for the products of ROS and the adducts of ROS action is one way to assess oxidative damage in the body and is commonly used in research studies on oxidative stress. Box B summarizes some common assays used for assessment of oxidative stress and includes examples of nutrient-dependent activity assessment and surrogate markers. The caveat for these tests is that they are not specific to the nutrient; however, they can be extremely useful in narrowing down a set of issues and, when taken together with clinical signs and symptoms, can provide information for developing a personalized intervention plan for a patient.

All of these types of tests are useful at different times; however, the best approach to use with a specific patient depends on the clinical situation. When using one of these tests, a clinician should carefully consider its strengths and limitations. An example of how to incorporate clinical and laboratory assessment in a functional medicine approach is provided in Box C, in which clinical signs and symptoms, static laboratory tests (e.g., blood glucose, triglycerides), challenge tests (e.g., postprandial blood glucose and insulin), and indirect markers of nutrient deficiency (e.g., inflammatory markers) are used.

KEY CONSIDERATIONS IN A FUNCTIONAL MEDICINE ASSESSMENT

Each clinical situation is different and the specific approaches to a patient depend on many issues—most important, the patient's presenting complaints and the initial clinical evaluation. However, a few areas of assessment are central to the theme of nutrition since they relate directly to how nutrients are received by the body and the body's response to those nu-

trients. The following section summarizes these areas: Assessment of food allergy and intolerance, and the gastrointestinal milieu.

Assessment of Food Allergy and Intolerance

Food allergy assessment has generated more controversy than nearly any other area of laboratory assessment, perhaps because the ways humans react adversely to foods are more complex than was previously assumed. A primary consideration in this area is understanding the differences between food allergies and food intolerance. Some individuals may show clinical symptoms or sensitivity related to ingestion of a particular food substance, but only those reactions that involve an immune response are true food allergies. This may seem irrelevant since symptoms are symptoms, but it does relate to how a clinician may test for a food reaction and also how it may be handled clinically.

By definition, an immune response only occurs when an antigen/antibody reaction first takes place (Table 10.2). Therefore, if individuals do not have antibodies against a specific food antigen, they cannot have an allergic reaction to the food. Instead, they have a food intolerance. For example, lactase insufficiency, which underlies lactose intolerance, would not be considered an allergic response, but is instead a food intolerance. However, the response that occurs after peanut ingestion in a person with sensitivity to peanuts is a food allergy because it involves the immune system.

BOX B

Assessment of Oxidative Stress

Oxidative stress often stems from an imbalance in antioxidant and prooxidant status and this imbalance is associated with many chronic diseases of aging, such as CVD, cancer, macular degeneration, chronic inflammatory conditions, dementia, and cognitive dysfunction. Prooxidant status results from excessive production of reactive oxygen species (ROS), which can react with proteins, RNA, and DNA resulting in tissue damage, genomic instability (e.g., mutations), and altered cellular processes. Assessment for oxidative stress is an active area of research and focus is turning toward understanding total antioxidant capacity as a health support factor. Test panels and types of test are constantly being modified in this arena to include the most recent data. Laboratories with a specialty in oxidative stress provide useful partners in identifying the best and most current means with which to assess an individual patient; however, some commonly used approaches are outlined below.

Common Biomarkers of Presence of (and Resulting Damage from) Oxidative Stress

Oxidative stress can occur in a variety of tissues and lead to many different effects; therefore, no single assay can rule out the presence of oxidative stress. However, some markers have been associated with damage from high levels of oxidative stress in patients. Such markers include lipid peroxides, formed from reaction of ROS with unsaturated fatty acids and prostaglandins. The compound 8-hydroxy-2'-deoxyguanosine (8OH-DG) is a by-product of degradation of DNA by ROS. Elevations of lipid peroxides and 8OH-DG have been associated with several chronic diseases that accompany aging.

Nutritional and Subclinical Assessment for Oxidative Stress

From a functional medicine perspective, assessment for oxidative stress should include understanding the subclinical imbalances in the pathways and nutrient levels that provide protection from oxidative stress. A functional laboratory assessment for oxidative stress should consider both the direct enzyme activities that protect from ROS and the status of key nutrients to support these protective pathways. Many nutrients are important in protecting from ROS, and much discussion is taking place in the research community with respect to optimal levels. For example, studies

Common Laboratory Methods used to Detect Oxidative Stress

Principal Analyte	Comments
Catechol and/or 2,3-dihydrobenzoate	Obtained from challenge test with salicylate. Elevation of 2,3-dihydroxybenzoate and/or catechol indicates increased hydroxyl radical activity.
Lipid peroxides (serum or urine)	Several methods are used for quantification, including TBARS. Elevated lipid peroxides indicate peroxidation of unsaturated fatty acids in cell membranes.
F_2-isoprostanes	A measure of peroxidation of prostaglandins and polyunsaturated fatty acids.
8-OH-2'-deoxyguanosine	Quantification of hydroxylated deoxyguanosine residues present in DNA. Elevated 8-OH-2'-deoxyguanosine is an indication of hydroxyl radical damage to DNA.
Antioxidant panels	Includes quantification of various antioxidants: vitamins A, C, and E; alpha- and beta-carotene; the minerals selenium, copper, zinc, and iron; reduced glutathione, coenzyme Q10 and lipoic acid. Antioxidants are often depleted in conditions of oxidative stress, and low levels can yield a picture of susceptibility to oxidative stress.

(continues)

BOX B, *continued*

suggest vitamin C intake of at least 100 mg per day is optimal.

Key nutrients that support protection from oxidative stress include:

- vitamin C
- vitamin E
- carotenoids
- glutathione (e.g., cysteine, sulfate reserves)
- copper
- zinc
- selenium
- iron (Too much *and* too little of iron can indicate imbalance.)

Many plant compounds (such as flavonoids and polyphenols) also provide protection, but these are not feasible to assay individually. However, investigating a patient's dietary regime with a 3-day diet diary can provide insight into the level of these protective phytonutrients since they are the substances that provide color to vegetables and fruits (e.g., orange, red, blue, purple).

Minerals are also important in supporting primary protective pathways, as shown below. Investigating these enzyme activities directly may also provide guidelines for personalizing an intervention to protect against the damage of oxidative stress.

Further Reading

Carr AC, Frei B. Toward a new recommended dietary allowance for vitamin C based on antioxidant and health effects in humans. *Am J Clin Nutr.* 1999;69: 1086–1107.

Fenech M. Recommended dietary allowances (RDAs) for genomic stability. Mutat Res. 2001;480-81:51-54.

Ghiselli A, Serafini M, Natella F, Scaccini C. Total antioxidant capacity as a tool to assess redox status: critical view and experimental data. Free Radic Biol Med. 2000;29:1106–1114.

Halliwell B. Can oxidative DNA damage be used as a biomarker of cancer risk in humans? Problems, resolutions and preliminary results from nutritional supplementation studies. Free Radic Res. 1998;29: 469-486.

Mayne ST. Antioxidant nutrients and chronic disease: use of biomarkers of exposure and oxidative stress status in epidemiological research. J Nutr. 2003;133 Suppl 3:933S-940S.

Antioxidant Enzymes

Cu, Zn-superoxide dismutase (requires Cu and Zn), and Mn-superoxide dismutase (requires Mn):

$$2O_2^{-\bullet} + 2H \rightarrow H_2O_2 + O_2$$

Glutathione peroxidase (requires Se):

$$H_2O_2 + 2GSH \rightarrow 2H_2O + GSSG$$

Catalase (requires Fe):

$$2H_2O_2 \rightarrow 2H_2O + O_2$$

Ceruloplasmin (requires Cu); oxidizes iron without forming hydrogen peroxide or oxygen radicals; may scavenge hydrogen peroxide, superoxide and hydroxyl radicals:

$$Fe^{+2} \rightarrow Fe^{+3}$$

TABLE 10.2   *Terms Used to Describe Food Allergy and Food Intolerance*

Food Allergy (Hypersensitivity): Immunologic reaction resulting from exposure to food; reactions occur in only some subjects; reaction is unrelated to physiological effect of food.

Food Intolerance: Abnormal physiologic response to food; reaction is not immunologic.

Adverse Reaction: Symptoms attributed to the ingestion of a food or other material without a recognized organic etiology.

Antibody: Protein produced by immune cells of the body in response to an antigen.

Antigen: Substance with which an antibody will bind specifically. Antigens can be high-molecular-weight proteins, peptides, carbohydrates, nucleic acids, lipids, and any number of other types of substances.

A complete description of the immune response and subsequent biochemical changes is beyond the scope of this book. Briefly, however, this section emphasizes that the immune response to an antigen may involve some or all of a host of antibody subtypes, including IgE, IgG, IgM, IgA, and IgD. Of particular importance to food allergy is the IgG antibody, which comprises about 80 percent of antibodies in human serum, and the IgE antibody, which constitutes only a small percentage of antibodies but is central to the allergic response.[6,7]

IgG antibodies interact with the complement system after binding to their respective antigens. IgE antibodies occupy receptors on mast cells and basophils and mediate the release of histamine and other inflammation-associated chemicals after binding to their respective antigens. IgE responses are very rapid in onset, whereas IgG responses are not rapid, but usually represent a delayed hypersensitivity. A food may elicit an IgE response without an IgG-delayed response, or an IgG response without an immediate IgE response.

Some controversy exists with respect to the actual definition of food allergy. Some definitions describe a true food allergy as only an IgE-mediated response, which is also called a Type I hypersensitivity. However, not all symptoms of allergic responses can be ascribed to IgE-mediated mechanisms.[8] Many allergic responses appear to involve some form of prolonged or delayed reaction to allergens.[9] For example, the antibodies of the IgG4 subclass are increased in atopic dermatitis and asthma.[10] Therefore, evidence seems to support the role of both IgE and IgG4 antibodies in the provocation of immediate and delayed symptoms due to immunological reactions to food allergens.

No direct assessment of food intolerance is available. Determination of intolerant foods is best performed by dietary elimination with subsequent reintroduction and challenge to see whether symptoms are related to that

---

BOX C

Assessment of Insulin Resistance and Metabolic Syndrome

Problems of carbohydrate intolerance, insulin resistance, and poor glycemic control are responsible for considerable disease in industrialized countries. As many as 63 million people in the US are estimated to have poor glycemic control, with 25% of those having diagnosable type 2 diabetes mellitus. Fasting glucose, the standard screening tool to assess glycemic problems, may indicate poor glycemic control but it represents only a crude assessment because it may not occur until late in the establishment of dysglycemia. Ideally, clinicians use assessment panels in which not only fasting blood sugar control, but also the early-stage indicators of imbalance and the metabolic consequences of dysglycemia are also investigated.

Clinical signs that may suggest dysglycemia include:

- family history of diabetes
- gestational diabetes
- polycystic ovary syndrome (PCOS)
- low birth weight
- sleep apnea
- sugar cravings and carbohydrate "addiction"
- sleepiness after a meal; insomnia relieved by snacking
- increased appetite, usually after a carbohydrate meal
- fatigue after a high-carbohydrate meal
- pattern of nighttime eating
- hypoglycemia
- dietary history of high-refined carbohydrate intake
- resistant weight loss
- hirsutism, acne, and menstrual irregularities

Metabolic syndrome (also called insulin resistance syndrome) is a condition that often precedes frank diabetes and identification of individuals with metabolic syndrome can identify those at a high-risk for developing diabetes. The third report of the National Cholesterol Education Program Expert Panel (2001) defines metabolic syndrome as present when a patient has 3 or more of the following:

- abdominal obesity [waist circumference: men >102 cm (40 in); women: >88 cm (34.5 in)
- hypertriglyceridemia [blood triglycerides $\geq$150 mg/dL]
- low HDL-cholesterol [HDL-C: men <40 mg/dL; women <50 mg/dL]
- high blood pressure [BP$\geq$130/85 mm Hg]
- high fasting glucose [blood glucose$\geq$110 mg/dL]

In addition, several other laboratory signs may suggest an individual at high risk for developing metabolic syndrome:

- elevated postprandial (2-hr) blood glucose and/or insulin
- elevated triglyceride to HDL-C ratio (>4.0)
- elevated serum uric acid
- elevated inflammation markers (e.g., C-reactive protein, PAI-1, fibrinogen)

Nutrition is a key factor in diabetes management. Moreover, early intervention with diet and lifestyle modifications can halt further progression from metabolic syndrome to frank diabetes with its associated significant health risks.

Further Reading

Executive summary of the third report of the National Cholesterol Education Program (NCEP) Expert Panel on Detection, Evaluation, and Treatment of High Blood Cholesterol in Adults (ATP III). JAMA. 2001;285:2486–2497.

Reaven G. Pathophysiology of insulin resistance in human disease. Physiol Rev. 1995;75:473–485.

Lukaczer D, Liska DJ. Recognizing Insulin Resistance Syndrome. Integrat Med. 2003;2:42–48.

food. Since food allergies involve generation of specific antibodies, laboratory tests for allergic foods may be useful with some patients; however, no single laboratory test provides an entirely accurate assessment of food allergy. Since the onset of IgE-mediated reactions is generally rapid, most clinicians can determine an IgE-mediated response by carefully reviewing a patient's history (in other words, the patient can identify this type of response). Laboratory assessment or confirmation can be performed with an IgE Food Antibody Panel, which is commonly done using a radioallergosorbent test (RAST) or enzyme-linked immunoassay (ELISA) method.

The IgG-mediated responses are delayed responses and more difficult to determine both clinically and in the laboratory. IgG Food Antibody Panels often employ either total IgG assessment or IgG4, the subfamily of IgG believed to react commonly with food antigens. IgG Food Antibody Panels can be useful in determining which foods should be avoided during an elimination diet; however, they can also be misleading. In particular, if an individual has not ingested the food in question in the recent past, IgG antibodies may not be present in high enough quantity to determine the response on a Food Antibody Panel.

Furthermore, how food allergies are viewed is confusing. Like the conventional focus on disease states, a food allergy is often considered to be a specific response to a specific food antigen that will recur over an individual's lifespan. In many cases, some assumed food allergies are the result of a clinical condi-

TABLE 10.3 *Clinical Conditions Associated with Increased Antigen Uptake by the Intestine*

Intestinal Disorders
Gastrointestinal food allergy
Celiac disease
Acute gastroenteritis
Chronic intestinal infections
Inflammatory bowel disease
Surgery
System Insults
Excessive radiation
Extensive burns
Septicemia shock
Hypovolumetric shock
Malnutrition
Drugs
Antiinflammatory drugs

tion that has led to an increased uptake of large molecules in the intestinal tract that have, in turn, induced an allergic response (as well as other responses such as detoxification) (Table 10.3). Supporting intestinal integrity and reestablishing the intestinal barrier function may help individuals digest these foods, or keep the large molecules from entering circulation. Thus, the barrier function serves as protection and allows an individual to ingest some foods that previously caused allergic responses. The question of whether one is "allergic" or "sensitive" to foods should prompt clinicians to ask questions about immunologic status, detoxification status, nutritional status, intestinal microecology, digestive efficiency, and intestinal mucosal integrity.

The Gastrointestinal Milieu

One of the most crucial features affecting nutritional status is proper functioning of the gastrointestinal (GI) tract, and healthy function of the GI tract requires a healthy microenvironment. Assessment of gastrointestinal function includes determining adequate digestion and absorption, investigating intestinal mucosa integrity, and evaluating the intestinal microecology. Stool is the ultimate end product of digestive activity and, therefore, a survey of various metabolic markers in stool can provide an overview of digestive function with which to guide further clinical evaluation and develop targeted therapy. In particular, stool analysis provides insight into intestinal microecology, which can indicate problems with absorption and digestion. The integrity of the small intestinal barrier is an important factor in healthy GI function as well. A brief description of the key areas to consider in reviewing intestinal function is provided below.

Evaluating digestion and absorption

Stool analysis can be useful in assessing underlying causes of poor digestion and/or absorption (which can, in turn, relate to a host of systemic signs and symptoms). The measurement of markers such as fecal chymotrypsin or pancreatic elastase 1 may help in the assessment of frank or subtle pancreatic insufficiency. For example, chymotrypsin may provide a measure of proteolytic enzyme activity.[11] The measurement of triglycerides, long chain fatty acids, cholesterol and total fecal fat can provide clues to impairments in absorptive and/or digestive capacity. For example, elevated total fecal amounts may reflect incomplete fat hydrolysis and suggest pancreatic insufficiency.

Intestinal barrier function

The GI mucosa has the paradoxical role of allowing or facilitating transport of some molecules while excluding others. Changes in intestinal permeability are important in a number of GI tract disorders that have systemic implications. For example, permeable GI mucosa may create a portal of entry for large food molecules, such as peptides and proteins, which may become antigenic when in circulation, causing a food allergic response.[12] (Figure 7.2 illustrates permeability dynamics.)

The most widely used method for assessing intestinal permeability is a challenge test using inert sugars in the 300–400 dalton range—both monosaccharides and disaccharides—to evaluate differential saccharide absorption.[13] In this test, a disaccharide that is not well absorbed by the healthy intestine is administered at the same time as a monosaccharide that is well absorbed. The most commonly used saccharides in this challenge test include cellobiose/mannitol, lactulose/mannitol, lactulose/l-rhamnose, and cellobiose/l-rhamnose. Gastric integrity has also been evaluated using some of these same intestinal probe methods.[14]

Differential saccharide absorption studies are typically administered by oral ingestion of a sugar solution containing known amounts of the disaccharide and monosaccharide sugars following an overnight fast.[15] Urine is collected, the total volume recorded, and a sample returned to the lab to determine the recovery of the probe molecules. This type of testing also offers the advantage of being a noninvasive, outpatient procedure.[16] While this is a useful assessment tool, care should be taken in interpretation, as the intestinal lining is a dynamic interface, and permeability may change rapidly depending on recent dietary intake.

Gastrointestinal microecology

Dysbiosis, as described in Chapter 7, is a condition of altered intestinal microecology that may have clinical consequences. It generally refers to a state in which populations of indigenous microbes have grown excessively, exogenous organisms have taken up residence in the intestinal tract, or colonic microbes have migrated beyond their normal environment into the small intestine, stomach, or esophagus. Assessment of dysbiosis is clinically important because of its relationship to intestinal and systemic disease. In addition, dysbiosis may compromise nutritional status as a result of two primary effects: microbial competition for dietary nutrients, and damage to the mucosal absorptive surface.[17]

In general, assessment involves direct measurement of microbes and metabolites, which include bacteria, yeast, fungi, protozoa, roundworms, and others. However, this method can be problematic in assessment of bacteria, yeast and fungi in particular because of the difficulty in culturing many of these microbes and the dynamic nature of the GI milieu. Protozoa and worms can be difficult to diagnose because of variability in shedding and difficulty in proper identification. Despite the limitations, microscopic stool analysis is vital to assessing dysbiosis and infection.

Assessment of metabolic markers is also useful for determining the presence of dysbio-

TABLE 10.4   *Stool Markers Suggestive of Intestinal Dysbiosis*

Absorption Markers	Digestion Markers
Total fecal fat	Chymotrypsin
Total short-chain fatty acids	Triglycerides
Long-chain fatty acids	Valerate
Cholesterol	iso-Butyrate
Markers of Colonic Microbiological Activity	
β-Glucuronidase	
n-Butyrate (as mmoles/g and as % of total short-chain fatty acids)	
Acetate	
Propionate	
pH	

Note: Pathogenic microbes such as those listed in Figure 7.3 are also indicative of intestinal dysbiosis.

sis (Table 10.4). The nature of the metabolites often provides clinicians a reasonable picture of the nature and extent of the dysbiosis and, often, of the particular organisms involved. For example, the presence of beta-glucuronidase in stool may be a sign of microbes that enzymatically deconjugate specific molecular bonds. The presence of an elevated stool pH may signify a prevalence of bacteria species that foster a more alkaline environment and therefore may be more inhospitable for the acid loving probiotics. (Figures 7.3 and 7.4 present information about the GI microbial environment.)

SUMMARY

This chapter presented a general discussion of the types of tests and approaches useful to assessing a patient's nutritional status from a functional medicine perspective. While the field of assessment is rapidly changing and new tests will continue to be developed, knowing the basics of proper nutrition assessment is important for many reasons. Nutrition is core to competent patient care. Proper functioning is supported by the many nutrients found in whole foods. Nutritional choices influence the body's activity, and consistently poor choices may compromise an individual's health.

Furthermore, information provided by nutrition assessment tests can only be meaningful when integrated into a broader picture of a patient's health. Such tests should be administered by skilled and well-informed practitioners who can account for potential sources of error and interpret the results in light of other assessment findings. Practitioners must also keep in mind that nutrients interact; an abnormal value for one nutrient does not, by itself, indicate that a problem exists. Each assessment method is useful only when considered as part of the entire picture of an individual's health.

CHAPTER 10 REFERENCES

1. Bralley JA, Lord RS. Laboratory Evaluations in Molecular Medicine. Norcross, GA: The Institute for Advances in Molecular Medicine; 2001.
2. Jeejeebhoy KN. Clinical and functional assessments. In: Shils ME, Olson JA, Shike M, eds. Modern Nutrition in Health and Disease. Vol. 1. Philadelphia, Pa: Lea & Febiger; 1994:805–811.
3. Shenkin A. Micronutrients and outcome. Nutrition. 1997;13:825-828.
4. Hutt AJ, Caldwell J. Amino acid conjugation. In: Mulder GJ, ed. Conjugation Reactions in Drug Metabolism. New York, NY: Taylor & Francis; 1990:273-305.
5. Jeejeebhoy KN. Clinical and functional assessments. In: Shils ME, Olson JA, Shike M, eds. Modern Nutrition in Health and Disease. Vol. 1. Philadelphia, Pa: Lea & Febiger; 1994:805–811.
6. Hefle SL. Immunoassay fundamentals. Food Technol. 1995;Feb:102–107.
7. Taylor SL. Chemistry and detection of food allergens. Food Technol. 1992;May:148–152.
8. Carini C, Brostoff J, Wraith DG. IgE complexes in food allergy. Ann Allergy. 1987;59:110–117.
9. Halpern GM, Scott JR. Non-IgE antibody mediated mechanisms in food allergy. Ann Allergy. 1987;58:14–27.
10. Rafei A, Peters SM, Harris N, Bellanti JA. Diagnostic value of IgG4 measurements in patients with food allergy. Ann Allergy. 1989;62:94–99.
11. Bode C, Bode JC. Usefulness of a simple photometric determination of chymotrypsin activity in

stools—results of a multicentre study. Clin Biochem. 1986;19:333–37.

12. Laudet, A, Arnaud, P, Napoly, A, Brion, F. The intestinal permeability test applied to the diagnosis of food allergy in paediatrics. West Indian Med J. 1994;43:87–88.

13. Travis S and Menzies I. Intestinal permeability: functional assessment and significance. Clin Sci. 1992;82:471–488.

14. Sutherland LR, Verhoef M, Wallace JL, et al. A simple, non-invasive marker of gastric damage: sucrose permeability. Lancet. 1994;343(8904): 998–100.

15. Laker MF, Bull HJ, Menzies I, et al. Evaluation of mannitol for use as a probe marker of gastrointestinal permeability in man. Eur J Clin Invest. 1982;12:485–491.

16. Willems D, Cadranel S, Jacobs W. Measurement of urinary sugars by HPLC in the estimation of intestinal permeability: evaluation in pediatric clinical practice. Clin Chem. 1993;39(5):888–890.

17. Keusch, S. Nutritional consequences of bacterial overgrowth syndromes. In: Effects of Microorganisms on GI Tract. 182–185.

INDEX

A

Abdominal distention, 198, 202

Abdominal pain, 192, 198, 202

Absorptive capacity, clues to impairments in, 278

Acetylation, 251

Acne rosacea, low gastric acidity as
        influencing, 194

Addison's disease, 166, 196

Adenosine diphosphate (ADP)
    conversion of ATP to, 216, 218
    conversion to ATP of, 223–24

Adenosine triphosphate (ATP)
    anaerobic vs. aerobic metabolism for, 219
    compromised synthesis of, 263
    depletion of neuronal, 247
    generating, 216
    impairment in, 226
    rates during exercise of, 234

Adequate Intake (AI)
    for minerals, table of, 153–56
    for vitamins, table of, 102–104
    as one base for DRIs, 101

AIDS and HIV, 60, 122
    intestinal permeability disrupted in, 201, 202
    zinc deficiency in patients having, 172

Alcoholism, 107, 111, 202, 213
    depletion of nutrients in, 161
    risk of hemochromatosis in, 178, 179

Alcohols, xenobiotic, 243

Alzheimer's disease, 133, 216, 227–28, 256
    associated with injury to neurons, 59
    excess excitatory neurotransmitters associ-
        ated with, 247
    reduced sulfate excretion in patients
        having, 61

American Diabetes Association (ADA) meal
    recommendations, 35

Amino acid derivatives, 45

Amino acid exchange, interorgan, 51

Amino acids, 41–67
    aromatic, 50
    branched-chain (BCAA), 49–50, 257
    classes of, 42
    "conditionally essential," 47, 51
    conjugation of, 45–47, 251
    essential (from food source), 42, 44, 58, 207
    excitatory, 52–53
    nitrogen balance studies of, 58
    nonessential (synthesized internally), 42–45
    protein absorbed as, 200
    protein structured by, 42
    quality of proteins affecting deficiencies
        of, 41
    in soy protein, 57
    structure of, 42, 43
    sulfur/sulfation, 44–45, 56, 58, 61–62

Amino acids by name
    alanine, 43, 51
    arginine, 43, 44, 47–49, 50
    asparagine, 43
    aspartate, 52
    aspartic acid, 43
    betaine, 42, 45
    carnitine, 42, 50–51, 52, 223, 229, 233
    citrulline, 42, 44, 47–49
    creatine, 42, 50–51, 223–24
    cysteine, 43, 44, 45, 56, 58, 61, 82, 177, 230,
        234, 240
    gamma-aminobutyric acid, 52
    glutamate, 52–53
    glutamic acid, 43, 82
    glutamine, 43, 44, 51–52, 58–61, 207
    glycine, 43, 44–47, 50, 52, 257
    histidine, 43, 56

Amio acids by name, *continued*
  homocysteine, 45–46, 60, 61
  isoleucine, 42, 43, 49–50, 56, 257
  L-glutamine, 207
  leucine, 42, 43, 49–50, 56, 257
  lysine, 42, 43, 50, 56, 58, 223
  methionine, 42, 43, 45, 56, 58, 240
  ornithine, 42, 44, 47–49
  phenylalanine, 42, 43, 56
  proline, 43
  serine, 43
  taurine, 42, 44–47
  threonine, 42, 43, 58
  tryptophan, 42, 43, 56
  tyrosine, 43, 44, 56
  valine, 42, 43, 49–50, 56, 257
Amyotrophic lateral sclerosis, 180, 228
  associated with injury to neurons, 59–60
  excess excitatory neurotransmitters associated with, 247
Anemia, 12, 120, 122, 125–26, 171–74, 177, 181, 196, 245, 266
Angina, 165
Ankylosing spondylitis, 200, 211
  intestinal permeability altered in, 200
Anorexia, 50, 107, 109, 115, 138, 161, 245
Antecedents as key component of patient's story, 7
Antibodies, 175, 177, 275, 277, 278
Antigens, 29, 203–4, 209, 275, 277–78
Antioxidants
  for detoxification, 257
  for mitochondrial function, 229, 231–33
  for permeability-related conditions, 208, 211
  protecting against production of reactive oxygen, 59
  protecting cell lipids, 80–83
  of selenium, conditions improved using, 183
  of vitamers of vitamin E, 131
Arachidonic acid (AA) cascade, 74–79

Arsenic, toxic exposure to, 245. *See also* Heavy (toxic) metals, xenobiotic
Arthritis, 99, 112, 241. *See also* Immune-related arthritis, Osteoarthritis, *and* Rheumatoid arthritis
Ascorbate. *See* Vitamin C (ascorbate)
Asthma, 118, 122, 165, 183, 194, 196, 248, 275
  induced by MSG, 61
  possible magnesium deficiency in patients having, 165
  selenium to decrease symptoms of, 183
Ataxia, 60, 107, 122, 127, 227, 229, 241, 266
Atherogenesis, 45, 46
Atherosclerosis, 81, 84, 119, 122
Atopic skin disorders, atopy, 57, 91, 201, 203, 211, 275
Autism, 60, 118, 202
  diet-responsive, 61
  elevated metabolites in patients having, 243
Autoimmune disorders and dysfunction, 36, 133, 194, 205, 245–46

B

B-vitamins and B-complex vitamins. *See also* individual vitamins by name
  biochemical differences among humans for, 6
  in mitochondrial efficiency, 220, 223, 233
Bacteria
  aerobic and anaerobic, 199
  bifidobacteria, 22, 23–24, 206–7, 210
  in birth, 242
  Campylobacter jejuni, 205
  Chlamydia trachomatis, 205
  Clostridium perfringens, 23, 199–200, 207
  in colon, 199, 243
  "food" for growth of, 26, 199
  gastrointestinal, 206
  gut lumen, 242–43
  Helicobacter pylori, 196
  intestinal, 205

lactobacilli, 22, 206–7, 210
overgrowth of unwanted, 194, 196, 204, 211, 243
reintroduction of desirable, 210
Salmonella, 199–200, 205
Shigella flexneri, 205
streptococci, 206
thermophilized, 205
Yersinia enterocolitica, 205
Bacterial imbalance
development of chronic disease linked with, 204–8
intestinal permeability disrupted by, 203–4
nutritional support strategies to treat, 205
relationship of diet to, 204
Behavioral changes in eating habits, 193
Bernard, Claude, homeostasis defined, 8
Bile acids, sulfation of, 61
Bile secretion, 192, 197
Biochemical individuality in nutrition, 5–8, 244, 246–47, 258
Bioenergetics defined, 3
Biological inhalants, effects on total load of, 239
Biotin, 126–28
absorption of, 126–27
functional medicine considerations for, 128
functions of, 127
safety and toxicity of, 128
sources of, 127
structure of, 126
therapeutic considerations for, 127–28
Bladder cancer, 252
Bloating, 196, 198
carbohydrate intake related to, 29
conditions leading to, 30, 198
cooking techniques to minimize, 30
foods associated with, 30
Blood sugar regulation
carbohydrate metabolism and, 31–36
meal planning and, 36

Body mass index (BMI) calculation, 264–65
for individual deficiencies, table of, 266
Body temperature, homeostasis of, 8–9
Bone remineralization and resorption, 10–11
Boron, 186
absorption of, 186
functional medicine considerations for, 186
functions of, 186
RDA/AI and UL for, 156
safety and toxicity of, 186, 246
sources of, 186
therapeutic considerations for, 186
Bowel disorders, 9, 21
Bowel movements, difficult or painful, 29
Breast cancer, 87, 204
Brush border enzymes, 195

C

Cadmium, toxic exposure to, 245. *See also* Heavy (toxic) metals, xenobiotic
Calciferol. *See* Vitamin D
Calcium, 10, 11, 152–53, 156–60
absorption and regulation of, 152, 156, 161, 186, 194, 248
functional medicine considerations for, 159–60
functions of, 152, 157
RDA/AI and UL for, 153
safety and toxicity of, 159
sources of, 157, 158, 159
therapeutic considerations for, 157
Cancer anorexia, 50
Cancer (carcinoma), 5, 27, 45, 50, 74, 81, 87, 105, 137, 142, 179, 181, 183–84, 204, 205, 208, 238, 252, 254, 257, 273, 274. *See also* individual types
Carbohydrates, 17–40. *See also* Starch, and individual types of Carbohydrates
absorption of, 35, 200
classes of, 17, 18–27

Carbohydrates, *continued*
    complex, 19
    construction and conversion of, 18–19
    digestibility of, 17
    functional approach to, 29–36
    future directions in research about, 36
    metabolism of, 29–36
    simple, 18, 19, 21
Cardiac arrhythmia, possible magnesium defi-
        ciency in patients having, 165
Cardiomyopathy, possible magnesium deficiency
        in patients having, 165
Cardiovascular accident (CVA), 163
Cardiovascular disease, 34, 45, 48–49, 69, 74, 81,
        93, 109, 129–30, 138, 193, 230, 240,
        244–47, 250, 258
    chronic mercury ingestion as possible risk
            factor for, 245
    excess iron associated with, 179
    inadequate nutrient intake associated
            with, 100
    possible magnesium deficiency in patients
            having, 165
    prevention and treatment of, 18, 31, 35,
            57, 183
    risk factors for, 271
Celiac disease, 196, 198, 201–2, 211, 277
Cellular metabolism, influence of GSH on, 54
Cephalic phase analyses of digestion, 192–93
Cervical dysplasia, 124, 126
Challenge tests
    of detoxification, 257–58
    development of, 270
    of insulin level, 12
    nutritional assessments using, 270–1
    postprandial glucose/insulin, 270
    stress, 271
Cheilosis, 11, 112, 115, 119, 266
Chloride, 165–69
    absorption and regulation of, 166
    functional medicine considerations for, 169

functions of, 165, 166
    safety and toxicity of, 168–9
    sources of, 166
    therapeutic considerations for, 166–68
Cholesterol
    absorption of, 26
    HDL, 12, 34
    hormone synthesis from, 88
    LDL, 57
    as lipid type, 85–87
    mineral supplementation to lower, 185
    structure of, 86
    total, 57
Chromium, 169–71
    absorption and regulation of, 169
    functional medicine considerations for,
            170–71
    functions of, 169–70
    RDA/AI and UL for, 154
    safety and toxicity of, 170
    sources of, 170
    therapeutic considerations for, 170
Chronic fatigue immune deficiency syndrome
        (CFIDS), 256
Clinical imbalances underlying diseases or condi-
        tions, 3
    categories of, 3–4
    core, 4, 8
    readjusting, 5
Clinical nutrition, negative focus of traditional, 11
Cobalamin. *See* Vitamin B12 (cobalamin)
Coenzyme Q10 (ubiquinone)
    in detoxification, 257
    lipid protection from, 84–85
    in mitochondrial function, 229, 232
Colitis, 27, 116, 202
Colon cancer, 27, 208
Colon transit time. *See* Intestinal transit time
Colonic food, carbohydrates functioning as, 22
Colorectal cancer, dietary fiber linked with mini-
        mizing, 208

Conditionally essential nutrients, 13
Congestive heart failure (CHF), possible magnesium deficiency in patients having, 165
Constipation
    caused by increased fiber intake without more water, 29
    low gastric acidity causing, 196
Copper, 172–75
    absorption of, 173
    as detoxification support nutrient, 257
    functional medicine considerations for, 174
    functions of, 173
    RDA/AI and UL for, 154
    safety and toxicity of, 173–74, 246
    sources of, 173, 174
    therapeutic considerations for, 173
Coronary artery disease (CAD), 74, 105, 269
Cow's milk substitutes, 57
Creatinine excretion rate, 50
Crohn's disease, 201, 208, 211
Cystic fibrosis, 90, 197, 201, 211

D

Dementia, 107, 113, 122, 227, 229, 273
    associated with injury to neurons, 59–60
Depression, 107, 109, 112–13, 115, 119, 122, 124, 127–28, 165, 176, 228, 243
Dermatitis, 112, 113, 115, 127–28, 186, 196, 202, 245, 266, 269, 275
Detoxification. *See also* Toxicants *and* Xenobiotics
    amino acids' role in, 45–46, 51, 61
    assessment of, 257–58
    biochemistry of, 249–52
    challenge test of, 257–58
    defined, 249
    gastrointestinal system's function in, 5
    idiopathic disease and, 256
    importance of, 248–49
    neurologic disease affected by, 256
    nutritional support for, 256–57

phases of, 249–51, 256, 258
    regimes for, 248
Detoxification pathways
    influence of drugs on, 252–56
    supportive nutrients for, 254, 256
    under-functioning, 263
Detoxification reserve, assessing, 258
Diabetes mellitus, 36, 112–13, 119, 133, 138, 142, 167, 169, 196, 216, 227, 229, 270, 276
    blood glucose and insulin level increases in patients having, 21
    complications of, 31, 35
    fiber supplementation for, 34, 35
    inadequate nutrient intake associated with, 100
    increased need for vitamin C in, 7
    insulin-dependent (IDDM) (type 1), 31
    metabolic syndrome and development of type 2, 12
    non-insulin-dependent (NIDDM) (type 2), 31, 34, 35, 163, 184, 276
    nutrition in management of, 276
    possible magnesium deficiency in patients having, 163, 165
    prevention of, 18, 31
    resistant starch (RS) in management of, 26
    serum triglyceride increases in patients having, 20
    treatment of, 31. *See also* Blood sugar regulation *and* Insulin level
    vanadium in management of, 184
    vitamin A deficiencies in patients having, 138
Diarrhea, 112–13, 126, 165–69, 171, 186, 192, 198, 202, 205–6
    excess copper causing, 174
    fiber and water increases causing, 29
    infantile, 206
    lactose intolerance causing, 198
    low gastric acidity causing, 196
    mineral deficiencies caused by, 167, 168
    supplemental minerals causing, 165, 186

Diet diary
  analyzing patient's, 27
  to assess nutrient intake, 265
  to confirm vitamin deficiency, 11–12
Diet quality, shortcuts in evaluating, 27
Dietary influences on development of diseases, 5
Dietary intake, software for analyzing, 1
Dietary pattern, evaluating entire, 35
Dietary Reference Intakes (DRIs)
  development by FNB of, 101
  for minerals, table of, 153–56
  for vitamins, table of, 102–104
Digestion, 191–214
  cephalic phase of, 192–93
  in colon, 199–200
  evaluating, 278
  functional approach to, 200–211
  functional relationships among absorption,
    dysfunction, and, 192
  gases produced during, 29–30
  impaired, 197–99
  lifestyle factors affecting, 192–93
  in mouth, 193–94
  physiology of, 193
  in small intestine, 197
  in stomach, 194, 196
Digestion time of meals, 30
Digestion-related disorders, 192. *See also*
    individual conditions
Digestive tract
  active transport of nutrients through, 199
  ecological network of, 192
Disaccharides as simple carbohydrates, 19
Diverticulitis, 27
Drug/nutrient interaction, 247–48
Drugs
  increased antigen uptake by intestine
    for, 277
  influence on detoxification pathways of,
    252–56
  types of xenobiotic, 243, 247–48

Dry skin, 112, 138, 176
Dynamic balance
  body temperature in, 9
  for range of changes body experiences every
    day, 9
Dysbiosis, 211
  assessment using stool markers of, 279
  defined, 279
  nature and extent of, 280
  organisms associated with, 243
Dysglycemia and dysglycemic conditions,
    11, 19
  clinical signs of, 276
Dysmenorrhea, possible magnesium deficiency in
    patients having, 165

E

Eczema, 73, 87, 118, 196, 198, 201–203, 211
Eicosapentaenoic acid (EPA), 207
Electrolytes. *See* Chloride, Potassium, *and* Sodium
Electron transport chain (ETC), 217, 218, 225,
    230, 234
Elimination diet
  CFIDS treated using, 256
  in food allergy testing, 58, 277
  in treatment of inflammation, 194
  modified, 62–64
Energy, 215–36
  absorption of nutrients and, 224–25
  effects of impaired detoxification systems
    on, 252
  functional approach to, 229–34
  relationship of nutrition to, 223–25
  roles of creatine and carnitine in metabolism
    of, 50–51, 223–24
Energy production
  improving, 233
  role of mitochondria in, 216–18
Enteropathy, 134, 141, 198
Environment, effects of toxic factors in, 237–61

Environmental inputs
   assessing, 265
   key, 5
   in nutrition and functional medicine model, 4
Enzymatic cofactors, 223, 256
Enzyme-linked immunoassay (ELISA)
      assessment, 277
Enzymes
   antioxidant, 274
   digestive, major, 195
   digestive, replenishing, 210
   digestive, secretion of, 192, 193, 197–98
   effects of toxicity on, 244
   fiber not digested by, 26
   generation from genes of, 240, 242
   inadequate, 30
   inhibited, 13, 255
   Krebs cycle, 221, 225
   mitochondrial, 219, 221, 225
   oxidative, 82–83
   pancreatic, 197, 210
   protease, 198
   substrates of, 255
Enzymes by name
   aconitase, 221
   alpha-ketoglutaric dehydrogenase, 221
   amylase, 24, 198
   catalase (CAT), 55, 83, 274
   ceruloplasmin, 274
   citric synthetase, 221
   cyclooxygenase, 77
   fumarase, 221
   glucuronosyl transferase, 256
   glutathione peroxidase (GPO), 54–55,
      82, 274
   isocitric dehydrogenase, 221
   lactase, 198, 199
   lipase, 198
   lipoxygenase, 77
   malic dehydrogenase, 221
   P450, 252, 254–57

succinic dehydrogenase, 221
succinyl kinase, 221
sulfite oxidase, 61
superoxide dismutase (SOD), 54, 82
trypsin, 56
urease, 196
Epilepsy associated with injury to neurons, 59
Essential fatty acid deficiency (EFAD), 73–74, 83,
      85, 266, 269
Essential nutrients, 13
   vanadium one of, 184
Estimated Average Requirement (EAR) as one
      base for DRIs, 101
Exchange Lists for Meal Planning (American
      Diabetes Association), 17–18, 35
Excitotoxin concept for neuronal hyper-
      excitability, 247
Exercise
   in bone health, 10
   oxygen consumptive increased by some,
      81–82
   phosphocreatine resynthesis following, 234
   processing of, 3, 4
   type 2 diabetes initially treated with diet
      and, 31

F

Fanconi's syndrome, 216, 227
Fatigue, 107, 109, 112, 115–17, 119, 122, 126,
      128–29, 131–32, 134, 138, 163, 176,
      184, 202, 215–16, 227–29, 233, 245,
      256, 276
   causes of, 263
   iron deficiency causing symptoms of, 179
   possible magnesium deficiency in patients
      having, 165
Fats, 69–96
   bile secretions to break up, 197
   cell membranes and, 70–71
   dietary macronutrient balance and, 91–92

Fats, *continued*
    functions of, 69
    physical performance affected by, 93
    polyunsaturated, 80
    saturated, 69
Fatty acids
    cis, 79, 80
    classification of, 71–74
    clinical and laboratory assessments of insufficiencies in, 269
    derivative, 269
    essential (EFAs), assessment of deficiencies of, 269
    long-chain (LCFAs), 73
    measurement of plasma, 73–74
    medium-chain (MCFAs), 72, 73, 89
    nonessential, 208
    omega 3, 72, 74, 77, 78, 79, 207, 269
    omega 6, 72, 74, 77, 78, 79, 207, 269
    omega 9, 72, 74, 78
    plasma, 269
    ratios of, 73, 74, 77–78
    saturated, 72
    short-chain (SCFAs), 22, 29, 72, 73, 87–89, 207, 210, 242
    thyroid function and, 87
    trans, 73, 79–80
    transport into mitochondrial matrix of, 223, 225, 233
    types of, 71
    unsaturated, 72
    very-short-chain (VSCFA), 72
Fatty acids by name
    alpha-linolenic, 71–73
    butyric acid, 207–8
    linoleic acid, 72
    oleic acid, 72
    stearic acid, 72
Fiber, 26–29
    cereal, 27
    conversion to SCFAs of, 207, 242

    daily fluid intake increased while increasing intake of, 29
    evaluating intake of, 27, 29
    increasing dietary intake of, 29, 34
    insoluble, 19, 26–28
    physiological effects of types of, 27, 28
    soluble, 19, 22, 26–28, 29, 30, 34, 35
    tolerability of, 29
Fibromyalgia, 216
    possible magnesium deficiency in patients having, 165
Folic acid (folate), 122–26
    absorption of, 123, 194, 248
    as detoxification support nutrient, 256
    functional medicine considerations for, 126
    functions of, 123
    safety and toxicity of, 125–26
    sources of, 123–24
    structure of, 122–23
    therapeutic considerations for, 8, 11, 124–25, 242, 271
Follicular hyperkeratosis, 131, 138, 266
Food additives and dyes, xenobiotic, 243, 246–47
Food Guide Pyramid (USDA), 17
Food sensitivities, intolerance, and allergies
    antibodies generated in, 277
    assessment of, 272, 275, 276
    to dairy products, 198–99, 272
    delayed, 61
    elimination diet to manage, 62–64
    gluten/grain, 29, 62, 198
    impaired digestion associated with, 198–99, 209–10
    in infants, 203
    leading to bloating, 30, 198
    low gastric acidity as influencing, 194, 196
    protein intake evaluation and, 41
    to rice, 58
    statistics for children and adults having, 62
    terms for describing, 275

4R gastrointestinal support program
    Reinoculate, 208, 209, 210–11
    Remove, 208, 209–10
    Repair, 208, 209, 211
    Replace, 208, 209, 210
Free radicals
    oxidative stress and mitochondrial, 225–26
    production of, 80, 81, 178–79, 252
    scavenging by antioxidants of, 208
Fructooligosaccharides
    food sources of, 23, 25
    structure of, 23, 24
    as substrate for healthy bacteria, 207
Fructose
    glycemic index of, 33
    metabolism of, 19–21
    as simple carbohydrate, 18, 19
Fruit ripeness affecting GI, 36
Functional medicine
    body reserves examined in, 13
    context for laboratory or physical test results in, 9
    core principles in, 5
    defined, 3
    focus of, 2
    guiding principle of, 7
    imbalances in physiological processes under, 3
    integration of functional thinking with interventions in, 12
    model of nutrition and, 4
Functional perspective of nutrition, 1–15
    acknowledgment of nutrient deficiency in, 12
    for amino acids, proteins, and peptides, 58–64
    biochemical individuality in, 6
    for carbohydrates, 29–36
    "conditionally essential" nutrients in, 13
    for digestion, absorption, and intestinal permeability, 200–211
    for energy, 229–34

    estimating dietary fiber from, 27
    interconnections in, 10
    for laboratory assessment of nutrient status, 265, 267–72
    reasons for using, 2–3, 13
    for toxicity, 248–58
    uniqueness of physiological/biochemical life in, 6
    for vitamins, 101–105. *See also* individual vitamins

G

Galactose
    deposition of, 19
    as simple carbohydrate, 18
Gamma linolenic acid (GLA), 208
Gamma-oryzanol to support permeability-related conditions, 208
Gastric juice, 195
Gastrointestinal disease
    prevention and treatment of, 18
    in U.S. adults, 191–92
Gastrointestinal function, 192–200, 211
Gastrointestinal microbial metabolism, 242–43
Gastrointestinal microecology, 279–80
Gastrointestinal milieu, 278
Gastrointestinal tract
    common bacteria in, 206
    proper functioning of, 278
Genetic mutations and defects, 240
    in mitochondrial function, 263
    table of diseases attributable to, 241
Genetic tests of detoxification, 257
Gilbert's syndrome, 256
Gingivitis, 11, 131
Glaucoma, possible magnesium deficiency in patients having, 165
Glossitis, 11, 112, 115, 119, 266
Glucosaminoglycans (GAGs), 55

Glucose
    absorption of, 26–27
    branched-chain polymer of, 24
    conversion to phosphorus of, 161
    glycemic index of, 33
    glycolysis of, 219
    metabolism of, 184, 185, 207
    as simple carbohydrate, 18
Glucose level
    challenge tests of, 270
    classes of carbohydrates increasing, 21
    diet to maintain proper, 31
    exercise to improve, 31
    high fiber intake as regulating, 27
    high GL diets as increasing, 32
Glutathione (GTH)
    balancing other factors and cofactors with,
        229–30
    conjugation of, 251, 253
    decreased in aging process, 234
    as detoxification support nutrient, 257
    function and metabolism, 54–55
    in recycling vitamin E, 232
    as redox agent, 82, 232
    re-establishing proper cycle for, 230
Gluten, 29, 58, 62–64, 134, 141, 198, 203
Glycemic index (GI)
    calculation of, 32
    clinical conclusions about carbohydrates and,
        35–36
    factors affecting, 34–35
    food processing correlated with higher, 34
    to measure blood glucose response to
        food, 31
    problems with using, 36
Glycemic index table of commonly eaten foods, 33
Glycemic load (GL) of food, 32, 34
Glycobiology, 36
Glycoproteins, 55–56
Goiter, 175, 266
Gout, hyperuricemia in patients having, 20–21

Graves disease, 196
Gut-associated lymphatic tissue (GALT), imbal-
    anced activity in, 194

H
H2 receptor blockers, 194, 196
    detoxification inhibited by, 252, 255
Hair element analysis for toxic load, 244
Headaches and migraines, 109, 115, 138, 159,
    174, 181, 216, 227, 229, 245
    possible magnesium deficiency in patients
        having, 165
Health as positive vitality, nutritional support of,
    11–12
Health history questions, 27
Heart disease. See Cardiovascular disease
Heat treatment in soy food preparation,
    56–57
Heavy (toxic) metals, xenobiotic, 239, 244–46
    most common, 244
    signs and symptoms associated with excess
        amounts of, 244–45
Hemochromatosis, 131, 246
    excessive copper levels in, 174
    risk factors for, 178–79
Hemorrhoids, 27
Hepatic cancer, 252
Hepatitis, 122, 196
Herbicides, xenobiotic, 239, 243
High blood pressure. See also Hypertension
    as characteristic of metabolic syndrome, 12
    possible magnesium deficiency in patients
        having, 165
High carbohydrate diets, 18
High fat diet, bloating associated with, 30
High fiber diet, 35
High fructose corn syrup (HFCS), composition
    of, 21
High protein diet, accumulation of sulfite in,
    61–62

Homeostasis, 179, 182, 186
    calcium, 156
    defined, 8
Homocysteine
    in atherogenesis, 45, 46
    metabolism of, 125
    as risk factor for CVD, 271
Homocysteinemia, 105, 121, 125, 240, 242,
    258, 271
Hormonal aberration, effects on total load of, 239
Hormonal balance, 5
Hormone synthesis from cholesterol, 88
Hormone types
    parathyroid (PTH), 156
    thyroid, 61, 175
Hormone-dependent cancer, prevention of, 5
Hormones
    estrogen, 5, 160, 186, 204, 254
    glucagon, 193
    insulin. *See* Insulin level
    tests of, 268
Human milk, immunoglobulins in, 202–203
Huntington's disease, 60, 228
    associated with injury to neurons, 59
Hyperammonemia, 48
Hyperchlorhydria, 192, 194
Hypercholesteremia, 57, 85, 90
Hyperinsulinemia, 35, 91
Hyperkeratosis, 137, 139, 266
Hyperlipidemia, 31
Hypernatremic dehydration, 47
Hypertension, 31, 48, 134, 157, 159, 169, 205, 245
Hypertriglyceridemia, 20, 276
Hyperuricemia, 20–21
Hypochlorhydria, 177, 179, 194, 196
    leading to gas and bloating, 30
Hypoglycemia, 266, 276
    associated with injury to neurons, 59
    possible magnesium deficiency in patients
      having, 165
Hypothyroidism, 175–76, 196, 266

I

Immune-related arthritis, 204
Indigestion, 112, 115
    instigating causes of, 194, 196
Infections
    effects on total load of, 239
    excess stomach acid secretion allowing
      bacterial, 196
    increased need for vitamin C in, 7
    neonatal protection from, 202–203
    recurrent bacterial, low mineral levels and,
      174–75, 176
Inflammation and inflammatory conditions, 11,
    49, 51, 61, 74–77, 79, 94, 107, 112, 165,
    172, 179, 184, 204, 208, 228, 234, 250,
    269, 272–73, 275–76
    chronic, 194
    increased need for vitamin C in, 7
Inflammatory bowel disease, 171, 202, 276, 277
Insomnia, 99, 115, 126, 163, 245
Institute of Medicine's Food and Nutrition Board
    (FNB)
    RDAs developed by, 100
    RDAs revised as DRIs by, 101
Insulin level
    carbohydrate classes increasing, 21
    challenge test of, 12
    high GL diets affecting, 32
Insulin resistance, 31
    assessment of, 276
    increasing, 34
    in metabolic syndrome, 12
    possible magnesium deficiency in patients
      having, 165
Insulin resistance syndrome. *See* Metabolic syn-
    drome (Syndrome X, insulin resistance
    syndrome)
Intermittent claudication, possible magnesium
    deficiency in patients having, 165
Intestinal barrier function, assessment of, 278–79.
    See also Intestinal permeability

Intestinal cancer, 204

Intestinal disorders associated with increased antigen uptake, 277

Intestinal mucosa, nutritional supplements targeting, 205, 207–8

Intestinal permeability
  altered, 90, 200–211
  assessing, 278
  diseases associated with increased, 202
  dynamics of, 203
  events and agents disrupting, 200–1, 203–4
  4R gastrointestinal support program to normalize, 208–11
  in healthy individuals, 201
  stabilizing, 206
  symptoms associated with increased, 202

Intestinal transit time, 26–28, 30, 163, 203

Intracellular glycosylation, 36

Inulin
  breakdown into fructooligosaccharides of, 23
  food sources of, 22, 23
  structure of, 22

Iodine, 175–76
  absorption of, 175
  functional medicine considerations for, 176
  functions of, 175
  RDA/AI and UL for, 154–55
  safety and toxicity of, 176
  sources of, 175, 176
  therapeutic considerations for, 175

Iron, 11, 56, 131, 176–79
  absorption of, 176–77, 194, 248
  functional medicine considerations for, 179
  functions of, 177, 196
  RDA/AI and UL for, 155
  safety and toxicity of, 177–79
  sources of, 177, 178
  therapeutic considerations for, 177

Irritability, 99, 115, 118, 122, 126, 138, 163, 245, 266

Irritable bowel syndrome, 9, 21, 202, 208, 211

K

Kearns-Sayre syndrome, 232–33

Key subclinical imbalances, identifying, 12

Kidney stones and kidney diseases, 11, 31, 142, 168, 174, 216, 227, 238, 241, 245
  possible magnesium deficiency in patients having, 165

Krebs cycle, 217, 219–22, 225
  cofactors appearing in, 230
  intermediates in, 230

L

Lactose intolerance, 62, 198–99, 272
  in ethnic populations, 198

Lead toxicity, 11, 239, 245, 246

Leaky gut, 200

Learning disabilities, 11, 177

Legumes and beans
  contents of, as inhibiting digestion and absorption, 34
  cooking techniques to minimize bloating from, 30–31
  in elimination diet, 63

Lifestyle effects
  on detoxification systems, 257
  on digestion, 192–93
  on total load of, 239

Lifestyle questionnaires, 265

Lipid peroxides, 80–81, 245

Lipid protection, supplements offering, 83–85

Lipids
  categories of, 70–71, 85
  sulfation of, 61

Lipoic acid, 229, 231–33. *See also* Antioxidants

Low carb (Atkins) diet, 69

Low gastric activity
  common signs and symptoms of, 196
  diseases associated with, 196

Low-fat diet, effect on bone density of, 57

Low-fiber diet, 204
Lupus (systemic lupus erythematosus), 163

M

Macular degeneration, 133, 273
Magnesium, 161, 163–65
    absorption and regulation of, 161,
        163, 248
    conditions involving deficiency of, 165
    functional medicine considerations for, 165
    functions of, 163
    RDA/AI and UL for, 153
    safety and toxicity of, 165
    sources of, 164–65
    therapeutic considerations for, 163–64
Malabsorption, 11, 21, 30, 89, 134, 144, 179,
    191, 197–98
Maldigestion, carbohydrate metabolism and,
    29–31
Malnutrition, 211, 265, 277
Manganese, 179–81
    absorption of, 179
    as detoxification support nutrient, 257
    functional medicine considerations
        for, 181
    functions of, 179
    RDA/AI and UL for, 155
    safety and toxicity of, 180, 246
    sources of, 180
    therapeutic considerations for, 179–80
Mediators, 48, 126, 194
    as key component of patient's story, 7
Memory impairment, 107, 109, 113, 202, 269
Mercury toxic exposure to, 239, 245–46. *See also*
    Heavy (toxic) metals, xenobiotic
Metabolic patterns, restoring balance to, 10,
    11–12
Metabolic syndrome (Syndrome X, insulin resis-
    tance syndrome), 91
    development of, 12
    risk of developing diabetes in patients
        having, 276
    vanadium supplementation for symptoms
        of, 185
Metabolism
    enzyme family involved in, 255
    imbalanced, 240
    inborn errors of, 240
    influences on, 4, 6
    laboratory tests' role in assessing, 263–64
    roles of nonessential amino acids in, 44
Metabolite, static level determination of, 268, 270
Metals, toxic. *See* Heavy (toxic) metals,
    xenobiotic
Methylation, 251
Micelle formation, 197
Microflora balance and imbalance, 22–23,
    204, 207
Minerals, 151–90. *See also* individual minerals
    absorption of, 10
    antioxidant, 257
    bioavailability of, 56
    classification of, 152
    essential, 151, 184
    food sources of. *See* individual minerals
    functions of, 151
    intake of, 152
    lost in bedridden individuals, 10
    major, 152
    minor (trace), 152
    in mitochondrial metabolism, 225
    status tests of, 268
    supplementing, 56
Minimata disease, 244–45
Mitochondria
    ATP produced in, 216
    DNA mutations in, 275
    energy production and, 216–18
    number of, in body, 216
    nutritional support program for, 229–30
    structure of, 217, 219

Mitochondrial disorders, 59–60, 133–34, 215, 250, 263
    clinical conditions related to, 216
    clinical issues in, 226–29
Mitochondrial efficiency, nutrient substances for improving, 230–34
Mitochondrial matrix, 219
    transport of substrate into, 223, 225, 233
Mitochondrial metabolism, 50–51
    key cofactors in, 225–29
Mitochondrial myopathy, 263
Mitochondrial resuscitation, 229–30
Molybdenum, 181–82
    absorption of, 181
    functional medicine considerations for, 181–82
    functions of, 181
    insufficiencies and deficiencies of, 61
    RDA/AI and UL for, 155
    safety and toxicity of, 181
    sources of, 181, 182
    supplementation of, 174
    therapeutic considerations for, 181
Monosaccharides
    carbohydrates absorbed as, 200
    as simple carbohydrates, 19
    structure of, 18
Monosodium glutamate (MSG)
    umami taste produced by, 59, 61
    as xenobiotic flavor enhancer, 246–47
Mood disorders, 119, 121–22, 124
Multiple sclerosis, 122, 133, 243, 246
Muscle weakness, pain, or spasm, 109, 112, 115, 128, 157, 159, 163, 165, 166, 168–69, 228, 232–33, 241, 266
Myocardial infarction (MI), accumulation of mercury associated with risk of, 245
Myopathy, 60, 84, 133, 165, 183, 227–28, 233, 263, 266

N

N-acetylcysteine (NAC)
    as precursor to glutathione, 234
    supplementation of, 58
N-methyl-D-aspartate (NMDA) pathway, 58–61
Natural food components, xenobiotic, 243
Nausea, 115, 119, 127–28, 186, 196, 198
Nephropathy, 216, 229
    prevention of, 31, 35
Neural tube defects, 124
Neurodegenerative disease, 48, 59–61, 105, 228
Neurologic disorders
    associated with injury to neurons, 59
    detoxification impacting chronic, 256
    metabolites in urine of fungi and bacteria in patients having, 243
Neuropathy, 60, 107, 119, 133, 216, 227, 229, 266, 269
    prevention of, 31, 35
Neurotransmitters
    excitatory, overstimulation of, 247
    heavy and toxic metals impairing, 244, 246
    sulfation of, 61
Niacin. *See* Vitamin B3 (Niacin)
Night blindness, 105, 137–38, 266
Nitric oxide
    influences on body systems of, 49
    production of, increased, 58
    production of, inhibiting, 59
    synthesis of, 48
Nitric oxide signal transduction pathway, 48
Nonessential nutrients, 13–14
Nucleases, 195
Nutrient assessments, 263–81
    components of clinical, 264–65
    functional approach to, 265, 267–72
    indirect, 268, 271–72
Nutrient sufficiency/insufficiency continuum, 267

Nutrient transport in digestive system, 199
Nutrient-dependent activity assessment, 271
Nutritional status, 263–81
common analyses of, 268
"optimal," 263

O

Obesity, 5, 14, 276
Oligoantigenic diets, 209
Oligosaccharides
bloating associated with soy or legume, 30
food sources of, 25
nondigestible, 22
structure of, 19, 20, 21
as substrate for bifidobacteria, 23
Organ reserve, promotion of, 13–14
Osteoarthritis, 113
glucosamine sulfate for, 55–56
Osteomalacia, 141
Osteoporosis, 11, 119, 142–43, 157, 173, 196,
204, 266
possible magnesium deficiency in patients
having, 165
risk factors for, 159, 254, 256
Oxidative phosphorylation, 220, 222–23
impaired, 252
nutritional modulators of, table of, 231
Oxidative stress reactions, 58–59, 82–83, 112,
134–35, 184, 228–30, 232, 250, 263,
269, 271–74
assessment of, 273–74
defined, 80
mitochondrial free radicals and,
225–26, 230
mitochondrial function in, 230–32
relationship among mitochondrial dysfunction, Parkinson's disease, and, 228
role of vitamin E in, 135

under-functioning detoxification pathway
increasing, 263
Oxidative-stress studies, 58, 272

P

Pancreatic enzyme secretion, 197
Pancreatic juices, 195
Pancreatitis and pancreatic conditions, 91, 197,
202, 229, 278
Panel of tests, interpreting, 270
Pantothenic acid. *See* Vitamin B5 (pantothenic
acid)
Paracellular route of food into bloodstream, 200
Parasites, 196, 209, 239
Parkinson's disease, 133, 180, 216, 246, 256
associated with injury to neurons, 59
excess excitatory neurotransmitters associated with, 247
reduced sulfate excretion in patients
having, 61
relationship among mitochondrial dysfunc-
tion, oxidative stress, and, 228
Patient-centered nutrition, 7–8
Pearson's syndrome, 216, 227
Pediatric gastroenterology, 201–203
Pediculicides, xenobiotic, 243
Peptides
biological activity of, 53
conjugation of, 253
gut, increasing release of, 193
sulfation of, 61
transport by M cells in healthy individuals of,
201–202
Periodontal disease, 133
Peripheral neuropathy, 60, 122, 266
Personalized nutrition, 8
Pesticides, xenobiotic, 239, 243
Phenylketonuria, 240–41

Phosphocreatine, ADP converted to ATP by, 224
Phosphorus, 160–61
    absorption and regulation of, 160
    functional medicine considerations for, 161
    functions of, 160
    RDA/AI and UL for, 153
    safety and toxicity of, 161
    sources of, 161, 162
    therapeutic considerations for, 161
Phosphorus-to-calcium ratio, 161
Plant foods
    fiber in, 17
    protein in, 56
Plant oils
    fat content of, 92
    hydrogenation of, 79–80
    inflammation inhibited by, 79
    in nuts and seeds, 92–93
Polysaccharides, nonstarch
    as colonic foods, 22
    as complex carbohydrates, 19
    in dietary fiber, 26
    structure of, 21
Polycystic ovary syndrome, 276
Polymorphisms, 242
Positive vitality, evaluating, 12
Potassium, 165–69
    absorption and regulation of, 166
    functional medicine considerations for, 169
    functions of, 165, 166
    safety and toxicity of, 168–69
    sources of, 166, 167
    therapeutic considerations for, 166–68
Prebiotics, 205, 209, 249, 280
    carbohydrates functioning as, 19, 22
    to promote bacterial balance, 205, 206–7
    as substrate for SCFAs, 22–23
Premenstrual syndrome (PMS), 91, 119
    possible magnesium deficiency in patients
        having, 165

Preservatives, xenobiotic, 246–47
Pritikin-type diets, 18
Probiotic supplements, 205, 209, 249, 280
Processed foods, GL higher in, 34
Prostate cancer, 73
Protease inhibitors, 56
Proteins, 53–67
    absorption of, 200
    animal, 57
    average consumption of, 41
    classes of, 55
    dairy, 198–99
    digestion of, 41, 202
    functions of, 53
    grain, gluten sensitivity from, 62
    leaking into bloodstream from gut wall,
        197–98
    plant, 56
    quality of, 41, 56
    rice, 57–58
    soy, 56–57
    synthesizing, 55
    vegetable, 53
Proteoglycans, 55–56
Proton pump inhibitors, 194
Provitamin carotenoids, 136
Psoriasis, 91, 138, 171, 196, 202
Psychosocial factors, effects on total load of, 239
Pyridoxine. See Vitamin B6 (pyridoxine)

R

Radiation, processing of, 4
Radioallergosorbent test (RAST), 277
Reactive oxygen species (ROS), 77, 80–82,
    271, 273
Recommended Dietary Allowances, 7
    development of, 100
    of minerals, table of, 153–56
    of protein, 41

Redox agents, molecular, 82–83
Rheumatoid arthritis, 11, 61, 113, 116, 171,
    173, 179, 184, 194, 196, 200, 203–4,
    211, 256
Riboflavin. *See* Vitamin B2 (riboflavin)
Rickets, 138, 141, 157, 161, 266

S

Saccharide absorption studies, 278–79
Saliva enzymes, 195
Scurvy, 97, 100, 129, 131
Second meal effect to improve glucose
    tolerance, 35
Seizures, 10, 127, 216, 227, 229, 266
Selenium, 58, 182–84
    absorption and regulation of, 182
    as detoxification support nutrient, 257
    functional medicine considerations
        for, 184
    functions of, 182–83
    RDA/AI and UL for, 156
    safety and toxicity of, 184
    sources of, 183
    therapeutic considerations for, 183–84
Serum metabolites, study of vitamins and, 6
Shock, 48
Single nucleotide polymorphisms (SNPs), 8
Sjögren's syndrome, 196
Sodium, 165–69
    absorption and regulation of, 166
    functional medicine considerations
        for, 169
    functions of, 165, 166
    safety and toxicity of, 168–69
    sources of, 166, 168
    therapeutic considerations for, 166–68
Sodium chloride, foods with high amounts of
    added, 169
South Beach Diet, 69

Starch. *See also* Carbohydrates
    amylopectin, 24, 25, 34
    amylose, 24–25, 32, 34
    digestion of, 24
    phytate affecting digestibility of, 34–35
    rapidly digestible (RDS), 25–26
    in raw foods, 34
    resistant (RS) (nondigestible), 22, 24–26,
        28, 34
    slowly digestible (SDS), 25–26
    structure of, 21, 24, 25
Static level determination of nutrient or metabo-
    lite, 268, 270
Steroids, sulfation of, 61
Sterols, 85–87
Stimulants, xenobiotic, 246–47
Stomach acid secretion, 30
Stool surveys, 278
Stress
    amelioration of digestion-related disorders by
        reducing, 192
    challenge to optimal health of, 13
    effects on health of, 9
    nutritional support for, 9, 50
    oxidative, 58, 80
    permeability of intestine altered by, 200
    processing of, 4
Stress tests as challenge tests, 271
Stroke, 48, 192–93, 216, 227, 229
    associated with injury to neurons, 59–60
    possible magnesium deficiency in patients
        having, 165
Subclinical nutrient deficiencies, 265
Sucrose
    absorption of, 36
    glycemic index of, 33
Sulfation cycle, 45, 253
Sweeteners, xenobiotic, 246–47
Syndrome X. *See* Metabolic syndrome (Syndrome
    X, insulin resistance syndrome)

T

TBARS test, 81, 83
Thiamin. *See* Vitamin B1 (thiamin)
Thyroid function, role of fatty acids in, 87
Thyrotoxicosis, 196
Tocopherols. *See* Vitamin E.
Tolerable Upper Intake Level (UL) as one base for DRIs, 101
Total load
    defined, 238
    of xenobiotics, 238–40
Toxic element exposure, 238–39, 244–46
Toxicants. *See also* Detoxification
    actions on organisms of, 237–39
    determining exposure of patients to, 244
    effects on total load of, 239
    endogenous, 240–43, 253
    exogenous, 243–48
    functional approach to, 248–58
Trans sulfuration-sulfate pathways, 44
Transcellular route of food into bloodstream, 200
Trauma
    associated with injury to neurons, 59
    body's processing of, 3
Triene-to-tetraene ratio, 73
Triggers, 198
    as key component of patient's story, 7
Triglyceride concentrations
    associated with low GL diets, 34
    lowered with soy rather than animal protein intake, 57
    in metabolic syndrome, 12
Triglycerides, medium-chain (MCTs), 89–91

U

Ubiquinone. *See* Coenzyme Q10 (ubiquinone)
Ulcer, 191–92, 196, 208
Upper Limit (UL) for minerals, table of, 153–56
Upstream medicine, 12
Urea cycle, 47–49

V

Vanadium, 183–85
    absorption of, 184
    functional medicine considerations for, 185
    functions of, 184
    RDA/AI and UL for, 156
    safety and toxicity of, 185
    sources of, 185
    therapeutic considerations for, 185
Vegetarian diet, 174, 179
Vitamers, 97
    vitamin E tocopherols as, 131
Vitamin A, 134, 136–38
    absorption of, 134, 136, 197, 248
    functional medicine considerations for, 138–39
    functions of, 136
    safety and toxicity of, 138
    sources of, 137
    structure of, 134, 136
    therapeutic considerations for, 137–38, 257
Vitamin B1 (thiamin), 105–9
    absorption of, 105, 107
    functional medicine considerations for, 108–9
    functions of, 107
    safety and toxicity of, 108
    sources of, 107
    structure of, 105, 106
    therapeutic considerations for, 107
Vitamin B2 (riboflavin), 109–12
    absorption of, 109–10
    as detoxification support nutrient, 256
    functional medicine considerations for, 112
    functions of, 110–11
    safety and toxicity of, 112
    sources of, 111
    structure of, 109
    therapeutic considerations for, 11, 111–12
Vitamin B3 (niacin), 112–15
    absorption of, 112–13
    as detoxification support nutrient, 256

functional medicine considerations for,
114–15
functions of, 113
safety and toxicity of, 114
sources of, 113, 114
structure of, 112
therapeutic considerations for, 113
Vitamin B5 (pantothenic acid), 115–17
absorption of, 115
functional medicine considerations for, 117
functions of, 115, 211
safety and toxicity of, 116–17
sources of, 116
structure of, 115
therapeutic considerations for, 116
Vitamin B6 (pyridoxine), 117–19
absorption of, 117, 194
as detoxification support nutrient, 256
functional medicine considerations
for, 119
functions of, 117–18
safety and toxicity of, 119
sources of, 118
structure of, 117
therapeutic considerations for, 118–19
Vitamin B12 (cobalamin), 119–22
absorption of, 120, 194, 248
as detoxification support nutrient, 256
functional medicine considerations for, 122
functions of, 120–21
safety and toxicity of, 122
sources of, 121–22
structure of, 119–20
therapeutic considerations for, 122, 197
Vitamin C (ascorbate), 128–31
absorption of, 10, 128
environmental effects on need for, 7
functional medicine considerations for, 131
functions of, 83, 128–29
iron absorption enhanced by, 176–77
in recycling vitamin E, 232

as redox agent, 82
safety and toxicity of, 131
sources of, 129, 130
structure of, 128
therapeutic considerations for, 11, 129–31,
233, 257
Vitamin D (calciferol), 139–42
absorption of, 139, 197
functional medicine considerations for,
141–42
functions of, 139, 141
metabolism of, 140
safety and toxicity of, 141
sources of, 141
structure of, 139
therapeutic considerations for, 11, 141
Vitamin deficiency as traditional focus of clinical
nutrition, 11–12
Vitamin E (tocopherols), 131–34
absorption of, 131–32, 197
functional medicine considerations for, 134
functions of, 83, 132
recycling of, 232
as redox agent, 82
role in oxidative stress reactions of, 135, 233
safety and toxicity of, 134
sources of, 132–33
structure of, 131, 132
therapeutic considerations for, 133–34, 257
Vitamin K (K1–K3), 142–44
absorption of, 142, 197
functional medicine considerations for, 144
functions of, 142
safety and toxicity of, 144
sources of, 142, 144
structure of, 142, 143
therapeutic considerations for, 142–44,
233–34
Vitamins, 97–149. *See also* individual vitamins
classification of, 98
deficiencies of, traditional focus on, 11–12

Vitamins, *continued*
  DRIs for, 102–104
  in energy production, 220
  fat-soluble, 98, 131–44, 197
  food sources of. *See* individual vitamins.
  functional approach to, 101–105
  insufficiencies of, interindividual, 6, 98–100
  life circumstances affecting individuals' requirements for, 100
  in mitochondrial metabolism, 225
  pioneers in identification of, 97–98
  status tests of, 268
  structure and function of, 98
  water-soluble, 98, 105–31
Vitiligo, 196
Volatile organic compounds (VOCs) as xenobiotics, 243–44

W

Wilson's disease, 10
  excessive copper levels in patients having, 174, 246
Wolff-Parkinson-White syndrome, 216, 227
Wound healing, impaired, 130–31, 134, 138, 171–72, 265

X

Xenobiotics, 44, 49, 51, 54, 110, 112, 115, 136, 138, 209, 226–27, 237–40, 250–51, 256, 258, 270
  bio-reactive mechanisms for, table of, 253
  defined, 237
  detoxification of. *See* Detoxification
  functional changes induced by exposure to, 238
  processing of, 4
  studies of, 238–39
  sulfation of, 61
  types of, 243–44

Z

Zinc, 10, 56, 171–72
  absorption and regulation of, 171, 248
  as detoxification support nutrient, 257
  functional medicine considerations for, 172, 174
  functions of, 171
  RDA/AI and UL for, 154
  safety and toxicity of, 171–72
  sources of, 171, 172
  therapeutic considerations for, 171